Neonatal Opioid Withdrawal Syndrome

This collection synthesizes perspectives on Neonatal Opioid Withdrawal Syndrome (NOWS), providing a comprehensive resource for those in speech-language pathology and healthcare providers working within an interprofessional approach to treat and support infants, children, parents, caregivers, and families impacted by NOWS.

The volume responds to the growing challenge faced by SLPs and healthcare providers to develop new, evidence-based strategies to meet the needs of the emerging population of infants with NOWS, children prenatally exposed to opioids, their mothers, families and caregivers, in light of the growing opioid crisis in the US. Through a holistic approach, the book features contributions from researcher-clinicians across healthcare professions and from different countries. It brings together research on the impact of NOWS on child neurodevelopment, causes of neurodevelopmental alterations due to NOWS, interprofessional team care to optimize outcomes for this population, feeding, communication, sensory and motor issues, long-term outcomes into adolescence and adulthood, as well as best practices for addressing these. The volume also explores the impact of NOWS on families and effective strategies for supporting them. The Trauma Informed Care approach features throughout. The collection looks ahead to address research gaps toward enhancing evidence-based strategies from a strength-based perspective.

This book will be of interest to students and researchers in speech-language pathology, occupational therapy, physical therapy, nursing, pediatric medicine, and other related fields, as well as clinicians and instructors in these same disciplines.

Brenda Louw is a Professor Emerita of Speech-Language Pathology in the Department of Audiology and Speech-Language Pathology at East Tennessee State University, USA.

Routledge Research in Speech-Language Pathology
Series Editor: Louise Cummings

Routledge Research in Speech-Language Pathology looks beyond traditional areas of study within the discipline to showcase topics historically underserved in research on communication disorders, highlighting fresh perspectives on issues of key importance in speech-language pathology. The series offers comprehensive treatments of communication disorders and the work of speech-language pathology with an eye toward pushing the field forward, critically examining challenges in addressing disparities in speech-language pathology and exploring the latest developments in related disciplines with implications for the future of research on communication disorders. Volumes in this series will be of particular interest to students, scholars, and clinicians in speech-language pathology, speech and language therapy, and clinical linguistics, as well as related fields such as special education, psychology, neurology, psychiatry, social work, and nursing.

COVID-19 and Speech-Language Pathology
Louise Cummings

Communication and Sensory Loss
Global Perspectives
Edited by Kathryn Crowe

Language Research in Post-Traumatic Stress
Edited by Yvette D. Hyter

Neonatal Opioid Withdrawal Syndrome
Speech-Language Pathologists and Interprofessional Care
Edited by Brenda Louw

For more information about this series, please visit: www.routledge.com/Routledge-Research-on-Speech-Language-Pathology/book-series/RRSLP

Neonatal Opioid Withdrawal Syndrome

Speech-Language Pathologists and Interprofessional Care

Edited by Brenda Louw

Routledge
Taylor & Francis Group

NEW YORK AND LONDON

First published 2025
by Routledge
605 Third Avenue, New York, NY 10158

and by Routledge
4 Park Square, Milton Park, Abingdon, Oxon, OX14 4RN

Routledge is an imprint of the Taylor & Francis Group, an informa business

Library of Congress Cataloging-in-Publication Data
Names: Louw, Brenda, editor.
Title: Neonatal opioid withdrawal syndrome : speech-language pathologists and interprofessional care / edited by Brenda Louw.
Other titles: Routledge research in speech-language pathology.
Description: New York, NY : Routledge, 2024. |
Series: Routledge research in speech-language pathology |
Includes bibliographical references and index. |
Identifiers: LCCN 2024008041 | ISBN 9781032484051 (hardback) |
ISBN 9781032501895 (paperback) | ISBN 9781003397267 (ebook)
Subjects: MESH: Neonatal Abstinence Syndrome | Analgesics,
Opioid–adverse effects | Opioid-Related Disorders–therapy |
Communication Disorders–therapy | Patient-Centered Care | Infant, Newborn
Classification: LCC RJ520.P74 N46 2024 | NLM WS 421 |
DDC 618.92/869–dc23/eng/20240507
LC record available at https://lccn.loc.gov/2024008041

ISBN: 9781032484051 (hbk)
ISBN: 9781032501895 (pbk)
ISBN: 9781003397267 (ebk)

DOI: 10.4324/9781003397267

Typeset in Sabon
by Newgen Publishing UK

Contents

Contributors

Dr. Brenda Louw is a Professor Emerita in the Department of Audiology and Speech-Language Pathology, East Tennessee State University, USA as well as in the Department Speech-Language Pathology and Audiology, University of Pretoria, South Africa. She has extensive clinical experience in early communication intervention and craniofacial differences. Her areas of research interest are cleft lip and palate, Neonatal Opioid Withdrawal Syndrome (NOWS), pediatric HIV/AIDS, culturally responsive care, and leadership in speech-language pathology. She has over 90 peer-reviewed publications and co-edited a unique textbook on HIV/AIDS and related communication, hearing, and swallowing disorders. She has presented her research internationally on six continents. She is a Fellow of both the American Speech-Language Hearing Association (ASHA) and of the South African Speech-Language Hearing Association (SASLHA) and a member of the American Cleft Palate-Craniofacial Association (ACPA); the Tennessee Association of Audiology and Speech-Language Pathology (TAASLP); and the International Society on Early Intervention (ISEI).

Dr. Martha Velez is a pediatrician who performs neurobehavioral assessments and interventions for infants of mothers/caregivers attending treatment for substance use disorders at the Center for Addiction and Pregnancy, Johns Hopkins University. As part of an interdisciplinary treatment team, she conducts individual and group parenting sessions to support mothers/caregivers in understanding their history and the role of their recovery in promoting healthy physical and mental development of their children. Dr. Velez's research interests include the development and implementation of a program for parents with substance use disorders exposed to abuse/trauma, and the exploration of fetal and infant neurobehaviors in substance-exposed pregnancies.

Dr. Lauren Jansson is a developmental pediatrician, Professor of Pediatrics at Johns Hopkins University School of Medicine, and Director of Pediatrics at the Center for Addiction and Pregnancy. In that capacity she provides comprehensive healthcare and developmental assessment to substance-exposed infants/children through adulthood in the context of parental addiction and mental health concerns, and the often-difficult environment in which the dyad resides. Dr. Jansson's principal research interests involve exploring the effects of in-utero opioid/other substance exposures on the developing fetus/infant, neonatal abstinence syndrome, optimizing treatment for women with opioid use disorders, opioid-exposed infants/dyads, and lactation among women with substance use disorders.

Dr. Hendrée Jones is a licensed psychologist and an international expert in the development and examination of both behavioral and pharmacologic treatments for pregnant women and their children in risky life situations. She a Professor in the Department of Obstetrics and Gynecology at the UNC-Chapel Hill School of Medicine and a Senior Advisor to the UNC Horizons Division. She has received continuous NIH funding since 1994 and authored more than 250 peer-reviewed publications.

Dr. Kim Andringa is an Instructor in the Department of Obstetrics and Gynecology at the UNC-Chapel Hill School of Medicine and the Director of Research and Evaluation at the UNC Horizons Division. Prior to coming to UNC Horizons Dr. Andringa worked at the Center for Women's Health Research at UNC where she led or co-led large program evaluation projects, worked as a grant writer, and conducted research related to reproductive health, postpartum depression, and breastfeeding.

Senga Carroll is a Clinical Assistant Professor in the Department of Obstetrics and Gynecology at the UNC-Chapel Hill School of Medicine and Senior Clinical and Policy Advisor at the UNC Horizons Division. Ms. Carroll's current responsibilities include support of grant-funded research and writing on topics related to attachment, resource mapping for women leaving incarcerated settings, and care of pregnant people diagnosed with a substance use disorder.

Dr. Evette Horton is an Assistant Professor in the Department of Obstetrics and Gynecology at the UNC-Chapel Hill School of Medicine and the Director of Child Clinical Services for the UNC Horizons Division. Dr. Horton is also a Licensed Professional Counselor and Supervisor and a Nationally Certified Counselor. She has over 20 years of experience working with children and families in both school and community settings.

Dr. Lori Devlin is a practicing Neonatologist in the Norton Children's Medical Group and a professor of pediatrics at the University of Louisville School of Medicine. She is a lead study investigator for two multicenter trials supported by the National Institutes of Health Helping to End Addiction Long-Term – Advancing Clinical Trials in Neonatal Opioid Withdrawal Syndrome (NIH HEAL ACT NOW) Collaborative. Dr. Devlin is also a primary investigator for the NIH HEAL Evaluation of Limited Pharmacotherapies for Neonatal Opioid Withdrawal Syndrome (HELP for NOWS) research collaborative and the NIH Environmental Influences on Child Outcomes Institutional Development Award States Pediatric Clinical Trials Network (ECHO ISPCTN).

Dr. Lenora Marcellus is a Professor in the School of Nursing at the University of Victoria, British Columbia. She has practiced as a Registered Nurse in a range of maternal-infant and academic settings and roles. Her research interests include perinatal substance use, neonatal opioid withdrawal, and supporting infants in foster care. She is a member of the Canada FASD Partnership Network Action Team on FASD Prevention from a Women's Determinants of Health Perspective. Dr. Marcellus has been involved in launching an integrated women's program in her community and developing an education and support program for foster care providers caring for infants prenatally exposed to substances.

Dr. Catherine Ringham is an Assistant Professor in the School of Nursing at Thompson Rivers University, British Columbia. She is a Registered Nurse with many years of clinical practice and research experience in the field of maternal and neonatal care. Dr. Ringham has a passion for qualitative approaches to health systems inquiries that show how people's work is organized within quality improvement, implementation, and evidence-informed discourses. Research and teaching interest wrap around the critical analysis of the social organization of work and healthcare systems with focus on Cannabis Use in Pregnancy and infant/child neurodevelopment, Family Integrated Care, and Mentorship in academia.

Dr. Karen McQueen, is a Professor in the School of Nursing at Lakehead University. She has extensive experience in the areas of perinatal and women's health as an educator, researcher, and nurse. Her research interests in breastfeeding include interventions to increase breastfeeding self-efficacy and the relationship between infant feeding methods and Neonatal Opioid Withdrawal Syndrome.

Dr. Alison Thompson is a Nurse Practitioner and Assistant Professor with the Lakehead University School of Nursing. She is a clinician-researcher with expertise in the areas of pediatric health and knowledge translation for parents. She is passionate about finding ways to ensure parents and caregivers have reliable, relevant, and accessible health information to make decisions about their child's health.

Dr. Pam Holland is an Associate Professor, Chair and Graduate Program Director for the Department of Communication Disorders at Marshall University. She is board certified in swallowing and swallowing disorders and founder of the Marshall University Pediatric Feeding and Swallowing Clinic. She is a part of Healthy Connections, a multi-agency coalition focused on improving outcomes for children with a history of prenatal opioid exposure. She is the coordinator for the University's Interprofessional Education Initiative and served on the CAPCSD IPE/IPP Committee. Her private practice, Family First Feeding, LLC provides family-centered services in the West Virginia Birth to Three program.

Dr. Jenene Craig lives in metro Atlanta, GA and is the Program Director of the Infant and Early Childhood Mental Health and Development PhD and MA degrees at Fielding Graduate University. She has been in practice for over 40 years, received her NIDCAP training under the tutelage of Dr. Heidelise Als and has specialized in the NICU since 1985, serves in leadership with the National Association of Neonatal Therapists, and is a certified neonatal therapist. Her advocacy and research are for neuroprotective care of premature infants and parent–infant outcomes for families embattled in the stressful environment of the NICU.

Dr. Christy Gliniak is a Neonatal Occupational Therapist and Associate Professor in the IECD Program at Fielding Graduate University who resides in the Pacific Northwest. She's passionate about advancing neuroprotective, trauma-informed, developmental care for medically fragile infants worldwide. Christy serves in leadership with the National Association of Neonatal Therapists and as a National Perinatal Association Board Member. Her clinical work, research, and advocacy target improvements in infant mental health, feeding, and neurodevelopmental outcomes of high-risk infant–parent dyads. Utilizing interprofessional collaboration and innovation, Christy aims to enhance services for marginalized communities, particularly families who are indigenous, rural, and affected by substance use.

Dr. Dana McCarty is an Assistant Professor of Physical Therapy at the University of North Carolina Chapel Hill and a board certified pediatric clinical specialist. Dr. McCarty conducts research examining the efficacy of physical therapy interventions on parent and infant outcomes and has published physical therapy guidelines for Neonatal Opioid

Withdrawal Syndrome (NOWS) in the American Physical Therapy Association's flagship journal, *Physical Therapy*. Dr. Dana McCarty has received funding from the NIH and Foundation from Physical Therapy Research. Within the UNC DPT program, Dana teaches pediatric content, directs UNC's Pediatric PT Residency Program, and coordinates the Neonatal PT Fellowship at UNC Health.

Dr. Kara Boynewicz is a board-certified pediatric specialist with over 21 years of clinical experience in hospital, early intervention, and outpatient settings. She is an assistant professor in the Department of Physical Therapy at East Tennessee State University (ETSU) and a core faculty member in the Vanderbilt Consortium LEND (Leadership Education in Neurodevelopmental Disabilities) (VCL) program. She provides clinical physical therapy services in the NICU, and Baby Steps Prenatal Drug Exposed Follow Up Clinic through ETSU Pediatrics. Her research focus is understanding early brain development with early identification and prevention of infants and children at risk for developmental delays.

Dr. Ju Lee Oei is a Neonatologist at the Royal Hospital for Women, Sydney, Australia, a Conjoint Professor of Pediatrics at the University of New South Wales, and a research associate at the NHMRC Clinical Trial Centre, University of Sydney. She is the Chair of the Pediatric Research Committee, member of the Executive Council and pediatric representative of the Royal Australian and New Zealand College of Physicians (2022–2025), and Chair of the Australian and New Zealand Perinatal Substance Use Special Interest group. Her research interests are in the impact of prenatal drug exposure on the mother and child and on the use of oxygen for the care of the newborn infant. She has special interest in clinical trials and the use of big data. She is lead author of the New South Wales Substance Use in Pregnancy and Parenting guidelines (2023).

Dr. Lynn Kemp is a Distinguished Professor and Director of the Translational Research and Social Innovation group in the School of Nursing and Midwifery at Western Sydney University and Ingham Institute. Prof. Kemp conducts a significant program of community-based child health research including world- and Australian-first intervention studies such as the Maternal Early Childhood Sustained Home-visiting (MECSH) study and the subsequent right@home randomized trial of sustained nurse home visiting, and the Volunteer Family Connect study, the world's largest trial of volunteer home visiting. She has been awarded over $16.5 million in career research funding, and published five book chapters and over 100 peer-reviewed works.

Dr. Stacy Blythe is a Registered Nurse, Professor and Head of Discipline (Nursing) in the School of Nursing and Midwifery, in the Faculty of Health at the University of Technology Sydney, and an authorized foster carer. Her research focuses on the health and well-being of children in out-of-home care and their families (biological/foster/adoptive). Using her skills as a nurse, knowledge as a researcher, and experience as a carer, Prof. Blythe provides training to health and social service providers, educators, foster/kinship carers, and adoptive parents working with children who have been prenatally substance exposed.

1 Introduction to Neonatal Opioid Withdrawal Syndrome (NOWS)

An Emerging Population for Speech-Language Pathologists

Brenda Louw

1.1 The NOWS Epidemic

An uncontrollable opioid epidemic is raging in the United States. It continues to grow in scope and complexity in the population at large, and there is an alarming increase in opioid use and opioid use disorder among pregnant women (Patrick et al., 2020). Prenatal substance use poses important health risks for the developing fetus (Behnke et al., 2013; Conradt et al., 2019; Patrick et al., 2020). A sequela of the opioid epidemic is Neonatal Opioid Withdrawal Syndrome (NOWS), in which infants exhibit a cluster of postnatal withdrawal symptoms due to the sudden discontinuation of fetal exposure to opioids used or misused by the mother during pregnancy. Opioids (and other substances) pass through the placenta and the infant becomes addicted together with the mother. Increases in maternal opioid use reflect a concomitant upsurge in the number of neonates experiencing NOWS (MacMullen & Samson, 2018; Patrick et al., 2020). However, whilst not all infants who are prenatally exposed to opioids experience NOWS, upwards of 50% to 100% of those newborns do develop NOWS (Conradt et al., 2019).

NOWS is a significant public health problem in the United States (Benninger et al., 2020) and is also now a global public health problem (Oei et al., 2023). High-income countries such as Canada, United Kingdom, Australia, and New Zealand have had significant increases in opioid use during pregnancy. While global efforts are made to make access to opioid analgesics available as a basic treatment in low- and middle-income countries (LMICs), misuse is increasing as access to these drugs increases. One unintended health consequence has been an increase in the incidence of Neonatal Abstinence Syndrome (NAS) (Marcellus, 2018). Although there is limited information on the prevalence of NAS in LMICs, healthcare professionals and policy makers need to be proactive about the effects on mothers and newborns and collaborate with professionals who have experience with NAS (Marcellus, 2018). Jones et al.

DOI: 10.4324/9781003397267-1

(2014) and Marcellus (2018) recommend international collaboration to guide research and evidence-based clinical practice related to opioid use during pregnancy. Moreover, the global problem of NOWS necessitates holistic and culturally appropriate practices for this population in a variety of contexts and countries.

1.1.1 Terminology

NOWS was traditionally known as Neonatal Abstinence Syndrome (NAS). NAS was a more general term that included exposure to nonopioids (e.g. benzodiazepines). However, recently the US Food and Drug Administration and other federal agencies renamed it NOWS due to evidence that the recent growth of neonatal drug withdrawal is primarily the result of opioid exposure, in isolation or in combination with other substances (Patrick et al., 2020). In this chapter the term NOWS will be used to reflect the current terminology. However, when discussing the work of other authors, the term used in their work will be referred to, whether it be NAS or NOWS.

1.1.2 Epidemiology

The Substance Abuse and Mental Health Services Administration (SAMHSA) sponsors a National Survey on Drug Use and Health (NSDUH) (SAMHSA, n.d.) providing national and state level information on the use of alcohol, tobacco, and illicit drugs. According to the 2022 report, approximately 8.9 million people aged 12 years and older misused opioids (heroin or prescription pain relievers) in the past year. The Center for Disease Control's (2023) 2019 self-reported data showed that about 7% of women reported using prescription opioid pain relievers during pregnancy, and 1 in 5 reported misuse of prescription opioids (getting them from a non-healthcare source or using them for a reason other than to relieve pain). The increased prevalence of opioid use disorder (OUD) in pregnant women places them in the midst of this public health challenge, and their infants are at high risk for developing NOWS and possible later long-term risk for adverse neurodevelopmental and academic problems. According to the National Institute for Drug Abuse (2023), approximately every 15 minutes a newborn experiences opioid withdrawal and every hour a baby is diagnosed with NOWS in the United States.

There are disproportionately higher rates of OUD in rural areas of the country, e.g. rural Appalachia. According to Jaekel et al. (2021) researchers have documented high rates of mental health problems, intimate partner violence, high rates of poverty and a lack of access to education and health services among women in rural Appalachia, which places them at an increased risk for substance use disorder. West Virginia is reported to have a significantly higher incidence rates of NOWS (44.1 in 1,000 births) than the national average (6.8 in 1,000 births) (Rutherford et al., 2022), which exacerbates the impact of NOWS on the infant, child, family, and caregivers.

1.1.3 Clinical Presentation of NOWS

The clinical presentation of NOWS may vary depending on opioid type, potency, maternal drug history, maternal metabolism, net transplacental transfer of drugs, placental metabolism, infant metabolism, and the addition of other substances such as tobacco and benzodiazepines. These factors can influence the onset, severity, or duration of the withdrawal (Patrick et al., 2020). NOWS is a complex, multisystem disorder and clinical presentation includes a constellation of symptoms associated with the central nervous system (e.g. high-pitched excessive crying, disrupted sleep, hyperactive Moro reflex, increased muscle tone, irritability, seizures), the autonomic nervous system (e.g. sweating, frequent yawning, hyperthermia, mottling, nasal stuffiness, sneezing, nasal flaring, increased respiratory rate), and the gastrointestinal system (e.g. excessive sucking, infrequent/uncoordinated suck, reflux or vomiting, diarrhea, weight loss) (Kocherlakota, 2014). Infants prenatally exposed to opioids may exhibit dysregulated behavior, high levels of stress, and have difficulty in modulating arousal, which affects the infant's interaction with caregivers and the environment (Velez et al., 2018). The symptomatology of infants with NOWS may be further influenced by maternal stress, nutrition, environmental factors, prematurity, and infections (Proctor-Williams & Louw, 2022). Benninger et al. (2020) reported that neurobehavioral functioning in exposed infants generally improves within the first four weeks of life, but stress and abstinence symptoms may persist. Despite this evidence, there is a dearth of published recommendations for screening, early identification of developmental delays, referrals for intervention, and follow-up (Benninger et al., 2020).

A body of research over the past three decades connects neurobehavioral differences related to prenatal opioid exposure with later developmental delays, but there are inconsistencies among the findings (Benninger et al., 2020). It is important to note that some of these studies reflected the early investigative nature of the research often using small numbers of research participants, inconsistent report of NOWS status, inconsistent descriptions of maternal drug use, and confounding variables including, but not limited to, potency, dose, timing, and duration of polydrug use (Proctor-Williams & Louw, 2022).

Contextual factors (such as environmental and social) also influence long-term outcomes of these children (Rutherford et al., 2022). Children prenatally exposed to opioids may have experienced adverse childhood experiences (ACEs) which are known to impact developmental outcomes (Maxwell et al., 2022). Conradt et al. (2019) reviewed the literature on the neurodevelopmental consequences of NOWS and highlighted the need for larger prospective studies with a longitudinal design and consideration of important confounding factors. These researchers unfolded an agenda for research that would address methodological gaps in the current literature with the goal of accurately identifying the children most at risk for adverse neurodevelopmental outcomes.

Despite these limitations, there do appear to be trends in the literature suggesting that the long-term adverse neurodevelopmental outcomes in children prenatally exposed to opioids should be of concern to all healthcare providers (Oei et al., 2023; Proctor-Williams & Louw, 2022). Studies show that children prenatally exposed to opioids have a high risk for cognitive differences; developmental delays; speech and language delays; hearing disorders; mental health symptoms associated with attention deficit/hyperactivity disorder (ADHD); autism spectrum disorder (ASD); visual and motor impairments; poor academic performance from elementary through high school; and difficulties with literacy and math (Benninger et al., 2020; Maxwell et al., 2022; Proctor-Williams & Louw, 2022). Some of these problems may persist into adulthood (Oei et al., 2017). Recent research (Benninger et al., 2022; Langa et al., 2021; Proctor-Williams & Louw, 2021) revealed that infants prenatally exposed to opioids have an increased prevalence of isolated cleft lip and palate and Pierre Robin sequence. Children with craniofacial differences and prenatal exposure to opioids are particularly at risk and require social support to cope with craniofacial differences and cleft-related speech and language disorders that are further compounded by the sequelae of NOWS and the complex social and home environments (Langa et al., 2021).

1.1.4 *Clinical Management of NOWS*

Clinical management for infants with NOWS includes pharmacologic and nonpharmacologic therapies. It is widely accepted that essential to the care of infants with opioid exposure is effective nonpharmacologic care, which engages the mother. Nonpharmacologic care needs to be individualized and tailored to the behavioral and physiologic symptoms the infant is experiencing. Regardless of the need for pharmacologic intervention, nonpharmacologic care needs to be provided at birth and throughout the hospitalization and thereafter (Patrick et al., 2020). It includes a variety of supportive care approaches that focus on decreasing sources of stimulation that trigger irritable behaviors and implementing soothing and calming techniques such as gentle handling, swaddling, minimal stimulation with low lighting and low noise levels, and parental rooming-in (Kocherlakota, 2014; Maguire et al., 2015). In infants with severe opioid withdrawal, both medication and nonpharmacologic care are often needed to improve clinical signs of withdrawal, pain, minimize complications from withdrawal, and manage their symptoms so that the infant can rest and feed sufficiently. Although morphine is the most common first-line therapy, other longer-acting opioids such as methadone, phenobarbital, clonidine, and buprenorphine may be used (Kocherlakota, 2014; Patrick et al., 2020). Pharmacological care has been associated with shorter hospital stays and lower morbidity (Kocherlakota, 2014). Because these infants are at higher risk for developmental problems, they should be closely monitored in the Neonatal Intensive Care Unit (NICU) follow-up clinics or by primary care pediatricians for early assessment and identification of developmental differences and the need for referral for appropriate early intervention (Benninger et al., 2020; Patrick et al., 2020). Oei et al. (2023) underscore the need for continued focus on these developmental challenges even after the infant has been withdrawn from the opioid. Recent research on the long-term effects of NOWS and pre-natal exposure to opioids suggests that neurodevelopmental outcomes in this vulnerable population calls for long-term treatment using a holistic, interprofessional approach, that can continue throughout adulthood (Benninger et al., 2020; Oei et al., 2017).

1.1.5 Challenges to Clinical Practice

Despite the current literature on neurodevelopmental outcomes and the fact that children prenatally exposed to opioids are increasingly entering healthcare and school systems, there are no known guidelines or position statements in speech-language pathology (SLP) to guide intervention for infants with NOWS, children prenatally exposed to opioids, and children with NOWS and other conditions. However, Proctor-Williams and Louw (2022) recommended such guidelines for infants with NOWS and children prenatally exposed to opioids with cleft lip and palate. They described the importance of an interprofessional team approach to care and the role of the SLP regarding feeding, communication intervention, advocacy, and education for this new population on SLP caseloads. Other healthcare disciplines such as physical therapy (PT) have responded to the opioid crisis and strongly advocated for physical therapy as a safe alternative to pharmacological pain management through the "#ChoosePT" cam-paign and the dedication of a special issue in the *Physical Therapy* journal (McCarty et al., 2019). Discipline-specific recommendations for the phys-ical therapist's examination and plan of care, including pharmacological management considerations, are outlined (McCarty et al., 2019). Research on NOWS is emerging among healthcare disciplines, but still there are gaps that affect the understanding of NOWS, equitable care, and development of evidence-based practice.

SLPs and other healthcare professionals face an ever-changing practice landscape which requires new knowledge and evidence-based strategies to meet the needs of this emerging population of infants and children who are becoming part of their caseloads. This growing population requires an interprofessional, holistic approach that is coordinated to improve care and short- and long-term outcomes. The complexity of NOWS is layered in, for example, mother–child dyads, families, caregivers, the impact of NOWS on multiple systems, comorbidity of disorders, socio-economic and cultural issues, and epigenetics, which all need to be addressed. To be knowledgeable about NOWS, to develop attitudes and skills regarding NOWS, to provide evidence-based care, and to improve the outcomes of this new population, pre-professional clinical and didactic preparation of NOWS should be required for SLPs and other healthcare professionals. Although SLPs are already competent in providing services to individuals with communication disorders and their families, continuing education (CE) can address knowledge gaps on NOWS and provide evidence-based interventions for this population.

In the United States, the healthcare and public systems are overburdened by the increasing number of infants with NOWS in the NICU, and by children prenatally exposed to opioids who are enrolled in early intervention and the school systems. These burdens include costs of longer NICU stays (Kocherlakota, 2014) and larger caseloads for healthcare and school-based providers (Maxwell et al., 2022; Proctor-Williams & Louw, 2022), which also translates into administrative burdens (Rutherford et al., 2022). Oei et al. (2023) make an urgent call for more effective research on treatments and long-term outcomes, and to direct funding to address the lifelong sequelae of NAS. These efforts will provide critical direction for mental, physical, and educational services to optimize these children's outcomes (Oei et al., 2023).

The following sections of the chapter address the basic tenets that should be regarded as general guidelines for interprofessional teamwork; for education and training of SLPs regarding NOWS; the research challenges posed by NOWS in speech-language pathology; and, finally, an overview of the purpose and organization of this volume is presented.

1.2 Basic Tenets of an Interprofessional Approach to Neonatal Opioid Withdrawal Syndrome (NOWS)

NOWS requires an interprofessional approach to gain insight from a variety of disciplines regarding the development of infants with NOWS and children prenatally exposed to opioids, and how their lives develop in the context of family and community. As healthcare professionals collaborate in interprofessional NOWS teams, it is important for them to consider some basic tenets in approaching the care of these infants, children, their families, and caregivers. These basic tenets reflect the values and practices of different fields such as early intervention, and child development, and professions such as speech-language pathology (SLP), physical therapy (PT), occupational therapy (OT), and pediatrics. The basic tenets discussed below are by no means exhaustive, but may act as general guidelines and a starting point for interprofessional collaboration. They can provide guidance regarding the way in which assessments are conducted, intervention is provided, team members interact with one another, relationships are established with the family, caregivers, and with the community, and importantly professionals' understanding of the child as a developing individual within their context (Guralnick, 2000). Seven basic tenets are proposed.

1.2.1 Participating in Interprofessional Collaboration

Infants with NOWS, children prenatally exposed to opioids, and their families and caregivers present as a complex combination of medical and social dynamics during a vulnerable time. Interprofessional teamwork promotes a collaborative partnership between families and healthcare team members across healthcare settings (McDaniel et al., 2021). Interprofessional collaboration (IPC) is propagated by the World Health Organization (WHO, 2010) in order to strengthen health systems and improve patient outcomes (Bornman & Louw, 2023).

Multiple teams and team members are required to provide services in different settings across the lifespan, which includes teams in the NICU, high-risk follow-up clinics, early intervention teams, educational teams, and, in cases of comorbidity such as cleft lip and palate, craniofacial teams (Langa et al., 2021; Proctor-Williams & Louw, 2022). SLPs and other healthcare professionals may also serve as community service providers and liaise closely with the interprofessional teams.

Irrespective of their roles, healthcare professionals need specific knowledge and skills to practice interprofessional collaboration. A set of core competencies have been used to define this knowledge and skills base within four domains of interprofessional practice (IPP) (Johnson, 2016). First, Values/Ethics refers to working with individuals of other professions to maintain a climate of mutual respect and shared values. Second, Roles/Responsibilities refers to using the knowledge of one's own role and those of other professions to appropriately assess and address the healthcare needs of patients and populations served. Third, Interprofessional Communication encompasses communication with patients, families, communities, and other health professionals in a responsive and responsible manner that supports a team approach to the maintenance of health and the treatment of disease. Fourth, Teams and Teamwork requires the application of relationship-building values and the principles of team dynamics to perform effectively in different team roles to plan and deliver person-centered care that is safe, timely, efficient, effective, and equitable. In addition, interprofessional collaboration and care makes collaborative leadership an essential skill (Iachini et al., 2022; Bornman & Louw, 2023). It is essential to respect each discipline's contribution to the overall process, as well as the perspective that each contribute to the holistic approach (Guralnick, 2000).

The interprofessional team approach to NOWS has been described and researched in recent literature. McCarty and Braswell (2022) found that the implementation of interprofessional rounds reduced the length of stay for infants with NAS. Education of team members on the impact of trauma of mothers with substance use disorder and trauma-informed care (TIC) was determined to promote collaboration between team members and mothers (Linn et al., 2021). McDaniel et al. (2021) identified important structures, processes of care, and meaningful outcomes to enhance and evaluate team care for infants with NAS. The authors called for further research to improve the quality of care for this population through interprofessional team care.

1.2.2 Applying the International Classification of Functioning, Disability and Health (ICF)

The International Classification of Functioning, Disability and Health (ICF) (WHO, 2001) provides a biopsychosocial framework which is a holistic approach to health and focuses on the individual as a whole. The ICF is an integration and interaction of the biological and social models of health in a unitary manner (de Camargo et al., 2019). The framework considers the biological impairment in both body structure and function experienced by the individual and how that impairment impacts their activity and participation in daily events. Contextual factors are considered, which include social attitudes and beliefs about impairment and barriers to well-being, as well as the personal characteristics of an individual. It is a strength-based model, emphasizing functioning (de Camargo et al., 2019).

The ICF has multiple applications to help healthcare providers view individuals within the broader context. It serves as a powerful tool for evidence-based advocacy and for health policies. The ICF can also be used as an educational tool for all healthcare professions. Healthcare providers can apply the ICF for personalized documentation of infants with NOWS and children prenatally exposed to opioids; to identify their strengths, barriers or issues, needs, and goals and, importantly, identify windows of management and evaluations of specific management (de Camargo et al., 2019). Based on the results of their focus group study regarding SLPs' perceptions of their role in service provision in the opioid epidemic, Maxwell et al. (2022) proposed a shift in practices to focus on the whole child and the environmental context in which the child lives. Applying the ICF framework would be a practical way to achieve these recommendations.

Considering the interaction between all the components of the ICF, an understanding of the many factors that contribute to the effects of NOW on the functioning and participation of these infants and children is strengthened. The ICF guides assessment, clinical decision making, and intervention. Developing a Functional Profile for a child and their family provides a holistic view of the infant and child within their environment to inform intervention. The American Speech-Language-Hearing Association (ASHA) recommends the use of the ICF and has adopted this framework in its policy document, the Scope of Practice for Speech-Language Pathology (2016), which serves as a guideline for delivering quality of care. Finally, the implementation of the ICF facilitates interprofessional collaboration and family-centered care (FCC).

1.2.3 Following a Family-Centered Care (FCC) Approach

Recently, in healthcare, there has been a shift in research and clinical practice toward a more holistic perspective that emphasizes Family-Centered Care (FCC). This approach is grounded in collaboration between families and healthcare providers for the planning, delivery, and evaluation of healthcare as well as in research and education of healthcare professionals (American Academy of Pediatrics, 2012). However, mothers, families, and caregivers of infants with NOWS and children prenatally exposed to opioids are a socially complex population. Extreme challenges may be posed by contextual factors such as abusive and neglectful relationships, chaotic homes, unstable housing, and residential programs for mothers and children. Mothers themselves may experience ongoing trauma and behavioral brain changes due to their substance use disorder (SUD) and, in some cases, their own prenatal substance exposure (Velez et al., 2021).

The core elements of FCC are crucial and need to be used in combination with other approaches. These core elements are: respect for all team members (including families as team members); a focus on family strengths and resources; cultural competence; a balanced and trusting relationship between families and providers; active partnerships between families and team members; empowerment; and individual goal-orientated and community-focused services (Braun et al., 2017). The American Academy of Pediatrics (AAP) provides principles to guide practitioners in collaborating with families to modify practices to improve families' experiences (American Academy of Pediatrics, 2012). Some of these core elements will be discussed in more detail due to their importance as basic tenets in the interprofessional approach to NOWS proposed in this text.

The benefits of the FCC approach have been extensively researched and include increased family involvement in care, improved caregiver well-being, more positive parental perceptions of their children, increased parental confidence in supporting their child's needs, and improved parental self-management (Braun et al., 2017). This approach ensures that families and children have a choice in services and that families and professionals work collaboratively.

Together, the ICF (WHO, 2001) and FCC provide an evidence-based framework for interprofessional team members to develop a holistic view of infants with NOWS, children prenatally exposed to opioids, and their mothers, caregivers, and families. However, it is clear that the FCC approach alone is not sufficient, or always appropriate, for the NOWS population and needs to be supplemented by other approaches such as trauma-informed care (Marcellus, 2014).

1.2.4 Implementing Trauma-Informed Care (TIC)

Women's substance use is often linked to personal experiences of trauma and violence. Infants with NOWS and children exposed prenatally to opioids are most likely to experience some type of trauma during childhood and suffer from ACEs (Maxwell et al., 2022). According to Forkey et al. (2021), research in multiple fields such as genetics, neuroscience, and epidemiology provide evidence that these experiences have effects at the molecular, cellular, and organ level, with consequences on physical, emotional, developmental, and behavioral health across the lifespan. Trauma-informed care (TIC) addresses trauma and promotes resilience (Forkey et al., 2021).

TIC is used by different disciplines such as pediatrics, nursing, and social work, and is emerging in other healthcare professions, e.g. in SLP (Roberson & Lund, 2022). It is viewed to be an effective evidence-based approach to supporting mothers of infants with NOWS, children prenatally exposed to opioids, and their families and caregivers. TIC involves realizing the impact of trauma; recognizing the signs of trauma and how trauma affects all individuals in the organization (clients, families, and team members); responding by integrating this knowledge about trauma into policies, procedures, and practice; and actively resisting re-traumatization of the child and family (SAMHSA, 2014).

The caregiver's role in promoting regulation and resilience is encouraged. Integrating TIC to prevent and reduce the impact of trauma so that all members of the care team feel supported and valued is an integral part of TIC. It promotes a culture of safety, empowerment, and healing within the team approach that decreases stress responses, and promotes the building of resilience (Forkey et al., 2021). In addition to the FCC approach, TIC provides a complementary way in which to address the unique caregiving requirements of mothers of infants with NAS and children prenatally exposed to opioids, and their families and caregivers (Marcellus, 2014).

1.2.5 Focusing on a Strength-Based Approach

The APA lists family strengths as a core element of FCC (American Academy of Pediatrics, 2012). Interprofessional team members need to recognize and build on the strengths of individual children and families and empower them to discover their own strengths, build confidence, and participate in making choices and decisions about their own healthcare (American Academy of Pediatrics, 2012). Clinicians need to move away from a deficit-focused approach that focuses on risk and vulnerability and work from a strength-based approach. This approach recognizes the inherent and learned attributes that individuals have rather than the individual's deficits (Ezell et al., 2023). It focuses on the strengths, resources, and competencies of a child and family and moves away from the pathology and disorder. Ezell et al. (2023) proposed the Integrated Strengths-Based Engagement Framework (ISBEF) to be used with individuals who misuse drugs. Their model consists of four steps: discuss client strengths and establish strength-based goals; select socio-culturally appropriate co-participants; implement processes in a culturally humble and affirmational manner; and measure program satisfaction and self-efficacy outcomes (Ezell et al., 2023). This model is appropriate for implementation by interprofessional NOWS team members.

The strengths of infants with NOWS and children prenatally exposed to opioids can also be described by using the ICF to create an individual profile (de Camargo et al., 2019). For each ICF component (personal factors, environmental factors, participation and activities, and body structure and functions) strengths and facilitators are identified as well as barriers and issues. A profile can be created jointly by the interprofessional team members to provide a holistic view and identify areas of support needed. The interprofessional NOWS team members would then reflect upon the strengths-based approach using verbal language that identifies strengths and positive qualities, encourages participation from all team members, and focuses on goals and solutions. Such language then needs to be used in diagnostic reports and other written communication (Braun et al., 2017).

The concepts of resilience and protective factors dovetail with the strength-based approach. Resilience is a dynamic process and is the capacity of a system to adapt successfully to challenges that threaten the function, survival, or future development of the system, despite significant adversities (Forkey et al., 2021; Masten & Barnes, 2018). According to Masten and Barnes (2018) the capacity to adapt to challenges depends on an individual's connections to other people and systems external to the individual through relationships and other processes. Werner (2000) describes protective factors as being within the child (infancy, early childhood, middle childhood, adolescence, and adulthood), within the family and within the community.

Interprofessional NOWS team members need to promote and build resilience both within the child and the family. Forkey et al. (2021) suggest that anticipatory guidance about development and safety can be used to promote relational health and positive childhood experiences, including achievements at home, at school, and in neighborhoods. When mothers, caregivers, and families raise concerns about development, these challenges can be framed with resilience and positive experiences as the goal. Educating mothers, caregivers, and families on the importance of childhood for nurturing lifelong capacities for health and well-being is important and these messages can be tailored to age and context. In addition, referrals for normative developmental resources can be made available as well (Masten & Barnes, 2018).

1.2.6 Integrating Cultural Responsiveness, Cultural Competence, and Cultural Humility Into Service Provision

As the demographics in the US continue to change, the opioid crisis affects an increasingly diverse population, which introduces a variety of health beliefs, values, and behaviors that are influenced by cultural backgrounds. Interprofessional team members are required to understand and relate to infants with NOWS, children prenatally exposed to opioids, and their families and caregivers, whose cultural backgrounds differ from their own. Honoring racial, ethnic, cultural, and socio-economic backgrounds is listed as a core element by the AAP's policy on FCC (American Academy of Pediatrics, 2012).

Cultural competence, cultural humility, and culturally responsive services are all vital components to each professional interaction and are dynamic, complex, and lifelong practices (American Speech-Language-Hearing Association [ASHA], n.d.a) that fall under Cultural Responsiveness. ASHA (n.d.a) describes cultural responsiveness as understanding, appropriately including, and responding to the combination of cultural variables and the full range of dimensions of diversity that an individual brings to an interaction. It requires valuing diversity and seeking to further cultural knowledge. Cultural competence is a dynamic and complex process requiring ongoing self-assessment, continuous cultural education, openness to others' values and beliefs, and willingness to share one's own values and beliefs. It evolves over time and begins with an understanding of one's own culture, continues through reciprocal interactions with individuals from various cultures, and extends through one's own lifelong learning (ASHA, n.d.a). Cultural humility is the process of being aware of how people's culture can impact their health behaviors and using this awareness to cultivate sensitive approaches in treating individuals (ASHA, n.d.a). Hughes et al. (2020) state that embracing and incorporating cultural humility is essential to creating a comprehensive and individualized plan of care.

Integrating cultural competence, cultural humility, and culturally responsive care is essential for the accuracy of assessments and establishing effective collaborations with the mother, family, and caregivers affected by NOWS. When developing a plan and pathway of care, the needs and expectations of mothers, families and caregivers need to be considered with respect to their cultural values and beliefs. Specifically, SLPs need to consider linguistic diversity in intervention (Hyter & Salas-Provance, 2019).

1.2.7 Including Community Providers

To ensure that the interprofessional NOWS teams' recommendations are implemented, it is essential that community providers are involved in care. Teams should consult key providers in the community regarding the infant with NOWS or child prenatally exposed to opioids. Active participation of early intervention specialists and educators is also critical. Follow-up communications with community providers, such as the child's service coordinator identified as part of the Individualized Family Service Plan (IFSP) or Individual Education Program (IEP) process, is extremely important and valuable to care (Guralnick, 2000).

Interprofessional teams need to develop a common vision and advocate for supportive attitudes regarding mothers of infants with NOWS and children prenatally exposed to opioids (Proctor-Williams & Louw, 2022). Mothers of infants with NOWS often have to contend with the challenges of overcoming stigma and they may be ostracized, diminished, and alienated. They may become discouraged and may even altogether cease to interact with or visit their infants and forgo efforts that facilitate their recovery (Recto et al., 2020). Recto et al. (2020) recommend education and direct contact to change attitudes and behavioral intentions. Team members should advocate for, promote, and model non-stigmatizing attitudes when collaborating with community providers (Proctor-Williams

& Louw, 2022). Community providers and administrators need to be educated on NOWS and its detrimental effects on the child and his/her chances to overcome adverse early life exposures and to understand the need for longitudinal service needs (Oei et al., 2023).

1.3 Implications of NOWS for Education and Training of Speech-Language Pathologists

Infants with NOWS and children prenatally exposed to opioids are on the caseloads of SLPS in a wide variety of clinical settings including NICUs (Craig & Smith, 2020; Proctor-Williams & Louw, 2017; Proctor-Williams & Louw, 2022); interdisciplinary NICU follow-up clinics (Benninger et al., 2022); specialty clinics such as cleft lip and palate clinics (Langa et al., 2021) and in schools (Rutherford et al., 2022). The question arises: how prepared are the SLPs in managing these infants, children, their mothers, families, and caregivers? Maxwell et al. (2022) indicated that SLPs across the United States have expressed concerns regarding the need to provide appropriate services for children with a history of opioid exposure.

The need for education and training regarding the NOWS population, their mothers, caregivers, families, and communities continues to grow, but there has been a limited response to this need in the field of speech-language pathology specifically. Many different reasons are posited for the current gap in professional preparation. First, the rapid growth and development in the field of speech-language pathology which currently overburdens academic and clinical curricula (Knollhoff, 2023) makes additions to curricula challenging. Second, Oei et al. (2023) state that research during the past two decades has shown that withdrawal is only the tip of the iceberg and that there may be lifelong sequelae, which need to be addressed in more effective research. The implication is that services to these individuals and mothers, families, and caregivers are required beyond the NICU with a longitudinal emphasis, and that this population needs to be included in the professional preparation of SLPs and other healthcare professionals. Third, the training dilemma is exacerbated by scant evidence-based research on the assessment and treatment of communication for infants with NOWS and children prenatally exposed to opioids (Proctor-Williams & Louw, 2022). In spite of extensive research on neurodevelopmental outcomes and comorbid conditions in this population, true understanding of the complexities of NOWS remains elusive. The result is a lack of evidence for appropriate and effective assessment and intervention of this diverse population, which is a major challenge to education. Maxwell et al. (2022) point out that, although SLPs are well equipped to provide services to a wide range of populations, children with a history of opioid exposure are a heterogenous group, often with comorbid conditions and adverse social contexts, that renders service provision challenging. Given the magnitude of the opioid crisis in the United States (Patrick et al., 2020) and globally (Oei et al., 2023), SLP and other healthcare professions have an ethical responsibility to conduct research, educate, and train pre-professionals and professionals alike to provide effective, evidence-based intervention services to infants with NOWS, children prenatally exposed to opioids, and their mothers, families, and caregivers to meet their needs and ensure optimal outcomes. On the other hand, it may be the case that SLP programs are in fact preparing students to provide services to this population, but have yet to disseminate their efforts widely.

There are promising approaches to address this gap in training. First is developing course work on a graduate level. Programs seeking to address NOWS in the curriculum could consider the following suggestions to guide their efforts. Maxwell et al. (2022) conducted a focus group study which informed the development of a graduate level course with the title *Effects of the Opioid Epidemic on Student Language Skills*. This course focuses on the impact of the opioid epidemic on speech and language development and provides intervention suggestions. This model could be followed by other programs. However, research needs to be conducted to determine what pre-professional training on NOWS is provided and to identify the best solution for expanding curricula without overburdening students. Second, Knollhoff (2023) advocated for training in pediatric dysphagia in SLP graduate programs and suggested that programs need to be creative in order to support the growing needs for pediatric swallowing and feeding disorders. There is also growing concern for the limited number of programs that offer course work on cleft lip and palate (CLP) (Mills & Hardin-Jones, 2019). Feeding issues in infants with CLP are one of the first challenges to parents and teams. Furthermore, infants with NOWS are also characterized by feeding disorders, albeit of a different nature. Instead of competing for space in overfull curricula, it is suggested that proponents of these topic areas collaborate in advocating for course work additions and infuse content on pediatric swallowing and feeding to include feeding issues in the CLP and NOWS populations.

Third, the Council on Academic Accreditation in Audiology and Speech-Language Pathology standards include interprofessional education/interprofessional collaborative practice (IPE/IPC) that needs to be addressed by training programs through academic and clinical curricula (Council on Academic Accreditation, n.d.). Since infants with NOWS, children prenatally exposed to opioids, and their mothers, families, and caregivers require an interprofessional approach to assessment and intervention (Craig & Smith, 2020; Patrick et al., 2020; Saunders et al., 2016), case studies on infants with NOWS and children prenatally exposed to opioids can be used in teaching. Simulation representing family and primary caregivers could be used to develop knowledge about NOWS and insight of the various professionals on the team. At the same time students would be preparing for IPC post-graduation. Shrader et al. (2015) emphasize the importance of faculty development in the sustainability of an IPE program. Faculty training could enhance their knowledge and skills for teaching and clinical supervision. These academic endeavors would ensure that future professionals would be better equipped to provide services to this population in future without over-burdening the curriculum and students and creating anticipation for more information on NOWS in SLP course work.

Fourth, IPC has been propagated by the World Health Organization (WHO) to strengthen health systems and improve patient outcomes (WHO, 2010). As mentioned earlier, the ICF framework (WHO, 2001) provides a biopsychosocial and holistic structure for conceptualizing the human experience of health and health service provision and is recommended for enhancing patient-centered interprofessional care. Embedding the ICF framework within curricula of health professions programs supports interprofessional education (IPE) and collaborative practice (CP) (Moran et al., 2020). Snyman et al.(2015) explored the experiences of medical students and their preceptors using the ICF in IPE and CP, and how patients perceived the care they received by using an associative group analysis methodology. They concluded that the value of integrating IPE and CP as an authentic learning experience was demonstrated clearly, as was the ICF as a catalyst in pushing boundaries for change. The ICF can therefore be applied in both IPE and coursework on NOWS to approach this population holistically, enhance teamwork, and provide training in evidence-based services.

Fifth, there is an increased focus on student satisfaction in higher education and by determining the education needs as perceived by graduate students, curricula may be designed from the bottom up (Busch & Ma, 2023). Training programs can give students a voice in developing didactic content by exploring students' perception of their knowledge, attitudes, and confidence and comfort levels related to NOWS. Konstanty et al. (2023) examined 67 SLP graduate students' perspectives of NOWS and their education needs through a national survey. Although the response rate was low (N 67), important information was gained. Overall respondents expressed a range of confidence levels (from extremely confident to not confident all) regarding their clinical skills of assessment and intervention of feeding, communication, and interprofessional teamwork with this new population. They were less confident in the ability to provide resources to mothers, families, and caregivers. All the respondents agreed that NOWS should be included in the graduate curricula (Konstanty et al., 2023).

Improved understanding of this topic from a student perspective may be used to inform training to better equip and prepare future SLPs to address the needs of this new population.

Sixth, clinical supervisors and instructors need to share their efforts and exchange information. Platforms such as the annual conferences of the Council of Academic Programs in Communication Sciences and Disorders (CAPCSD) and ASHA's national conventions may be utilized to establish a foundation for the scholarship of teaching and learning, formal research, and evidence-based education. Lastly, clinical practice guidelines based on NOWS research are needed by SLPs and are crucial to inform the content of training and to define the role of the SLP. Based on their focus group study, Maxwell et al. (2022) stated their intention to suggest guidelines for SLPs serving this population. Currently some examples in the literature may be expanded upon and followed. It is evident that major curriculum changes need to occur to equip future professionals to change long-term outcomes of infants with NOWS and children prenatally exposed to opioids.

Lifelong learning is a professional responsibility of SLPs (ASHA, n.d.b) and is required for SLPs to keep abreast of changes and new developments in the field. According to ASHA (n.d.b) it is essential that SLPs seek out and engage in continuing education experiences to update their knowledge base and hone their skills. CE on NOWS is another opportunity that needs to be addressed forthwith. A national survey of school-based SLPs was conducted by Ratliff (2017) to explore the prevalence of children post-NAS on their caseloads and to examine their perceptions of these children's speech, language, literacy, and any comorbidities. Three hundred respondents from 40 states participated in the research and 95.6% reported that they had not received any specific education on NAS. Those 4.4% who had received training listed continuing education events, in-service training, a certificate program, and a graduate course as sources. More recent focus group research with school-based SLPs in West Virginia validated these findings (Maxwell et al., 2022; Rutherford et al., 2022). These authors identified four areas of training and education to better equip SLPs for service provision to children with prenatal opioid exposure their families, namely understanding psychological variables that affect learning; sensitivity to appropriately address issues of safety and well-being; dealing with the challenges posed by case management; and understanding the social consequences often associated with substance use disorder. A small pilot study that explored SLPs' perspectives and experiences of NOWS and CLP co-occurring in infants and children prenatally exposed to opioids with CLP on their caseloads determined that only three of five participants were interested in learning more about the topic (Brandon et al., 2023). It is possible that SLPs do not seem to be aware of the importance of NOWS and CLP co-occurring and do not fully understand the consequences of this new population. Infants with NOWs, children prenatally exposed to opioids, their mothers, families, and caregivers require clinicians to adjust their clinical practices, and develop new strategies for assessment and intervention to best serve this population. CE efforts need to be promoted creatively to stimulate the interest of SLPs.

There are exciting strategies to approach the development of CE opportunities to ensure that newfound knowledge is applied. An evidence-based approach to professional development called Participatory Adult Learning Strategy (PALS) was proposed by Dunst and Trivette (2009) based on several meta-analyses of adult learning methods. PALS places emphasis on active learner involvement in all aspects of the training opportunities and instructor/trainer-guided learner experiences. The use of PALS is associated with improved learner knowledge, use, and mastery of different types of intervention practices. A novel manner of evaluating CE offerings can also be applied. A Personal Commitment to Change Statement (PCS) was developed by Bornman and Louw (2019). They explored using it in a case study using a purposive sampling technique, to determine its impact on the integration of new knowledge and skills with previous knowledge and clinical practice. Thirty-two participants (SLPs, audiologists, physical therapists, and occupational therapists) turned in a PCS with a total of 71 text statements at the end of a one-day interprofessional continuing education event on the introduction of assessment tools developed within the ICF framework. The PCSs of the participants reflected their intention to make changes to their clinical practice and in their workplace environments. It was concluded that PCSs guide health practitioners to reflect on the implementation of change to their knowledge, skills, or performance in practice. CE events on NOWS can be planned within the PALS framework to enhance the effectiveness of the training, followed by a PCS to encourage application to clinical practice, which would enhance the skill set of SLPs working with infants with NOWS in, e.g. the NICU and early intervention, with children prenatally exposed to opioids in schools and their families.

Last, SLPs also need to prioritize education of mothers, families, caregivers, colleagues, and administrators. Topics such as, e.g. neurodevelopmental outcomes, social complexities, stigma, and TIC need to be addressed (Proctor-Williams & Louw, 2022). The enduring nature of the problem needs to be stressed to address the lifelong sequelae and service needs (Oei et al., 2023). According to Rutherford et al. (2022) more education and training is needed to better understand the psychological variables; to develop sensitivity to address issues of safety and well-being; to deal with case management challenges; and to understand the social consequences associated with NOWS.

1.4 Challenges Posed by NOWS to Research in Speech-Language Pathology

Conducting and participating in research is a specific professional practice domain of SLPs according to ASHA's Scope of Practice (2016). Nelson and Gilbert (2021) describe research as having many roles in the field of SLP such as satisfying scientific curiosity; guiding clinical practice; evidence-based practice; program evaluation and support; and developing public policy.

Research on NAS and NOWS abounds in fields such as pediatrics (e.g. Benninger et al., 2020; Velez et al., 2021); nursing (e.g. McGlothen-Bell et al., 2021; McQueen et al., 2019); public health (e.g. Conradt et al., 2019; Kolodny et al., 2015); and psychology (e.g. Jones et al., 2019; Lee et al., 2020) and many other health-related fields. Topics addressed are directly relevant to SLP assessment and intervention practices for this population, of which examples include: elemental role of the SLP in a team within the NICU serving infants with NAS (Craig & Smith, 2020); long-term outcomes of infants with NAS (Joseph et al., 2020); neurodevelopmental outcomes of NAS (Shearer et al., 2018); feeding issues in infants with NAS (Liu et al., 2015); preschool language development in infants of mothers with opioid use disorder (Kim et al., 2021); the effect of NAS on language delay (Miller et al., 2020); cognitive development in children of children born to mothers with opioid use (Nygaard et al., 2015); fMRI study on working memory-selective attention task (Sirnes et al., 2017); attention deficit/hyperactivity disorder (ADHD) associated with prenatal opioid exposure (Graham et al., 2019; Schwartz et al., 2021); autism spectrum disorder (ASD) and autism features in children prenatally exposed to opioids (Rubenstein et al., 2018); mental health issues (Conner et al., 2020); health and educational outcomes in children after NAS (Fill et al., 2018; Rees et al., 2020); and high school performance in children with NAS (Oei et al., 2017).

However, in the field of SLP to date research has been conducted on NOWS in a limited and desultory manner and topics are scattered to include, e.g. comorbidity of NOWS and cleft lip and palate (Proctor-Williams & Louw, 2021; Proctor-Williams & Louw, 2022); perceptions of SLPs service provision to children with a history of opioid exposure (Maxwell et al., 2022); and perceived characteristics of children with a history of opioid exposure (Rutherford et al., 2022). Research on opioid-induced hearing loss in audiology is scant as well (Creel et al., 2020; Rigg & Rigg, 2020; Hite et al., 2024), but nonetheless important to SLPs.

Due to the dearth of research in the field, it is important to take gray literature into account when reviewing research on NOWS in SLP. Gray literature is produced outside of traditional publishing channels and can include conference abstracts, conference presentations, theses, reports, policy literature, working papers, newsletters, government documents, etc. It can assist applied researchers and practitioners to understand what interventions exist for a particular problem, the full range of evaluations (if any) that have been conducted, and where further intervention development and evaluation are needed (Adams et al., 2016). Conference presentations such as those by Holland et al. (2021), Proctor-Williams and Louw (2021), and Fabrize et al. (2019) introduced this population to SLPs and provided an overview of research and clinical strategies, whilst Horstman et al. (2019) reviewed which infants with NAS receive services in the NICU. Master's theses on topics such as SLPs' perceptions of children diagnosed with NAS on their school caseloads (Ratliff, 2017); NICU SLPs' perceptions of infants with NAS (Fabrize, 2019); and the relationship between respiration and feeding in NAS (Rice, 2020). Such gray literature has contributed to SLPs' knowledge with suggestions for clinical application.

The paucity of research on NOWS in SLP poses a dilemma to clinicians, since they not only have to search outside of the field of SLP for literature and evidence for best practice, but need to consider and evaluate the scientific merit of gray literature as well. Evidence-based practice (EBP) is the integration of clinical expertise, internal and external evidence, and client/patient perspectives. This enables clinicians to make informed evidence-based decisions to provide high-quality professional services which take the interests, values, needs, and choices of individuals with communication disorders into account (ASHA, n.d.b). Thome et al. (2020) surveyed SLPs regarding their understanding and use of EBP and concluded that their participants would benefit from increased training on EBP and require more time during the workday to engage in EBP. Furthermore Rutherford et al. (2022) pointed out that research in other disciplines on speech and language in children with a history of opioid exposure did not present specific patterns of speech and/or language differences or delays and, as a result, SLPs lack clinical guidance in caring for this population. Research on NAS and NOWS in other fields has been subjected to critique, limiting their application value for SLPs. Rutherford et al. (2022) identified that some studies used a retrospective design and based conclusions regarding outcomes from data obtained in medical charts, and data collected retrospectively from the 1990s did not address the needs of the infants and children affected by the current opioid crisis. Conradt et al. (2019) reviewed the state of the literature on neurodevelopmental outcomes in NOWS according to developmental periods: newborn, infancy, and beyond three years of age. They identified a number of key methodological shortcomings, such as small sample sizes, which make it difficult to adjust for confounding variables; the actual method used to assess and diagnosis of NOWS; the lack of a neurodevelopmental risk-monitoring marker at birth to identify newborns at risk for NOWS and track their neurodevelopmental outcomes; how the timing of opioid exposure during pregnancy can influence neurodevelopmental outcomes; and the impact of maternal genetic or epigenetic factors or addiction liability, as confounding variables (Conradt et al., 2019). It is clear that currently the research evidence regarding NOWS in the field of SLP is limited, and lacks cohesiveness, which has important implications for the communication outcomes of children prenatally exposed to opioids, since there is not a strong external evidence base for true EBP with this population.

Several areas of research needs in SLP have been identified by different authors: feeding and swallowing; communication speech, language literacy, hearing and behavioral characteristics of children prenatally exposed to opioids to expand SLPs' basic knowledge of the population; and how to support these children (Maxwell et al., 2022; Fabrize, 2019; Rutherford et al., 2022); the types of systematic supports needed for SLPs and other team members serving this population (Maxwell et al., 2022); the relationship between NOWS and comorbidities such as cleft lip and palate (Proctor-Williams and Louw, 2022); identifying service needs (Rutherford et al., 2022); guidelines for SLPs in providing services to this population (Rutherford et al., 2022); and the andragogical aspects of implementing NOWS into SLP curricula.

Researchers in other fields also identified research needs which SLPs can participate in addressing, such as guidelines for the follow-up of infants with NOWS to facilitate screening and timely identification of developmental impairment and referral for appropriate services, as well as larger prospective and comprehensive follow-up studies (Benninger et al., 2020); and treatment and long-term outcomes (Oei et al., 2023). Conradt et al. (2019) call for rigorously designed studies for both short- and long-term neurodevelopmental consequences of children with prenatal opioid exposure. They proposed a solution-oriented research agenda to address existing limitations in the literature which would lead to more rigorous tests of how prenatal opioid exposure could impact neurodevelopmental outcomes from infancy to adolescence and provide specific suggestions for research topics.

The research–clinical gap is a barrier to EBP in SLP as the knowledge generated by research is not immediately or always applied in clinical settings (Olswang & Prelock, 2015). Clinical practice research could effectively address this barrier. Researchers and clinicians are encouraged to collaborate to close the research–practice gap and develop clinical practice research projects. Spencer (2022) states that one purpose of science is to create new knowledge, but informing clinical practice is another. Clinical practice research is an emerging type of research in SLP. Clinical practice research is clinical research, but maximizes the relevance and application of research for practice. It specifically addresses the evaluation of methods of prevention, assessment, intervention, and implementation and is informed by current need and barriers to practice, and regards clinicians as the primary audience (Spencer, 2022). SLP researchers and clinicians also need to seek opportunities to collaborate on interprofessional research projects, given the complexity of NOWS.

With the growing NOWS population on SLP caseloads and the current lack of research-based guidelines for clinical practice, SLPs have multiple opportunities to address the significant gaps in knowledge and understanding of this population, and, importantly, to fulfill their professional practice requirement of research and contribute to the outcomes of infants with NOWS and children with prenatal opioid exposure. It is crucial that SLPs share their research findings, not only by publishing and presenting the results, but also by using social media to inform colleagues via a wider platform due to the limited knowledge of infants with NOWS and children prenatally exposed to opioids.

1.5 Purpose and Organization of This Volume

The purpose of this volume is to provide an accessible, comprehensive, and evidence-based resource on NOWS for students, clinicians, instructors, and researchers in SLP and other healthcare professions working within an interprofessional approach to treat infants with NOWS, children prenatally exposed to opioids, their mothers, caregivers, and families.

Bringing together the accumulated experience and knowledge of nationally and internationally recognized researcher-clinicians from different disciplines and from different countries, this text applies concise updates on theoretical underpinnings, current research, and personal experience to clinical settings.

Infants with NOWS and children prenatally exposed to opioids may demonstrate multiple complex issues, which necessitate a holistic team-based approach. The background chapters serve as a general orientation for an all-inclusive approach to the field and to the interprofessional approach propagated by the volume. A chapter on the understanding of the dyad – as opposed to the infant and child only – affected by NOWS is presented as a necessary pathway to the provision of optimal care. This is followed by a chapter on the neurodevelopmental outcomes of children prenatally exposed to opioids, emphasizing past and recent research, identifying limitations, and providing recommendations for future research to improve care to this population. Next, a chapter on the multidisciplinary collaborative approach based on an integration of high-quality evidence, from the prenatal period through the newborn hospital stay and into childhood, is presented. The focus is on empowering parents and primary caregivers and guiding team members in working with this vulnerable population. Mothers of infants diagnosed with NOWS and of children prenatally exposed to opioids experience great stress, as do their families and caregivers. A chapter on trauma-informed care as a foundational approach for interprofessional team members to support this population is presented. These chapters are of fundamental relevance to all interprofessional team members.

Feeding issues characteristic of infants diagnosed with NOWS are one of the first challenges experienced by mothers, caregivers, and team members and a cause of anxiety in mothers. Evidence-based clinical recommendations for feeding infants with NOWS, and children prenatally exposed to opioids, are presented in a chapter which addresses feeding issues that prevail in this population in a practical manner.

The perspectives of three specific disciplines, namely speech-language pathology (SLP), occupational therapy (OT), and physical therapy (PT), follow in separate chapters. The role of each of these professionals regarding NOWS is addressed by describing the specific problems in developmental domains addressed by each discipline, research needs and clinical strategies for managing this population, and how each of these disciplines collaborates interprofessionally to serve infants with NOWS, children prenatally exposed to opioids, their mothers, families and caregivers.

Emerging evidence that NOWS has a long-term, multisystem impact on infants diagnosed with NOWS necessitates clinical intervention, support, and research across the lifespan. A chapter describes the impact of NOWS on older children and young adults. Strategies for research, healthcare pathways, and policy to innovate outcomes of this complex and growing population are discussed. Coming full circle, the environment of this population is highlighted. Families, including fathers, are emphasized. A chapter focusing on the needs of families in non-stigmatizing, non-judgmental service environments – to promote positive outcomes – is presented. Finally support for foster/kinship and adoptive parents of infants with NOWS, and children prenatally exposed to opioids, is described. Novel aspects and approaches regarding each of the chapter topics are presented throughout the text.

The combination of this content in a single text makes it the first comprehensive and all- inclusive reference and clinical resource on NOWS to provide holistic, multidimensional, strength-based, and evidence-based care to improve the outcomes of these children and their families.

1.6 Summary

The United States is experiencing an opioid crisis as a result of the increase of opioid use and opioid-related complications such as NOWS. Opioid misuse is on the upsurge globally, from low-income to high-income countries. This highlights the importance of future research and developing evidence-based practices for this growing population in a variety of contexts and countries. The complexity of NOWS requires a coordinated, interprofessional, holistic approach to improve care and short-term and long-term outcomes. Basic tenets may act as general guidelines for interprofessional team members to collaborate and plan services. Education on NOWS for SLPs and other healthcare professionals needs to be prioritized in pre-professional training and as part of ongoing CE to ensure that healthcare providers are prepared to provide appropriate care and meet the needs of this population. Continued research is required to address the gaps in current knowledge which informs the understanding of NOWS, the lifelong impact, and longitudinal service needs to improve child and family outcomes.

References

Adams, J., Hillier-Brown, F. C., Moore, H. J., Lake, A. A., Araujo-Soares, V., White, M., & Summerbell, C. (2016). Searching and synthesising 'grey literature' and 'grey information' in public health: Critical reflections on three case studies. *Systematic Reviews*, *5*(1), 164. https://doi.org/10.1186/s13643-016-0337-y

American Academy of Pediatrics. (2012). Patient- and family-centered care and the pediatrician's role. *Pediatrics*, *129*(2), 394–404. https://doi.org/10.1542/peds.2011-3084

American Speech-Language-Hearing Association. (n.d.a). *Cultural Responsiveness*. https://www.asha.org/practice-portal/professional-issues/cultural-responsiveness

American Speech-Language-Hearing Association. (n.d.b). *Evidence-Based Practice (EBP)*. https://www.asha.org/Research/EBP/

American Speech-Language-Hearing Association. (2016). *Scope of Practice in Speech-Language Pathology*. https://www.asha.org/policy/code-of-ethics-2016/

Behnke, M., Smith, V. C., Levy, S., Ammerman, S. D., Gonzalez, P. K., Ryan, S. A., Smith, V. C., Wunsch, M. M. J., Papile, L.-A., Baley, J. E., Carlo, W. A., Cummings, J. J., Kumar, P., Polin, R. A., Tan, R. C., & Watterberg, K. L. (2013). Prenatal substance abuse: Short- and long-term effects on the exposed fetus. *Pediatrics*, *131*(3), 1009–1024. https://doi.org/10.1542/peds.2012-3931

Benninger, K. L., Borghese, T., Kovalcik, J. B., Moore-Clingenpeel, M., Isler, C., Bonachea, E. M., Stark, A. R., Patrick, S. W., & Maitre, N. L. (2020). Prenatal exposures are associated with worse neurodevelopmental outcomes in infants with Neonatal Opioid Withdrawal Syndrome. *Frontiers in Pediatrics*, *8*, 462. https://doi.org/10.3389/fped.2020.00462

Benninger, K. L., Richard, C., Conroy, S., Newton, J., Taylor, H. G., Sayed, A., Pietruszewski, L., Nelin, M. A., Batterson, N., & Maitre, N. L. (2022). One-year neurodevelopmental outcomes after Neonatal Opioid Withdrawal Syndrome: A prospective cohort study. *Perspectives of the ASHA Special Interest Groups*, *7*(4), 1019–1032. https://doi.org/10.1044/2022_PERSP-21-00270

Bornman, J., & Louw, B. (2019). Personal commitment statements: Encouraging the clinical application of continuing professional development events for health practitioners in low- and middle-income countries. *Journal of Continuing Education in the Health Professions*, 39(2), 86–91. https://doi.org/10.1097/CEH.0000000000000248

Bornman, J., & Louw, B. (2023). Leadership development strategies in interprofessional healthcare collaboration: A rapid review. *Journal of Healthcare Leadership*, 15, 175–192. https://doi.org/10.2147/JHL.S405983

Brandon, E., Burton, H., Clark, T., Evans, C., & Louw, B. (2023, Nov. 16–18). *SLPs' perceptions of Neonatal Opioid Withdrawal Syndrome co-occurring with Cleft Palate: A pilot study* [Poster presentation]. ASHA 2023 Conference, Boston, MA, United States.

Braun, M. J., Dunn, W., & Tomchek, S. D. (2017). A pilot study on professional documentation: Do we write from a strengths perspective? *American Journal of Speech-Language Pathology*, 26(3), 972–981. https://doi.org/10.1044/2017_AJSLP-16-0117

Busch, C. M., & Ma, T. (2023). Speech-language pathology graduate students' perception of satisfaction, confidence, and interpersonal skill development during simulated experiences amid COVID-19. *Perspectives of the ASHA Special Interest Groups*, 8(1), 134–150. https://doi.org/10.1044/2022_persp-22-00073

Center for Disease Control. (2023). *Data and Statistics About Opioid Use During Pregnancy, 2019.* [Data set]. https://www.cdc.gov/pregnancy/opioids/data.html

Conner, K. L., Meadows, A. L., Delcher, C., & Talbert, J. C. (2020). Neonatal Abstinence Syndrome and childhood mental health conditions, 2009–2015: Commercial versus Medicaid populations. *Psychiatric Services*, 71(2), 184–187. https://doi.org/10.1176/appi.ps.201900180

Conradt, E., Flannery, T., Aschner, J. L., Annett, R. D., Croen, L. A., Duarte, C. S., Friedman, A. M., Guille, C., Hedderson, M. M., Hofheimer, J. A., Jones, M. R., Ladd-Acosta, C., McGrath, M., Moreland, A., Neiderhiser, J. M., Nguyen, R. H. N., Posner, J., Ross, J. L., Savitz, D. A., ... Lester, B. M. (2019). Prenatal opioid exposure: Neurodevelopmental consequences and future research priorities. *Pediatrics*, 144(3). https://doi.org/10.1542/peds.2019-0128

Council on Academic Accreditation. (n.d.). *Standards for Accreditation.* ASHA. https://caa.asha.org/reporting/standards/

Craig, J. W., & Smith, C. R. (2020). Risk-adjusted/neuroprotective care services in the NICU: The elemental role of the neonatal therapist (OT, PT, SLP). *Journal of Perinatology*, 40(4), 549–559. https://doi.org/10.1038/s41372-020-0597-1

Creel, L. M., Van Horn, A., Hines, A., & Bush, M. L. (2020). Neonatal Abstinence Syndrome and infant hearing assessment: A kids' inpatient database review. *The Journal of Early Hearing Detection and Intervention*, 5(1), 20–27. https://doi.org/10.26077/gdpm-at71

de Camargo, O. K., Simon, L., Ronen, G. M., & Rosenbaum, P. L. (Eds.). (2019). *ICF: A hands-on approach for clinicians and families.* Mac Keith Press.

Dunst, C. J., & Trivette, C. M. (2009). Let's be pals. *Infants & Young Children*, 22(3), 164–176. https://doi.org/10.1097/iyc.0b013e3181abe169

Ezell, J. M., Pho, M., Jaiswal, J., Ajayi, B. P., Gosnell, N., Kay, E., Eaton, E., & Bluthenthal, R. (2023). A systematic literature review of strengths-based approaches to drug use management and treatment. *Clinical Social Work Journal, 51*(3), 294–305. https://doi.org/10.1007/s10615-023-00874-2

Fabrize, L. (2019). *Neonatal Intensive Care Unit speech-language pathologists' perceptions of infants with Neonatal Abstinence Syndrome.* [Master's thesis, East Tennessee State University]. ProQuest Dissertations Publishing.

Fabrize, L., Proctor-Williams, K., & Louw, B. (2019, November 21–23). *Neonatal Intensive Care Unit Speech-Language Pathologists' perception of infants with Neonatal Abstinence Syndrome.* [Poster presentation] American Speech-Language-Hearing Association Annual Convention, Orlando, FL, United States.

Fill, M.-M. A., Miller, A. M., Wilkinson, R. H., Warren, M. D., Dunn, J. R., Schaffner, W., & Jones, T. F. (2018). Educational disabilities among children born with Neonatal Abstinence Syndrome. *Pediatrics, 142*(3). https://doi.org/10.1542/peds.2018-0562

Forkey, H., Szilagyi, M., Kelly, E. T., Duffee, J., Springer, S. H., Fortin, K., Jones, V. F., Vaden Greiner, M. B., Ochs, T. J., Partap, A. N., Davidson Sagor, L., Allen Staat, M., Thackeray, J. D., Waite, D., & Weber Zetley, L. (2021). Trauma-informed care. *Pediatrics, 148*(2). https://doi.org/10.1542/peds.2021-052580

Graham, S. (2019). *What is the prevalence of ADHD in children who were diagnosed with Neonatal Abstinence Syndrome? A retrospective chart review.* [Doctoral dissertation, University of Kentucky]. DNP Projects. https://uknowledge.uky.edu/dnp_etds/299

Guralnick, M. J. (Ed.). (2000). *Interdisciplinary clinical assessment for young children with developmental disabilities.* Brookes.

Hite, M. K., Chroust, A. J., Proctor-Williams, K., & Lowe, J. L. (2024). Newborn Hearing Screening Results for Infants With Prenatal Opioid Exposure in Southern Appalachia. *Journal of Speech, Language, and Hearing Research, 67*(4), 1268–1280. https://doi.org/10.1044/2024_JSLHR-23-00492

Holland, P., Fry, L., & Lankford, A. (2021, Nov. 18–20). *Perspectives and practices of speech-language pathologists treating children with a history of opioid exposure.* ASHA 2021 Conference, Washington, D.C.

Horstman, E., Sanders, K., Nava-Sifuentes, M., Townsend, S., Bowman, C. H., Proctor-Williams, K., & Carder, N. (2019). *Infants with Neonatal Abstinence Syndrome: Who receives SLP services in the NICU?* [Poster presentation]. East Tennessee State University. https://dc.etsu.edu/asrf/2019/schedule/195/

Hughes, V., Delva, S., Nkimbeng, M., Spaulding, E., Turkson-Ocran, R.-A., Cudjoe, J., Ford, A., Rushton, C., D'Aoust, R., & Han, H.-R. (2020). Not missing the opportunity: Strategies to promote cultural humility among future nursing faculty. *Journal of Professional Nursing, 36*(1), 28–33. https://doi.org/10.1016/j.profnurs.2019.06.005

Hyter, Y. D., & Salas-Provance, M. B. (2019). *Culturally responsive practices in speech, language and hearing sciences* (Second edition). Plural Publishing, Inc.

Iachini, A., Kim, J., Browne, T., Blake, E. W., & Dunn, B. L. (2022). A mixed-method longitudinal study of an interprofessional education course. *Journal of Interprofessional Care, 36*(1), 111–116. https://doi.org/10.1080/13561820.2021.1884052

Jaekel, J., Johnson, E. I., Reyes, L. M., Layton, K. N., & Harris, M. N. (2021). Conducting research with families of infants born with Neonatal Abstinence Syndrome: Recommendations from rural Appalachia. *Social Work Research*, 45(1), 63–68. https://doi.org/10.1093/swr/svaa024

Johnson, K. F. (2016). Interprofessional Education (IPE): Strategic questions. *Health & Interprofessional Practice*, 3(1). https://doi.org/10.7710/2159-1253.1095

Jones, H. E., Friedman, C. J., Starer, J. J., Terplan, M., & Gitlow, S. (2014). Opioid use during pregnancy. *Addictive Disorders & Their Treatment*, 13(1), 8–15. https://doi.org/10.1097/adt.0b013e318271c437

Jones, H. E., Kaltenbach, K., Benjamin, T., Wachman, E. M., & O'Grady, K. E. (2019). Prenatal opioid exposure, Neonatal Abstinence Syndrome/Neonatal Opioid Withdrawal Syndrome, and later child development research: Shortcomings and solutions. *Journal of Addiction Medicine*, 13(2), 90–92. https://doi.org/10.1097/adm.0000000000000463

Joseph, R., Brady, E., Hudson, M. E., & Moran, M. M. (2020). Perinatal substance exposure and long-term outcomes in children: A literature review. *Pediatric Nursing*, 46(4), 163–173. https://www.scopus.com/inward/record.uri?eid=2-s2.0-85098597415&partnerID=40&md5=f9554e076649df4c1118c6284acbb541

Kim, H. M., Bone, R. M., McNeill, B., Lee, S. J., Gillon, G., & Woodward, L. J. (2021). Preschool language development of children born to women with an opioid use disorder. *Children*, 8(4), 268. https://doi.org/10.3390/children8040268

Knollhoff, S. M. (2023). Pediatric dysphagia: A look into the training received during graduate speech-language pathology programs to support this population. *Language, Speech, and Hearing Services in Schools*, 54(2), 425–435. https://doi.org/10.1044/2022_lshss-22-00114

Kocherlakota, P. (2014). Neonatal Abstinence Syndrome. *Pediatrics*, 134(2), 547–561. https://doi.org/10.1542/peds.2013-3524

Kolodny, A., Courtwright, D. T., Hwang, C. S., Kreiner, P., Eadie, J. L., Clark, T. W., & Alexander, G. C. (2015). The prescription opioid and heroin crisis: A public health approach to an epidemic of addiction. *Annual Review of Public Health*, 36(1), 559–574. https://doi.org/10.1146/annurev-publhealth-031914-122957

Konstanty, K., Smith, H., & Louw, B. (2023, Nov. 16–18). *Graduate SLP students' perspectives of Neonatal Opioid Withdrawal Syndrome (NOWS) and their education needs* [Poster presentation]. ASHA 2023 Conference, Boston, MA, United States.

Langa, O., Cappitelli, A. T., & Ganske, I. M. (2021). Cleft lip and palate in infants with prenatal opioid exposure. *The Cleft Palate-Craniofacial Journal*, 59(4), 497–504. https://doi.org/10.1177/10556656211011896

Lee, S. J., Bora, S., Austin, N. C., Westerman, A., & Henderson, J. M. T. (2020). Neurodevelopmental outcomes of children born to opioid-dependent mothers: A systematic review and meta-analysis. *Academic Pediatrics*, 20(3), 308–318. https://doi.org/10.1016/j.acap.2019.11.005

Linn, N., Stephens, K., Swanson-Biearman, B., Lewis, D., & Whiteman, K. (2021). Implementing trauma-informed strategies for mothers of infants with Neonatal

Abstinence Syndrome. MCN: *The American Journal of Maternal/Child Nursing*, 46(4), 211–216. https://doi.org/10.1097/nmc.0000000000000728

Liu, A., Juarez, J., Nair, A., & Nanan, R. (2015). Feeding modalities and the onset of the Neonatal Abstinence Syndrome. *Frontiers in Pediatrics*, 3, 14. https://doi.org/10.3389/fped.2015.00014

MacMullen, N. J., & Samson, L. F. (2018). Neonatal Abstinence Syndrome: An uncontrollable epidemic. *Critical Care Nursing Clinics of North America*, 30(4), 585–596. https://doi.org/10.1016/j.cnc.2018.07.011

Maguire, D. J., Rowe, M. A., Spring, H., & Elliott, A. F. (2015). Patterns of disruptive feeding behaviors in infants with Neonatal Abstinence Syndrome. *Advances in Neonatal Care*, 15(6), 429–439. https://doi.org/10.1097/ANC.0000000000000204

Marcellus, L. (2014). Supporting women with substance use issues: Trauma-informed care as a foundation for practice in the NICU. *Neonatal Network*, 33(6), 307–314. https://doi.org/10.1891/0730-0832.33.6.307

Marcellus, L. (2018). Neonatal Abstinence Syndrome in countries with no to low medical opioid consumption: A scoping review. *International Nursing Review*, 66(2), 224–233. https://doi.org/10.1111/inr.12489

Masten, A., & Barnes, A. (2018). Resilience in children: Developmental perspectives. *Children*, 5(7), 98. https://doi.org/10.3390/children5070098

Maxwell, J., Rutherford, K., Holland, P., Fry, L., Rigon, A., & Lankford, A. (2022). Perceptions of speech-language pathologists' service provision in the opioid epidemic: A focus group study. *American Journal of Speech-Language Pathology*, 31(4), 1672–1686. https://doi.org/10.1044/2022_ajslp-21-00337

McCarty, D. B., Peat, J. R., O'Donnell, S., Graham, E., & Malcolm, W. F. (2019). "Choose physical therapy" for Neonatal Abstinence Syndrome: Clinical management for infants affected by the opioid crisis. *Physical Therapy*, 99(6), 771–785. https://doi.org/10.1093/ptj/pzz039

McCarty, T., & Braswell, E. (2022). Implementation of interprofessional rounds decreases Neonatal Abstinence Syndrome length of stay. *The Journal of Pediatric Pharmacology and Therapeutics*, 27(2), 157–163. https://doi.org/10.5863/1551-6776-27.2.157

McDaniel, C. E., Jacob-Files, E., Deodhar, P., McGrath, C. L., & Desai, A. D. (2021). Strategies to improve the quality of team-based care for Neonatal Abstinence Syndrome. *Hospital Pediatrics*, 11(9), 968–981. https://doi.org/10.1542/hpeds.2020-003830

McGlothen-Bell, K., Recto, P., McGrath, J. M., Brownell, E., & Cleveland, L. M. (2021). Recovering together: Mothers' experiences providing skin-to-skin care for their infants with NAS. *Advances in Neonatal Care*, 21(1), 16–22. https://doi.org/10.1097/anc.0000000000000819

McQueen, K., Taylor, C., & Murphy-Oikonen, J. (2019). Systematic review of newborn feeding method and outcomes related to Neonatal Abstinence Syndrome. *Journal of Obstetric, Gynecologic, & Neonatal Nursing*, 48(4), 398–407. https://doi.org/10.1016/j.jogn.2019.03.004

Miller, J. S., Anderson, J. G., Erwin, P. C., Davis, S. K., & Lindley, L. C. (2020). The effects of Neonatal Abstinence Syndrome on language delay from birth to 10 years. *Journal of Pediatric Nursing, 51*, 67–74. https://doi.org/10.1016/j.pedn.2019.12.011

Mills, B., & Hardin-Jones, M. (2019). Update on academic and clinical training in cleft palate/craniofacial anomalies for speech-language pathology students. *Perspectives of the ASHA Special Interest Groups, 4*(5), 870–877. https://doi.org/10.1044/2019_pers-sig5-2019-0023

Moran, M., Bickford, J., Barradell, S., & Scholten, I. (2020). Embedding the International Classification of Functioning, Disability and Health in health professions curricula to enable Interprofessional Education and collaborative practice. *Journal of Medical Education and Curricular Development, 7.* https://doi.org/10.1177/2382120520933855

National Institute for Drug Abuse. (2023). *Novel technologies for infants with Neonatal Opioid Withdrawal Syndrome.* https://heal.nih.gov/news/stories/technologies-neonatal-opioid-withdrawal

Nelson, L., & Gilbert, J. L. (2021). *Research in communication sciences and disorders: Methods for systematic inquiry.* Plural Publishing, Inc.

Nygaard, E., Moe, V., Slinning, K., & Walhovd, K. B. (2015). Longitudinal cognitive development of children born to mothers with opioid and polysubstance use. *Pediatric Research, 78*(3), 330–335. https://doi.org/10.1038/pr.2015.95

Oei, J. L., Blythe, S., Dicair, L., Didden, D., Preisz, A., & Lantos, J. (2023). What's in a name? The ethical implications and opportunities in diagnosing an infant with Neonatal Abstinence Syndrome (NAS). *Addiction, 118*(1), 4–6. https://doi.org/10.1111/add.16022

Oei, J. L., Melhuish, E., Uebel, H., Azzam, N., Breen, C., Burns, L., Hilder, L., Bajuk, B., Abdel-Latif, M. E., Ward, M., Feller, J. M., Falconer, J., Clews, S., Eastwood, J., Li, A., & Wright, I. M. (2017). Neonatal Abstinence Syndrome and high school performance. *Pediatrics, 139*(2). https://doi.org/10.1542/peds.2016-2651

Olswang, L. B., & Prelock, P. A. (2015). Bridging the gap between research and practice: Implementation science. *Journal of Speech, Language, and Hearing Research, 58*(6), 1818–1826. https://doi.org/10.1044/2015_jslhr-l-14-0305

Patrick, S. W., Barfield, W. D., Poindexter, B. B., Cummings, J., Hand, I., Adams-Chapman, I., Aucott, S. W., Puopolo, K. M., Goldsmith, J. P., Kaufman, D., Martin, C., Mowitz, M., Gonzalez, L., Camenga, D. R., Quigley, J., Ryan, S. A., & Walker-Harding, L. (2020). Neonatal Opioid Withdrawal Syndrome. *Pediatrics, 146*(5). https://doi.org/10.1542/peds.2020-029074

Proctor-Williams, K., & Louw, B. (2017, Nov. 9-11). *Infants and children prenatally exposed to drugs; Neonatal Abstinence Syndrome (NAS) and neurodevelopmental outcomes.* [Conference presentation]. ASHA 2017 Conference, Los Angeles, CA, United States.

Proctor-Williams, K., & Louw, B. (2021) Cleft lip and/or palate in infants prenatally exposed to opioids. *Cleft Palate Craniofacial Journal, 59*(4), 513–521. https://doi.org/10.1177/10556656211013687

Proctor-Williams, K., & Louw, B. (2022). When cleft lip and/or palate and antenatal opioid exposure intersect: A tutorial. *Perspectives of the ASHA Special Interest Groups, 7*(4), 1006–1018. https://doi.org/10.1044/2022_PERSP-21-00249

Ratliff, B. V. (2017). *Prevalence of communication disorders in children with Neonatal Abstinence Syndrome on school speech-language pathology caseloads: A national survey.* [Master's thesis, East Tennessee State University]. ProQuest One Academic. https://www.proquest.com/dissertations-theses/prevalence-communication-disorders-children-with/docview/1906663045/se-2

Recto, P., McGlothen-Bell, K., McGrath, J., Brownell, E., & Cleveland, L. M. (2020). The role of stigma in the nursing care of families impacted by Neonatal Abstinence Syndrome. *Advances in Neonatal Care, 20*(5), 354–363. https://doi.org/10.1097/anc.0000000000000778

Rees, P., Stilwell, P. A., Bolton, C., Akillioglu, M., Carter, B., Gale, C., & Sutcliffe, A. (2020). Childhood health and educational outcomes after Neonatal Abstinence Syndrome: A systematic review and meta-analysis. *The Journal of Pediatrics, 226.* https://doi.org/10.1016/j.jpeds.2020.07.013

Rice, P. (2020). *Neonatal Abstinence Syndrome and the relationship between respiration and feeding.* [Master's thesis, East Tennessee State University]. ProQuest Dissertations Publishing.

Rigg, K. K., & Rigg, M. S. (2020). Opioid-induced hearing loss and Neonatal Abstinence Syndrome: Clinical considerations for Audiologists and recommendations for future research. *American Journal of Audiology, 29*(4), 701–709. https://doi.org/10.1044/2020_aja-20-00054

Roberson, M. M., & Lund, E. (2022). School-based speech-language pathologists' attitudes and knowledge about trauma-informed care. *Language, Speech, and Hearing Services in Schools, 53*(4), 1117–1128. https://doi.org/10.1044/2022_LSHSS-21-00172

Rubenstein, E., Young, J. C., Croen, L. A., DiGuiseppi, C., Dowling, N. F., Lee, L.-C., Schieve, L., Wiggins, L. D., & Daniels, J. (2018). Brief report: Maternal opioid prescription from preconception through pregnancy and the odds of autism spectrum disorder and autism features in children. *Journal of Autism and Developmental Disorders, 49*(1), 376–382. https://doi.org/10.1007/s10803-018-3721-8

Rutherford, K., Maxwell, J., Fry, L., Holland, P., Rigon, A., & Lankford, A. (2022). Perceived clinical characteristics of children with history of opioid exposure: A speech-language pathology perspective. *American Journal of Speech-Language Pathology, 31*(4), 1801–1816. https://doi.org/10.1044/2022_ajslp-21-00336

Saunders, R., Singer, R., Dugmore, H., Seaman, K., & Lake, F. (2016). Nursing students' reflections on an interprofessional placement in ambulatory care. *Reflective Practice, 17*(4), 393–402. https://doi.org/10.1080/14623943.2016.1164686

Schwartz, A. N., Reyes, L. M., Meschke, L. L., & Kintziger, K. W. (2021). Prenatal opioid exposure and ADHD childhood symptoms: A meta-analysis. *Children, 8*(2), 106. https://doi.org/10.3390/children8020106

Shearer, J. N., Davis, S. K., Erwin, P. C., Anderson, J. G., & Lindley, L. C. (2018). Neonatal Abstinence Syndrome and neurodevelopmental health outcomes: A state of the science. *Journal of Neonatal Nursing, 24*(5), 242–246. https://doi.org/10.1016/j.jnn.2018.06.002

Shrader, S., Mauldin, M., Hammad, S., Mitcham, M., & Blue, A. (2015). Developing a comprehensive faculty development program to promote interprofessional education, practice and research at a free-standing Academic Health Science Center. *Journal of Interprofessional Care, 29*(2), 165–167. https://doi.org/10.3109/13561820.2014.940417

Sirnes, E., Oltedal, L., Bartsch, H., Eide, G. E., Elgen, I. B., & Aukland, S. M. (2017). Brain morphology in school-aged children with prenatal opioid exposure: A structural MRI study. *Early Human Development, 106–107*, 33–39. https://doi.org/10.1016/j.earlhumdev.2017.01.009

Snyman, S., Von Pressentin, K. B., & Clarke, M. (2015). International Classification of Functioning, Disability and Health: Catalyst for interprofessional education and collaborative practice. *Journal of Interprofessional Care, 29*(4), 313–319. https://doi.org/10.3109/13561820.2015.1004041

Spencer, T. D. (2022). Clinical impact of research: Introduction to the forum. *Perspectives of the ASHA Special Interest Groups, 7*(3), 647–650. https://doi.org/10.1044/2022_persp-22-00012

Substance Abuse and Mental Health Services Administration. (n.d.). *2022 National Survey on Drug Use and Health (NSDUH) releases.* https://www.samhsa.gov/data/release/2022-national-survey-drug-use-and-health-nsduh-releases

Substance Abuse and Mental Health Services Administration. (2014). *SAMHSA's Concept of Trauma and Guidance for a Trauma-Informed Approach.* HHS Publication No. (SMA) 14-4884. https://store.samhsa.gov/sites/default/files/sma14-4884.pdf

Thome, E. K., Loveall, S. J., & Henderson, D. E. (2020). A survey of speech-language pathologists' understanding and reported use of evidence-based practice. *Perspectives of the ASHA Special Interest Groups, 5*(4), 984–999. https://doi.org/10.1044/2020_PERSP-20-00008

Velez, M. L., Jordan, C., & Jansson, L. M. (2021). Reconceptualizing non-pharmacologic approaches to Neonatal Abstinence Syndrome (NAS) and Neonatal Opioid Withdrawal Syndrome (NOWS): A theoretical and evidence-based approach. Part II: The clinical application of nonpharmacologic care for NAS/NOWS. *Neurotoxicology and Teratology, 88.* https://doi.org/10.1016/j.ntt.2021.107032

Velez, M. L., McConnell, K., Spencer, N., Montoya, L., Tuten, M., & Jansson, L. M. (2018). Prenatal buprenorphine exposure and neonatal neurobehavioral functioning. *Early Human Development, 117*, 7–14. https://doi.org/10.1016/j.earlhumdev.2017.11.009

Werner, E. E. (2000). Protective factors and individual resilience. In J. P. Shonkoff & S. J. Meisels (Eds.), *Handbook of early childhood intervention* (Second edition). Cambridge University Press. https://doi.org/10.1017/CBO9780511529320

World Health Organization. (2001). Classification of Functioning, Disability and Health (ICF). *ICF full version.*

World Health Organization. (2010). *Framework for action on interprofessional education and collaborative practice.* World Health Organization. https://iris.who.int/handle/10665/70185

2 Understanding the Dyad Affected by NOWS as a Necessary Pathway to Provision of Optimal Care

Martha L. Velez and Lauren M. Jansson

2.1 Introduction

Neonatal abstinence syndrome (NAS) is a clinical diagnosis that includes a variety of physiological and neurobehavioral signs seen in a newborn as a result of prenatal chronic exposure to, and abrupt cessation of, prescribed and/or unprescribed psychoactive substances. More recently, the Food and Drug Administration has used the term neonatal opioid withdrawal syndrome (NOWS) to indicate prenatal opioid exposure specifically (U.S. Food and Drug Administration [FDA], 2013; FDA, 2016). Because most of the children are exposed to other psychoactive substances (e.g., nicotine) in addition to opioids, we will use the term NAS/NOWS. The cascade of neurobiological and neuroadaptive mechanisms that generate the diversity of signs and dysregulated neurobehaviors termed NAS/NOWS is very complex and still not well understood, but it is accepted that there is a dysregulation of several neurotransmitters systems (i.e., dopamine, serotonin) that affect the functioning of different biobehavioral systems (Kocherlakota, 2014); taken as a whole the resulting signs comprise the dysregulation that is the essence of NAS/NOWS.

The real incidence of NAS/NOWS cannot be accurately determined, but with the ongoing opioid epidemic and the concomitant increase in NAS/NOWS reported in several countries, awareness of this complex and consequential public health problem has increased (Brandt & Finnegan, 2017). Not all infants prenatally exposed to opioids develop signs of NAS/NOWS that require pharmacologic treatment. Studies report that up to 94% of infants show varying manifestations of signs after opioid discontinuation at birth, with smaller percentages requiring pharmacotherapy (Johnson et al., 2003). Because the neurobehavioral dysregulation caused by NAS/NOWS in the different neurobehavioral domains (wake/sleep control and attention, sensory processing, autonomic functioning, and motor/tone control) is so unique to each infant, non-pharmacologic care to mitigate these

DOI: 10.4324/9781003397267-2

dysregulatory features needs to be consciously applied to every opioid-exposed infant/dyad in an individualized and systematic way (Velez & Jansson, 2008). Non-pharmacologic care has been the first line and primary mainstay of treatment for all opioid-exposed infants for decades.

Although studies of long-term neurobehavioral outcomes of prenatally opioid-exposed children are inconclusive and are confounded by numerous bio-psychosocial issues frequently related with a maternal/parental opioid use disorder (OUD), there appears to be a trend toward poorer outcomes in different neurodevelopmental areas including attention, language, behavioral, and emotional (Azuine et al., 2019). Therefore, multisystem approaches may be necessary. Detection of and timely intervention for specific neurobehavioral dysfunction(s) associated with prenatal opioid exposure during sensitive developmental periods, when each ontogenetic accomplishment in each developmental area supports and interacts with subsequent ones, is important to future development. Any providers treating the opioid-exposed infant should understand the factors that affect NAS/NOWS presentation (see Figure 2.1), the infant's individual NAS/NOWS expression and non-pharmacologic and pharmacologic strategies used to treat the infant, and the importance of the mother/parent/caregiver and dyadic approaches.

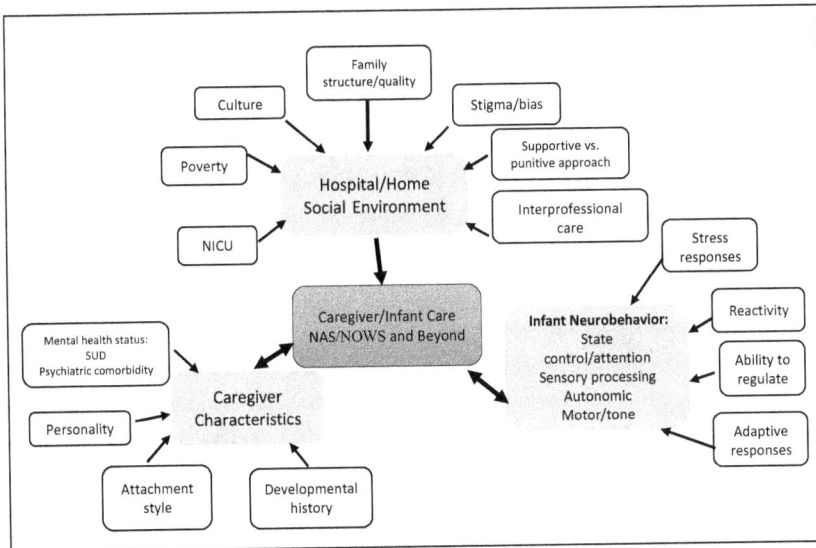

Figure 2.1 Caregiver, environmental, and infant factors that influence the presentation and care of NAS/NOWS

2.1.1 Factors That Determine the Presentation of NAS/NOWS

The physiopathology of NAS/NOWS and its impact on child neurodevelopment is complex due to myriad factors. In addition to the intrauterine opioid exposure, infants born to people with OUD are usually exposed to multiple stressors throughout gestation and after birth. NAS/NOWS is a disorder that is variably expressed both in type of dysregulated neurobehaviors and severity, between infants and in the same infant over time with development, and its expression is modified by many maternal, infant, and environmental factors, as described below.

2.1.1.1 Parental/Caregiver Factors

There are several genetic, developmental, and psychosocial conditions that determine the caregiver functioning in general and in particular in relation to the expression/evolution of the NAS/NOWS. Polysubstance use, which includes illicit and licit substances such as nicotine and alcohol, is more common than use of a single substance during pregnancy. Polysubstance exposures in general alter the expression and severity of NAS/NOWS, primarily increasing its severity. Pregnant people with OUD may use different types of opioids (prescribed or not) at different times in pregnancy and with different patterns of use with the potential for differential effects for the fetus. Concomitant nicotine exposure is very frequent, and many women report the additional use of Tetrahydrocannabinol (THC), alcohol, benzodiazepines, cocaine, and lately xylazine. Psychiatric comorbidity is common, as is the necessity of prescribed psychoactive medications, including benzodiazepines, selective serotonin reuptake inhibitors (SSRIs), and gabapentin. All these substances can alter NAS/NOWS expression and have the potential to interfere with the typical development of the various neurotransmitters and hormonal systems that orchestrate developmental processes (cell formation, proliferation, apoptosis, myelination, etc.), influencing the microstructure and functional connectivity that will determine the organization of the infant at birth and during different stages of development (Boggess & Risher, 2022; Tsai et al., 2019). Medications for OUD like methadone and buprenorphine predispose the infant to have NAS/NOWS, but their role in providing benefit to the mother/parent with OUD is paramount. Most researchers agree that NAS/NOWS severity is not related to maternal/parental methadone dose or cumulative methadone exposure in utero (Jones et al., 2013) and it has been indicated that a more stable maternal/parental serum methadone level, achieved by increased and more frequent doses of methadone over the course of pregnancy, may have a protective effect against NAS/NOWS (Brandt & Finnegan, 2017; McCarthy et al., 2015). In comparison to methadone, buprenorphine monotherapy or the combination of buprenorphine/naloxone exposure in utero is associated with shorter length of hospital stays for the neonate, and decreased frequency/duration of pharmacotherapy for NAS/NOWS symptoms (Goshgarian et al., 2022; Jones et al., 2010).

There are many other parental/maternal factors associated with the OUD condition that can be considered intrauterine stressors, including maternal physiology (Jansson et al., 2007) and comorbid medical conditions, maternal poor nutrition, homelessness, violence, excessive stress, isolation, and poverty. All these conditions have been linked to adverse effects for the pregnancy and fetus as well as the organization and functioning of the infant at birth and beyond. Common parental developmental histories of cumulative adverse experiences and/or an insecure attachment style, high level of distress, and lack of support likely interact in a unique manner within each individual pregnancy, are unique to each dyad, and may affect the NAS/NOWS expression individually or cumulatively. The quality of the parent/caregiver's responses, and their recovery and responses to the infant may facilitate or obstruct the process of postnatal adaptation, recovery from NAS/NOWS, and the successful accomplishment of the demands related to this important period of dyadic communication and child development. Finally, depression, guilt regarding the NAS/NOWS display in the infant, and feelings of shame or anxiety due to chronic and unresolved trauma or current abusive relationships can keep the mother in a state of hyper- or hypoarousal. These conditions can cause dysregulation in the mother/parent and can limit their ability to adjust the interactions in the necessary interactive and supportive processes that foster self-regulatory capacities between caregivers and infants (also known as coregulation). Postnatal parental substance use or unaddressed psychosocial adverse experiences of the caregiver (e.g., homelessness or involvement with children's services) can overwhelm their psychological resources and hinder their ability to identify, understand, and respond to the infant in a mindful way, with the unintended consequences of hampering the infant's wellbeing, the caregiver's recovery, and the trajectory of the caregiver–infant interaction, and hence, child development.

2.1.1.2 *Physical and Psychosocial Environmental Factors*

Physical and psychosocial environmental factors are also determinants of the dyad's health, wellbeing, and the developmental/interactional trajectory of the child. Physical environmental stimuli presented to the infant vary substantially in terms of type (auditory, visual, movement, touch) frequency, duration, and intensity, provoking more or less regulated responses from the infant. A loud, congested, stressful physical environment like the NICU can be physiologically, behaviorally, and/or emotionally overwhelming for the infant, parents, and providers (Maguire et al., 2016). Health care facilities where providers are warm, nonjudgmental and unbiased toward parents with OUD or psychiatric issues will decrease distress for the parent, increase compliance with treatment, and assist the parents in acquiring self-competence as nourishing caregivers. Stress initiated by difficult interactions or environments, housing problems, lack of transportation, and financial difficulties can impair the required focused attention, relaxation, and calm demeanor required to soothe, feed, and relax a motorically, physiologically, or sensory dysregulated neonate affected by NAS/NOWS.

2.1.1.3 Infant Factors

The infant also brings genetic, epigenetic, maturational, and temperamental factors that contribute positively or negatively to the severity and quality of the neurobehavioral expression of NAS/NOWS, as well as to their responses to non-pharmacologic and pharmacological interventions. Limited by small cohorts, studies have identified associations of variants in maternal and infant genes that encode the μ-opioid receptor (OPRM1), catechol-O-methyltransferase (COMT), and prepronociceptin (PNOC) with differences in NAS/NOWS pharmacologic treatment rates and length of hospitalization (Cole et al., 2017). Epigenetic changes like increased DNA methylation of the mu-opioid receptor gene (OPRM1) have been associated with more severe NAS/NOWS. In addition, pharmacologic treatment of NAS/NOWS has been associated with decreased DNA methylation of the OPRM1 gene and improved neonatal neurobehavior; epigenetic changes may play a role in these changes in neonatal neurobehavior (Camerota et al., 2022). It is expected that advances in knowledge regarding the role of genetic/epigenetic aspects of the presentation and evolution of NAS/NOWS can be used to provide a more precise approach to the treatment. Gestational age can also affect expression, with premature infants generally having less severe NAS/NOWS signs (Dysart et al., 2007). Whether this indicates decreased NAS/NOWS severity or physiological immaturity is currently uncertain.

Each infant has individual reactivity, defined as both their physiological and behavioral arousal in a tonic state along with their responses to the environment. Reactivity can be high for one child, negligeable for another, or disguised by stress signs. The unique set of the infant's innate reactivity and regulatory predispositions will influence the caregivers' responses (Jones & Sloan, 2018). This in turn may influence the expression and evolution of NAS/NOWS and the developing patterns of the infant's arousal responses, multisensory integration, and/or ability to manage attention and activity.

All of these parental, environmental, and infant factors, and their interrelationships, which influence the variability of the NAS/NOWS presentation, progress, and resolution, need to be considered when caring for the dyad affected by NAS/NOWS. The potential for the positive impact that can be provided by different professional disciplines and agencies supporting the dyad affected by parental OUD pre- and postnatally cannot be underestimated.

2.2 The Infant With NAS/NOWS

2.2.1 Understanding the Infant With NAS/NOWS

The evaluation and decisions regarding the NAS/NOWS diagnosis, non-pharmacologic strategies to promote the regulation of the infant, and pharmacologic treatment when needed should be based on a thorough observation of the infant and dyad functioning during unprompted or triggered circumstances and parental/caregiver responses (Velez & Jansson, 2008; Velez et al., 2021a; Velez et al., 2021b).

Regulation, a developmental construct, forms the basis for early functioning and development. The physiological and behavioral functioning of any newborn (such as having clear sleep–awake states, appropriate levels of arousal, maintaining vital signs within the normal rage) and the responses to any external (e.g., auditory, visual, touch) or internal (e.g., hunger, fatigue) stimuli depend on the integrity of the regulatory mechanisms that orchestrate strategies to maintain homeostasis and adaptive responses during spontaneous or provoked events. The infant's regulatory capacities of key biobehavioral systems such as *state control/attention*, *motor/muscle tone*, *autonomic control*, and *sensory processing* are an indication of the interaction of factors intrinsic to the infant with cumulative prenatal and postnatal experiences. Exposure to stressors or insults in the womb, such as substance exposure or unremitting stress, may persistently strain fetal neurobehavioral systems (e.g., autonomic, stress response, sensory, motor) as they are being organized, which may lead to lower levels of self-regulatory capacities in the infant after birth (Conradt et al., 2018). The infant's signs of dysregulation associated with NAS/NOWS can lead to unrestful or fragmented sleep, feeding difficulties, excessive irritability, failure to gain weight, and increased dysregulated autonomic/signs of stress responses (e.g., increased respiratory rate, avoiding eye contact, pull-down) to care routines (e.g., feeding, diaper changing) and interactional activities (e.g., giving cues to caregivers, responding to caregiver(s)).

A systematic and methodical observation of these domains of the infant's functioning is fundamental to understanding how NAS/NOWS is expressed in each infant and how that expression may be affecting their ability to regulate sleep/awake states and motor activity, feed and gain weight, maintain physiological parameters within normal ranges, and ability to focus/attend. All these domains functioning together in a synchronized way are needed for typical physical, cognitive, social, and emotional development. Signs of neurobiological dysregulation can indicate the environmental and interactional modifications (i.e., non-pharmacologic care) that are needed to prevent and/or ameliorate the physiological and/or behavioral dysregulation associated with NAS/NOWS. In addition, a routinary observation of these systems can detect areas of the newborn's functioning that need special attention to prevent developmental or behavioral problems at later stages (Velez et al., 2021a, Velez et al., 2021b). Figure 2.2 illustrates different signs of dysregulation associated to NAS/NOWS by domain of functioning.

Dysregulation in one domain can impact the functioning of a different domain(s). For example, an infant with excessive movement can have difficulty focusing on an object or person, and that may subsequently interfere with attentional/relational abilities. An infant with sensory processing difficulties can be easily dysregulated with visual, auditory, movement, or

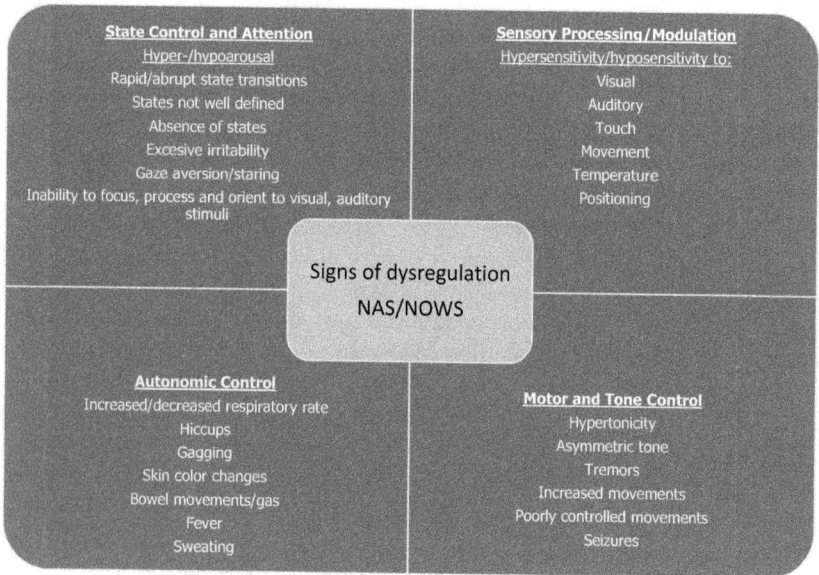

Figure 2.2 Four dimensional and interactional neurobehavioral domains – state control/attention, motor/tone control, autonomic control, and sensory processing/modulation – that are affected by NAS/ NOWS

tactile stimuli and display signs of hyperarousal or hypoarousal manifested by autonomic or physiological signs of stress (changes in skin color, tachypnea, bowel sounds or decreased movements). Understanding how the infant is functioning in each domain at different moments and how the domains influence each other is crucial to being able to understand and support the organization/maturation of the different systems and the integral functioning of the infant (Velez & Jansson, 2008).

2.2.2 Management of the Infant With NAS/NOWS

An infant without problematic predispositions, exposed to minimal distress during pregnancy, born to sensitive and well-regulated caregivers, is expected to have a smooth post-birth neurobehavioral adaptation leading to smooth sleep–awake transitions, periods of restful sleep and periods of quiet alert that allow a gratifying caregiver/infant interaction and adequate feeding according to the age. However, all infants having signs of NAS/NOWS require environmental changes and care strategies that are generally considered to be the essence of non-pharmacologic care. Non-pharmacologic care is applied to each infant and dyad beginning at birth (or ideally prenatally with education), regardless of the need or not for medication to manage NAS/NOWS signs, and should continue throughout hospitalization and beyond, as long as the infant has any dysregulatory features. Infants frequently respond with particular and sometimes similar signs of dysregulation to different aversive experiences at different stages of NAS/NOWS evolution, and the frequency and expression of the signs can change with maturation or interventions.

Atypical neurobehavioral signs or responses associated with prenatal opioid exposure need to be identified and managed during and after hospitalization until they subside due to resolution of NAS/NOWS expression or maturity.

2.2.2.1 Assessing Dysregulatory Features of NAS/NOWS

For several decades, hospitals have used scoring tools such as the Finnegan Neonatal Abstinence Scoring tool (Finnegan & Kaltenbach, 1992) or modified versions. The use of these tools led to concerns that this assessment tool may overestimate the need for pharmacologic treatment. Based on this concern, and especially due to the costs of prolonged hospitalization of the infant, a new assessment tool – Eat, Sleep and Console – has been widely promoted, but conclusive evidence to support its use is not yet available (Young et al., 2023). We have proposed a neurodevelopmental approach to NAS/NOWS assessment and treatment. This approach, based in neurodevelopmental theory, assesses the newborn through infant in four domains (state control and attention, motor, sensory integration, and autonomic functioning), providing for specific non-pharmacologic interventions by dysregulatory feature, and suggests medication only for those infants who have persistent dysregulation despite the application of maximal and specific non-pharmacologic care (Velez et al., 2021b).

While NAS/NOWS is a well-accepted clinical syndrome, it remains incompletely understood. However, the effects of NAS/NOWS and its management typically extend beyond the first days and weeks of life. Another assessment tool that has been used to evaluate neonatal neurobehaviors in relation to prenatal opioid exposure is the NICU Network Neurobehavioral Scales (NNNS) (Lester & Tronick, 2004). The NNNS is a comprehensive assessment tool to evaluate the neurobehavioral functioning of the at-risk newborns with or without a history of prenatal exposure to stressors. Neonatal neurobehavior is a useful indicator of NAS/NOWS severity, and the NNNS has been used to evaluate the evolution of NAS/NOWS symptoms during the first weeks of life, responses to pharmacologic treatment for NAS/NOWS, and long-term developmental outcomes of affected infants (Camerota et al., 2022; Coyle et al., 2012).

Each hospital determines the scoring tool used to initiate medication and the score thresholds defined for the application of pharmacologic treatment. After the initiation of pharmacotherapy for NAS/NOWS medication is adjusted with the goal of maintaining the neonate in a more organized state while sleeping or being alert, without sedation or overmedication. The parent/caregiver should understand the need for and goals of medication therapy beyond the dose required by the infant. Many caregivers only pay attention to the scores given to the infant after the evaluation with the Finnegan Neonatal Abstinence Scoring tool (Finnegan & Kaltenbach, 1992) or other tools used to determine pharmacologic treatment, but they do not know the signs of withdrawal and ways they may have to decrease their presentation. They may only focus on the amount of medication or number of days the infant will be hospitalized, and not in the modifications of environment and interactions that can contribute to the improvement of the signs of withdrawal. After identification of specific needs, providers can use discussions or modeling for the caregiver to support the parent's communication with the infant and to increase their self-confidence in the care of the infant. Many parents with OUD grew up in chaotic households where their own parents had substance use problems or mental health issues that prevented them from providing a healthy role modeling of parenting. It should be assumed that any parent with OUD may need additional support in sensitive parenting (Substance Abuse and Mental Health Services Administration [SAMHSA], 2020).

2.2.2.2 Managing Dysregulatory Features of NAS/NOWS in the Neonatal Period

Problems in one domain that interfere with functioning in that domain or others, as well as with developmental milestones at subsequent stages of development, need to be elucidated and interventions provided to address them. For example, excessive movement or increased muscle tone may interfere with smooth feeding or cause excoriations during the first days of life, but can also cause difficulty with eye contact, following objects or paying attention in the first months of life if regulatory techniques (e.g., holding hands, containing head, pacifier during interaction) are not implemented properly or the triggers are not identified and mitigated. Any specialized intervention provided at any developmental period should be mindful of the interconnection of these dysregulatory features and potentially be able to work with other subspecialists in providing care that affects change for the infant. Figure 2.3 shows specific non-pharmacologic interventions that can prevent or decrease problems observed in the different domains. (For a

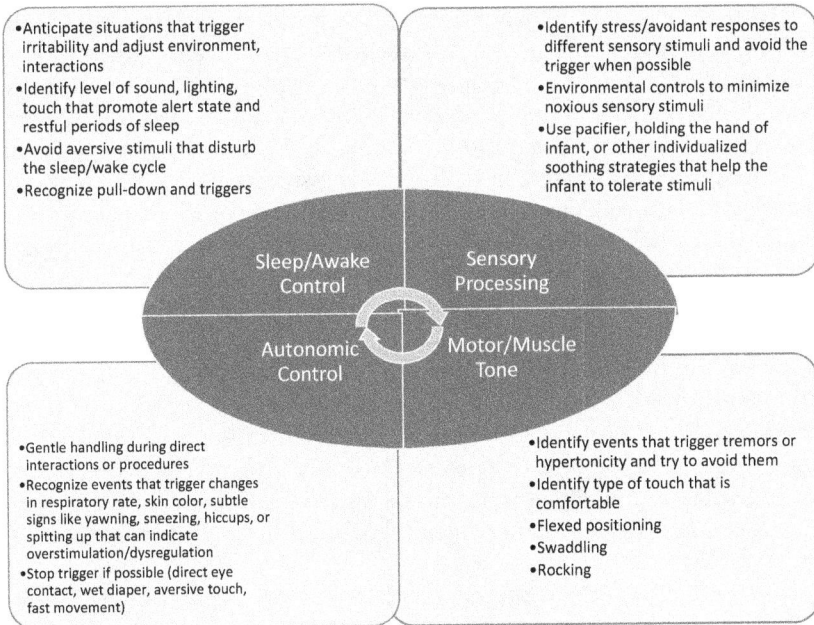

Figure 2.3 Non-pharmacologic strategies to prevent or address dysregulatory signs that can be triggered or amplified by NAS/NOWS in different domains of functioning

comprehensive and detailed description of non-pharmacologic approaches to the dyad affected by NAS/NOWS see Velez et al., 2021a; Velez et al., 2021b.)

There is no gold standard or ideal system to determine the need for pharmacological treatment for infants with NAS/NOWS. A judicious clinical observation coupled with the implementation of comprehensive and individualized non-pharmacologic treatment is necessary before the initiation of pharmacological treatment to avoid both under- and overmedication. Pharmacologic treatment is recommended for infants with neurobehavioral signs that *impair major physiological and behavioral functions* in one or different domains (state control/attention, motor/tone, autonomic, and sensory) that do not respond to well-implemented specific non-pharmacologic care.

2.2.2.3 Follow-Up Care for Infants Affected by NAS/NOWS

Most infants (requiring or not requiring pharmacologic treatment) go home with NAS/NOWS symptoms. Opioid-exposed infants require frequent visits to knowledgeable pediatric care to monitor residual symptoms, subacute presentation of symptoms, and/or problems related to the NAS/NOWS expression, and effects of these on growth, health, and development. Some infants may have difficulty initiating or maintaining adequate feeding and gaining weight, persistent sleeping difficulties, or may display gastrointestinal problems such as dysbiosis/dysbiotic gut syndrome (Maguire & Gröer, 2016). In addition, excessive movement, difficulty in focusing and making direct eye contact, hypertonicity, or other symptoms can last for several weeks and may impact dyadic interaction or initiate altered trajectories of development that can lead to future problems. It is necessary to pay attention to coping mechanisms to attempt self-regulation employed by the infant (gaze aversion, pulldown, self-clinging, irritability due to overstimulation) that will require environmental and interactional accommodations. Adaptation of the environment, interactional patterns, and appropriate soothing strategies adjusted to the infant's developmental capacities by the parent/caregiver and hospital staff should be continued after discharge, modifying intervention strategies according to the changing functioning of the infant related to maturation (such as longer periods of the awake state).

The potential for long-term harm related to NAS/NOWS and its treatments to the developing brain remains a poorly comprehended concern and findings are inconclusive. Neonatal neurobehavior can be an indicator of long-term developmental outcomes. Identifying infants with atypical neurobehavioral patterns could be one way to screen infants who could benefit from early intervention (Camerota et al., 2022), and early intervention may be particularly critical for infants who can have multiple risk factors (other substance exposure, poverty, racism) for developmental, emotional, and behavioral problems. Specialty follow-up clinical care, such as occupational, physical, and feeding therapies, can be considered on a case-by-case basis, ensuring that this involvement does not significantly interfere with parental SUD treatment. Recognizing that prenatal substance use with or without other psychiatric conditions may have consequences that extend or present beyond the neonatal period as affected neurosystems mature provides an enormous opportunity to support not only the infants but their families and communities (Hartgrove et al., 2019). A family-centered approach may require communication with child welfare, early intervention services, home visiting, or parental OUD treatment programs and other psychosocial assistance programs when necessary (e.g., housing, legal support, financial assistance, childcare).

2.3 Understanding the Mother With an OUD

Maternal/parental wellbeing should be thoroughly assessed, as multiple neurobiological and psychosocial risk factors may affect pregnant/post-partum people with OUD. The perinatal period is considered a "window of opportunity" for recovery, as most patients wish to have a healthy baby and become a healthy parent. In this section, various bio-psychosocial parental risk factors will be discussed. All of them need to be considered to address the specific needs of the parent caring for an infant with NAS/NOWS. In addition, the risk of returning to substance use and the risk of overdose increase during the first year post-delivery (Schiff et al., 2018) requiring non-judgmental screening for substance use at any encounter with any provider. Issues with relapse to substance use or lack of appropriate OUD or psychiatric treatment should be addressed with the provision of supportive care and assistance with returning to treatment rather than punitive responses, provided that the infant is not at imminent risk of harm.

2.3.1 Substance Use Disorders (SUD) and Stigma

Although there has been great interest in describing substance use disorders as chronic, relapsing conditions with distinct functional stages that reflect disturbances in major neurobiological circuits, pregnant and parenting people with a SUD, and especially on medications for OUD, encounter stigma by society, relatives, health care providers, and even themselves (Frazer et al., 2019). Stigma may be a contributing factor to maternal/parental engagement in their own and their infant's care. It has been shown that nurses or other health care providers view SUDs or requiring medication for OUD as a moral failing rather than a medical condition, and perceived judgments can interfere with breastfeeding, visits to the baby, or skin-to-skin care (Renbarger et al., 2023).

2.3.2 Psychiatric Comorbidity

Parenting people with OUD often face enormous challenges in their environment (such as generational substance use, abusive and neglectful relationships) and often struggle with other co-occurring medical and neuropsychiatric conditions such as anxiety, major depression, post-traumatic stress disorder, and personality disorders, and are at increased risk for postpartum depression and return to substance use after delivery (Campbell et al., 2021; Heller et al., 2023). Given the multiple variables that can determine the severity/course of NAS/NOWS, currently it is not possible to predict which infant will have functional and adaptive challenges that will require pharmacotherapy for NAS/NOWS which warrant prolonged hospitalization. A mother/parent with OUD who has several pregnancies can have one child who needs medication for NAS/NOWS and another with very mild neurobehavioral dysfunction who does not require pharmacological treatment. This resulting uncertainty and anxiety surrounding the neonate's functioning during the first weeks of life and the possibility of NAS/NOWS is a tremendous source of anxiety for the mother and can affect her OUD treatment. Psychiatric medication usage during pregnancy, like antidepressants, antipsychotics, both typical and atypical, have been implicated in causing independent or synergistic neonatal withdrawal signs and symptoms. Exploring beliefs and attitudes about their mental health status and reassuring the parent that their benefits regarding taking needed prescribed medications during pregnancy to maintain a functional mental status outweigh the discomfort of seeing the infant having withdrawal signs is frequently needed. This is a difficult discussion for the parents, but it is necessary, and the practice of self-compassion, acceptance, emotional regulation, and the use of safe coping skills should be encouraged and framed as part of a comprehensive recovery process and personal growth.

2.3.3 Compromised Maternal Behavior Neurocircuitry or Parental Caregiving Neural Network

During pregnancy, a shift occurs towards a new behavioral-motivational system, namely a caregiving system that underlies parental behavior, with a specific focus on attachment to and protection of the child. A healthy transition to parenthood depends on intact parental neurocircuits. However, studies have shown that molecular, structural, and functional changes in the brain and stress system responses due to chronic substance use, traumatic experiences, or an insecure attachment to primary caregivers can alter the neurobiological reward and parenting centers in the brain, resulting in reduced or distorted salience of infant cues (Rutherford et al., 2011). This may have an impact on how parents are able to process and respond to infant cues, especially infant distress. In turn, repeated impaired responses to infant distress impacts the infants' own self-regulatory capacities (Flykt et al., 2021; Lowell et al., 2022), creating a cycle that can portend problems with future development and parental engagement, negatively impacting both mother/parent and child for the current and future generations.

2.3.4 Parental Attachment and Responses to the Infant

Pregnant/parenting people with SUDs frequently have insecure or traumatic attachment styles themselves that can distort caregiver perceptions of infant cues and behavior. These distorted perceptions on many occasions induce and amplify painful emotions that lead to maladaptive responses such as avoiding the care of the infant, inappropriate behaviors toward providers, or use of substances. Frequently the parent or health care providers define a child as a "difficult child" if the infant has periods of crying, irritability, or difficulty modulating arousal (e.g., is difficult to calm or return to a quiet state). They may refer to a baby as a "good child" when using "pull down" as a defense in a loud/overwhelming environment, a "drowsy" infant due to sedation during pharmacologic treatment, or a lethargic infant with poor modulation of arousal or autonomic dysregulation. Some mothers report difficulty engaging with their infants with NAS/NOWS or return to use of substances due to guilt or remorse over NAS/NOWS symptoms (e.g., inconsolable crying, stiffness), the disruptive assessments related to the scoring of NAS/NOWS symptoms, an inability to nourish an infant with feeding difficulties, or the pejorative attitudes of the providers or family members who activate feelings of shame, lack of confidence, or anger. Caring for babies is not an innate ability but rather one learned through explicit and implicit ways, either from the parenting received or from a conscious effort by the parent to do things differently from their own experiences. Although many parents/caregivers with OUD wish to be nourishing parents, old negative patterns sculpted into their brains often emerge with the birth of an infant, especially during emotionally challenging situations. These patterns of maladaptive responses may be due to some combination of their own insecure attachments or childhood experiences of violence or neglect, or environments colored by their parent's substance use or psychiatric comorbidities.

2.3.5 Current or Past History of Trauma

Great proportions of parents/caregivers with SUDs have current or past experiences of physical, sexual, or emotional abuse by partners, relatives, or people close to them (Velez et al., 2006) that may not have been identified, treated, or resolved. Links between current trauma exposure or history of Adverse Childhood Experiences (ACEs) and parenting stress and psychiatric conditions are well established, leading to a person with frequent states of emotional dysregulation without the needed safe coping skills (e.g., self-awareness, healthy self-soothing, equanimity). All of these learned self-management skills are needed to navigate the stresses created by mother/parenthood, especially during events such as experiencing having an infant with NAS/NOWS. Infant behaviors of discomfort, irritability, poor feeding, or sleeplessness may reactivate representations of their own childhood experiences that can induce strong emotions of anxiety, fear, or anger, leading to avoidance or aggressive responses toward providers, relatives, or even the infant (Nair et al., 2003). Attachment and trauma-informed/based programs can be helpful in the healing process of the caregiver and can increase their emotional stability and sensitivity to the infant's needs during the infancy period and beyond. Validation of appropriate ways of managing challenging emotions and efforts to respond based on the needs of the infant will encourage the practice of reflective parenting, a practice that promotes attachment and supports self-regulatory skills in the child. A relationship-based reflective parenting intervention specifically designed for parents in recovery from SUDs demonstrated improvement in mother–child outcomes (Suchman et al., 2017).

2.3.6 Socio-Contextual Factors and Parenting Stress

Parental stress can contribute to less attentive, sensitive, and warm responses to the children. Socio-contextual risks, including poverty, legal, housing, lack of transportation, and racism can contribute to the experience of stress. An additional stress often experienced by this group is involvement with child protective services (typically precipitated by involvement with necessary treatment for OUD) and the fear of having the infant placed in the care of others. There are often additional stressors created by OUD treatment facilities, necessitating mothers to choose between requirements such as daily attendance for medication and the care of the infant, an unwinnable predicament. Despite the importance of resolving trauma and attachment issues, practical realities such as continued SUD treatment, housing, poverty, isolation, and unemployment issues often become primary needs and should always be addressed, prenatally if possible, or at hospital discharge with coordinated plans of safe care (Patrick et al., 2020).

2.3.7 Preparation Regarding NAS/NOWS and Useful Non-Pharmacologic Strategies

Comprehensive interventions for the pregnant person with OUD should include, in addition to medications for OUD and behavioral therapy, a thorough and repetitive psychoeducational preparation to identify and respond properly to spontaneous and/or provoked signs of physiological and/or behavioral dysregulation in the infant associated with NAS/NOWS.

Discussions with the caregivers regarding the specific behaviors or signs that could be related to NAS/NOWS, and their non-pharmacologic or pharmacologic interventions, is paramount. However, considering all the factors that can contribute to the functioning of the newborn, it is necessary to keep in mind that NAS/NOWS may mimic other conditions. Parents need to know that no clinical signs or common signs of stress seen in any newborn (e.g., yawning, sneezing, tremors, poor feeding) should be solely attributed to drug withdrawal without a careful assessment to exclude other causes. Without education, and according to their own psychological status and coping mechanisms, parents may attribute "everything" or "nothing" to NAS/NOWS. This amplification or denial of NAS/NOWS signs is not beneficial and can lead to inappropriate responses to the real needs of the child and parent. Caregivers need to be trained to identify the infant's internal or external environmental stimuli that trigger obvious or subtle signs of neonatal dysregulations and how to prevent or manage them. This observation will allow the caregivers to adjust the regular care activities, interactions, and environments to the specific biological/behavioral needs of the infant. This in turn will promote the scaffolding for healthy development, secure attachment, and a healthy dyadic interaction.

2.4 Providing Comprehensive Care to the Opioid-Exposed Dyad

While suggestions for specific modalities or areas of interventions are mentioned in this chapter, the broader argument is not for any particular intervention modality per se, but for providers encountering dyads affected by OUD or other SUD at any stage of life or setting (hospital, home, school) to more broadly consider the individual stories/experiences of each dyad, the social, structural, and interpersonal conditions that shape these experiences, and the contexts in which they develop to be able to elaborate appropriate plans of support and care. In most cases, these plans should be interprofessional, with each specialist providing a thoughtful component to an integrated plan of care for the dyad. As substance use patterns and histories, maternal/parental psychosocial histories, and infant and caregiver capacities are highly individual, these plans should be tailored to the unique needs of each dyad and considerate of the context in which the dyad resides. These plans should also be in place ideally as early as possible (i.e., prenatally) and extend beyond hospital discharge well into the child's life, necessitating extension over various modalities of care, including social services, parental OUD treatment, obstetric care, early infant hospitalization, early intervention (e.g., physical therapy, occupational therapy, speech-language pathologists), and ongoing pediatric care throughout the dyad's history together. Interprofessional approaches are needed where supportive caregiving environments for families and *strength-based strategies* (those that focus on individuals' strengths, community networks) and not those focused on their deficits (behaviors related to SUD or psychiatric concerns, past and current poor choices) (Ezell et al., 2023).

Interventions with parent–infant dyads typically provide parents with emotional support, coaching parents with strategies geared to the needs of the child and providing parallel parental self-management skills (i.e., skills used in both parenting and daily life). These interventions include: 1) *Helping the caregiver to frequently explore their own functioning* during interactions with the infant to manage difficult emotions (tiredness, anxiety, guilt, shame, fear) in a constructive way and to avoid impulses triggered by stressful situations. Health care providers can encourage the mother/parent/caregiver to spent time at the infant's bedside, which has been associated with decreased NAS/NOWS severity. Interactions should ideally occur when the dyad are both in a regulated state, with needed "breaks" or rest by either aspect of the dyad to avoid exhaustion or emotional overload. Caregivers' ability to engage in coregulating behaviors has been proposed to play a major role for the development of children's self-regulation. 2) *Helping the caregiver to understand the infant's behaviors* that indicate organization (restful sleep, calm quiet alert, making eye contact, smooth movements) or signs that indicate dysregulation (irritability, looking away during interaction, hypertonicity or tremors, excessive crying or grimacing, hiccups/spitting). 3) *Reassuring the mother/parent/ caregiver* when appropriately interpreting and using sensitive responses to the infant's cues. Nurses and other health care providers who are caring, understanding, and affirming toward mothers with SUDs are better poised to facilitate trusting relationships and improve health outcomes. 4) *Reducing parent stress,* when possible. This can be initiated during pregnancy during obstetric care and then during the pediatric care of the baby. NAS/NOWS is a frequent source of caregiver distress, and some parents are afraid to share with relatives and even partners that they are receiving medications for OUD, or they have a SUD due to shame, guilt, and pain of seeing the infant's signs of NAS/NOWS. This can be confounded if nurses, other health care providers, or relatives make pejorative comments or express their difficulty in calming the infant to the mother (Cleveland & Bonugli, 2014). 5) *Providing early, accessible and non-judgmental medical care immediately after hospital discharge*, so that the mother is provided with support and reassurance, or interventions should difficulties arise. Evidence indicates the importance of health care providers in discussing with the mother/parent their thoughts, questions, and feelings. Helping them to process them in a constructive and empowering manner may engage them in the care of the infant affected by NAS/NOWS. Supporting them and the family can facilitate understanding and treatment for NAS/NOWS, communication between the dyad, and maternal engagement in treatment and thereby improved outcomes for parents and children (Velez et al., 2021b).

2.5 Summary

The impact of the early life environment, broadly defined, on later child health and development is well recognized. The complex, dynamic systems that can adversely impact both the infant with substance exposure (and the situations that often accompany those exposures and NAS/NOWS) and their parent/caregiver require individualized, multisystem intervention approaches. Pharmacologic treatment or parenting instruction alone may not be sufficient. Interventions that are family-centered, that emphasize dyadic regulation during NAS/NOWS at the hospital and later at home, may be effective in reducing maternal/parental psychological symptoms and NAS/NOWS severity while increasing positive long-term attachment outcomes (Velez et al., 2021b).

Optimizing the hospital (newborn nursery, pediatric room or NICU) and home environment is likely to improve neurobehavioral outcomes for the infants. This approach would require a shift away from the current emphasis only on the caregiver's diagnosis of OUD and the infant with diagnosis of NAS/NOWS, looking more extensively at the social, economic, relational contexts which contribute to the physical and mental wellbeing of the dyad. Similarly, instead of the current focus on pregnancy and NAS/NOWS care only, a lifetime trajectories approach, extending from conception or preconception over the course of the child's lifetime, should be employed. Early screening, identification, and support from well-defined systems of care are needed to improve life trajectories (Tolan & Dodge, 2005). A holistic approach to working with opioid-exposed dyads ideally includes multidisciplinary work with social systems, communities, peer support from other mothers/parents, health care providers (including parental treatment providers, obstetricians, labor and delivery, newborn hospital staff, and following pediatricians), and subspecialists, each providing a necessary component towards optimizing parenting, maternal confidence and health, infant wellbeing, and synchrony for each unique dyad.

References

Azuine, R. E., Ji, Y., Chang, H.-Y., Kim, Y., Ji, H., DiBari, J., Hong, X., Wang, G., Singh, G. K., Pearson, C., Zuckerman, B., Surkan, P. J., & Wang, X. (2019). Prenatal risk factors and perinatal and postnatal outcomes associated with maternal opioid exposure in an urban, low-income, multiethnic US population. *JAMA Network Open*, *2*(6), https://doi.org/10.1001/jamanetworko pen.2019.6405

Boggess, T., & Risher, W. C. (2022). Clinical and basic research investigations into the long-term effects of prenatal opioid exposure on brain development. *Journal of Neuroscience Research*, *100*(1), 396–409. https://doi.org/10.1002/jnr.24642

Brandt, L., & Finnegan, L. P. (2017). Neonatal abstinence syndrome: Where are we, and where do we go from here? *Current Opinion in Psychiatry*, *30*(4), 268–274. https://doi.org/10.1097/YCO.0000000000000334

Camerota, M., Davis, J. M., Dansereau, L. M., Oliveira, E. L., Padbury, J. F., & Lester, B. M. (2022). Effects of pharmacologic treatment for neonatal abstinence syndrome on DNA methylation and neurobehavior: A prospective cohort study. *The Journal of Pediatrics*, *243*, 21–26. https://doi.org/10.1016/j.jpeds.2021.12.057

Campbell, J., Matoff-Stepp, S., Velez, M. L., Cox, H. H., & Laughon, K. (2021). Pregnancy-associated deaths from homicide, suicide, and drug overdose: Review of research and the intersection with intimate partner violence. *Journal of Women's Health*, *30*(2), 236–244. https://doi.org/10.1089/jwh.2020.8875

Cleveland L. M., & Bonugli, R. (2014) Experiences of mothers of infants with neonatal abstinence syndrome in the neonatal intensive care unit. *J Obstet Gynecol Neonatal Nurs*, *43*(3), 318–329. https://doi.org/10.1111/1552-6909.12306

Cole, F. S., Wegner, D. J., & Davis, J. M. (2017). The genomics of neonatal abstinence syndrome. *Frontiers in Pediatrics*, *5*, 176. https://doi.org/10.3389/fped.2017.00176

Conradt, E., Crowell, S. E., & Lester, B. M. (2018). Early life stress and environmental influences on the neurodevelopment of children with prenatal opioid exposure. *Neurobiology of Stress*, *9*, 48–54. https://doi.org/10.1016/j.ynstr.2018.08.005

Coyle, M. G., Salisbury, A. L., Lester, B. M., Jones, H. E., Lin, H., Graf-Rohrmeister, K., & Fischer, G. (2012). Neonatal neurobehavior effects following buprenorphine versus methadone exposure: Opioid-exposed neonatal neurobehavior. *Addiction*, *107*, 63–73. https://doi.org/10.1111/j.1360-0443.2012.04040.x

Dysart, K., Hsieh, H. C., Kaltenbach, K., & Greenspan, J. S. (2007). Sequela of preterm versus term infants born to mothers on a methadone maintenance program: Differential course of neonatal abstinence syndrome. *Journal of Perinatal Medicine*, *35*(4), 344–346. https://doi.org/10.1515/JPM.2007.063

Ezell, J. M., Pho, M., Jaiswal, J., Ajayi, B. P., Gosnell, N., Kay, E., Eaton, E., & Bluthenthal, R. (2023). A systematic literature review of strengths-based approaches to drug use management and treatment. *Clinical Social Work Journal, 51*(3), 294–305. https://doi.org/10.1007/s10615-023-00874-2

Finnegan, L. P., & Kaltenbach, K. (1992). Neonatal abstinence syndrome. *Primary Pediatric Care, 2,* 1367–1378.

Flykt, M. S., Salo, S., & Pajulo, M. (2021). "A window of opportunity": Parenting and addiction in the context of pregnancy. *Current Addiction Reports, 8*(4), 578–594. https://doi.org/10.1007/s40429-021-00394-4

Frazer, Z., McConnell, K., & Jansson, L. M. (2019). Treatment for substance use disorders in pregnant women: Motivators and barriers. *Drug and Alcohol Dependence, 205,* https://doi.org/10.1016/j.drugalcdep.2019.107652

Goshgarian, G., Jawad, R., O'Brien, L., Muterspaugh, R., Zikos, D., Ezhuthachan, S., Newman, C., Hsu, C. D., Bailey, B., & Ragina, N. (2022). Prenatal buprenorphine/naloxone or methadone use on neonatal outcomes in Michigan. *Cureus, 14*(8). https://doi.org/10.7759/cureus.27790

Hartgrove, M. J., Meschke, L. L., King, T. L., & Saunders, C. (2019). Treating infants with neonatal abstinence syndrome: An examination of three protocols. *Journal of Perinatology, 39*(10), 1377–1383. https://doi.org/10.1038/s41 372-019-0450-6

Heller, N. A., Logan, B. A., Shrestha, H., Morrison, D. G., & Hayes, M. J. (2023). Effect of neonatal abstinence syndrome treatment status and maternal depressive symptomatology on maternal reports of infant behaviors. *Journal of Pediatric Psychology, 48*(6), 583–592. https://doi.org/10.1093/jpepsy/jsad023

Jansson, L. M., DiPietro, J. A., Elko, A., & Velez, M. (2007). Maternal vagal tone change in response to methadone is associated with neonatal abstinence syndrome severity in exposed neonates. *Journal of Maternal, Fetal and Neonatal Medicine, 20*(9), 677–685. https://doi.org/10.1080/14767050701490327

Johnson, R. E., Jones, H. E., & Fischer, G. (2003). Use of buprenorphine in pregnancy: Patient management and effects on the neonate. *Drug and Alcohol Dependence, 70*(2), 87–101. https://doi.org/10.1016/s0376-8716(03)00062-0

Jones, H. E., Jansson, L. M., O'Grady, K. E., & Kaltenbach, K. (2013). The relationship between maternal methadone dose at delivery and neonatal outcome: Methodological and design considerations. *Neurotoxicology and Teratology, 39,* 110–115. https://doi.org/10.1016/j.ntt.2013.05.003

Jones, H. E., Kaltenbach, K., Heil, S. H., Stine, S. M., Coyle, M. G., Arria, A. M., O'Grady, K. E., Selby, P., Martin, P. R., & Fischer, G. (2010). Neonatal abstinence syndrome after methadone or buprenorphine exposure. *The New England Journal of Medicine, 363*(24), 2320–2331. https://doi.org/10.1056/NEJMoa 1005359

Jones, N. A., & Sloan, A. (2018). Neurohormones and temperament interact during infant development. *Philosophical Transactions of the Royal Society of London. Series B, Biological Sciences, 373*(1744). https://doi.org/10.1098/ rstb.2017.0159

Kocherlakota, P. (2014). Neonatal abstinence syndrome. *Pediatrics, 134*(2), 547–561. https://doi.org/10.1542/peds.2013-3524

Lester, B. M., & Tronick, E. Z. (2004). History and description of the Neonatal Intensive Care Unit Network Neurobehavioral Scale. *Pediatrics, 113*(3 Pt 2), 634–640. https://doi.org/10.1542/peds.113.S2.634

Lowell, A. F., Morie, K., Potenza, M. N., Crowley, M. J., & Mayes, L. C. (2022). An intergenerational lifespan perspective on the neuroscience of prenatal substance exposure. *Pharmacology Biochemistry and Behavior, 219.* https://doi.org/10.1016/j.pbb.2022.173445

Maguire, D., & Gröer, M. (2016). Neonatal abstinence syndrome and the gastrointestinal tract. *Medical Hypotheses, 97,* 11–15. https://doi.org/10.1016/j.mehy.2016.10.006

Maguire, D. J., Taylor, S., Armstrong, K., Shaffer-Hudkins, E., Germain, A. M., Brooks, S. S., Cline, G. J., & Clark, L. (2016). Long-term outcomes of infants with neonatal abstinence syndrome. *Neonatal Network, 35*(5), 277–286. https://doi.org/10.1891/0730-0832.35.5.277

McCarthy, J. J., Leamon, M. H., Willits, N. H., & Salo, R. (2015). The effect of methadone dose regimen on neonatal abstinence syndrome. *Journal of Addiction Medicine, 9*(2), 105–110. https://doi.org/10.1097/ADM.0000000000000099

Nair, P., Schuler, M. E., Black, M. M., Kettinger, L., & Harrington, D. (2003). Cumulative environmental risk in substance abusing women: Early intervention, parenting stress, child abuse potential and child development. *Child Abuse & Neglect, 27*(9), 997–1017. https://doi.org/10.1016/s0145-2134(03)00161-3

Patrick, S. W., Barfield, W. D., Poindexter, B. B., & Committee on Fetus and Newborn, Committee on Substance Use and Prevention (2020). Neonatal opioid withdrawal syndrome. *Pediatrics, 146*(5). https://doi.org/10.1542/peds.2020-029074

Renbarger, K. M., Phelps, B., Broadstreet, A., & Abebe, S. (2023). Factors associated with maternal engagement in infant care when mothers use substances. *Women's Health Reports, 4*(1), 48–64. https://doi.org/10.1089/whr.2022.0082

Rutherford, H. J., Williams, S. K., Moy, S., Mayes, L. C., & Johns, J. M. (2011). Disruption of maternal parenting circuitry by addictive process: Rewiring of reward and stress systems. *Frontiers in Psychiatry, 2,* 37. https://doi.org/10.3389/fpsyt.2011.00037

Schiff, D. M., Nielsen, T., Terplan, M., Hood, M., Bernson, D., Diop, H., Bharel, M., Wilens, T. E., LaRochelle, M., Walley, A. Y., & Land, T. (2018). Fatal and nonfatal overdose among pregnant and postpartum women in Massachusetts. *Obstetrics and Gynecology, 132*(2), 466–474. https://doi.org/10.1097/AOG.0000000000002734

Substance Abuse and Mental Health Services Administration. (2020, September) *TIP 39: Substance Abuse Treatment and Family Therapy.* U.S. Department of Health and Human Services. https://store.samhsa.gov/product/treatment-improvement-protocol-tip-39-substance-use-disorder-treatment-and-family-therapy/PEP20-02-02-012

Suchman, N. E., DeCoste, C. L., McMahon, T. J., Dalton, R., Mayes, L. C., & Borelli, J. (2017). Mothering from the inside out: Results of a second randomized clinical trial testing a mentalization-based intervention for mothers in addiction treatment. *Development and Psychopathology, 29*(2), 617–636. https://doi.org/10.1017/S0954579417000220

Tsai, S. A., Bendriem, R. M., & Lee, C. T. D. (2019). The cellular basis of fetal endoplasmic reticulum stress and oxidative stress in drug-induced neurodevelopmental deficits. *Neurobiology of Stress, 10.* https://doi.org/ 10.1016/j.ynstr.2018.100145

Tolan, P. H., & Dodge, K. A. (2005). Children's mental health as a primary care and concern: A system for comprehensive support and service. *American Psychologist, 60*(6), 601–614. https://doi.org/10.1037/0003-066X.60.6.601

U.S. Food and Drug Administration. (2013, September 10). *FDA announces safety labeling changes and postmarket study requirements for extended release and long-acting opioid analgesics.* [Press Release]. http://wayback.archive-it.org/ 7993/20170112130229/http:/www.fda.gov/NewsEvents/Newsroom/PressAn nouncements/ucm367726.htm

U.S. Food and Drug Administration. (2016, May 26). *Neonatal opioid withdrawal syndrome and medication assisted treatment with methadone and buprenorphine.* https://www.fda.gov/drugs/drug-safety-and-availability/neona tal-opioid-withdrawal-syndrome-and-medication-assisted-treatment-methad one-and-buprenorphine

Velez, M. L., & Jansson, L. M. (2008). Non-pharmacologic care of the opioid dependent mother and her newborn. *Journal of Addiction Medicine, 2*(3), 113– 120. https://doi.org/10.1097/ADM.0b013e31817e6105

Velez, M. L., Jordan, C. J., & Jansson, L. M. (2021a). Reconceptualizing non-pharmacologic approaches to neonatal abstinence syndrome (NAS) and neo-natal opioid withdrawal syndrome (NOWS): A theoretical and evidence-based approach. *Neurotoxicology and Teratology, 88.* https://doi.org/10.1016/ j.ntt.2021.107020

Velez, M. L., Jordan, C., & Jansson, L. M. (2021b). Reconceptualizing non-pharmacologic approaches to neonatal abstinence syndrome (NAS) and neo-natal opioid withdrawal syndrome (NOWS): A theoretical and evidence-based approach. Part II: The clinical application of non-pharmacologic care for NAS/NOWS. *Neurotoxicology and Teratology, 88.* https://doi.org/10.1016/ j.ntt.2021.107032

Velez, M. L., Montoya, I. D., Jansson, L. M., Walters, V., Svikis, D., Jones, H. E., Chilcoat, H., & Campbell, J. (2006). Exposure to violence among substance-dependent pregnant women and their children. *Journal of Substance Abuse Treatment, 30*(1), 31–38. https://doi.org/10.1016/j.jsat.2005.09.001

Young, L. W., Ounpraseuth, S. T., Merhar, S. L., Hu, Z., Simon, A. E., Bremer, A. A., Lee, J. Y., Das, A., Crawford, M. M., Greenberg, R. G., Smith, P. B., Poindexter, B. B., Higgins, R. D., Walsh, M. C., Rice, W., Paul, D. A., Maxwell, J. R., Telang, S., Fung, C. M., ... Devlin, L. A. (2023). Eat, sleep, console approach or usual care for neonatal opioid withdrawal. *New England Journal of Medicine, 388*(25), 2326–2337. https://doi.org/10.1056/NEJMoa2214470

3 Neurodevelopmental Outcomes of Children Prenatally Exposed to Opioids and Other Substances

Hendrée E. Jones, Kim Andringa,
Senga Carroll and Evette Horton

Box 3.1 Case Vignette

A young mother, who grew up in foster care due to her mother dying of a drug overdose and her father dying from suicide, reports initiating alcohol, tobacco, and cannabis use at age 13 and opioid use at age 17. She reports that her opioid use felt "out of control" for the three years leading up to her pregnancy, and at age 22 she made the decision to enter obstetrical care and substance use disorder treatment to stop using substances and "break the cycle of addiction" for herself and her baby to be. In foster care she experienced hunger and fear as her constant companions. Her medical records show her being underweight, having anaemia, and low levels of folic acid and vitamin D. She has also experienced low-level lead exposure, and battles asthma due to the air and water pollution she grew up with. She reports vaping tobacco daily and using alcohol. Her identified strengths include "being a survivor, a good friend, a hard worker at her job, and advocating for myself." During pregnancy she received methadone to treat her opioid use disorder, an SSRI to treat her depression, prenatal vitamins, and an inhaler for asthma. She gave birth to a baby at 36.3 weeks' gestation, weighing 5.6 pounds, and having mild withdrawal alleviated with non-pharmacological supports. At age 4, her child was diagnosed with language and speech delays and is currently being evaluated at the preschool for occupational therapy. She is working hard to get her child the services needed to thrive in development. She asked her pediatrician: "Did my opioid use during pregnancy cause my child's problems?" How should the provider respond? (See Box 3.2 for answers.)

DOI: 10.4324/9781003397267-3

3.1 Introduction

The current opioid crisis in the United States has had radiating harm for adults, children, and society. This crisis, like past opioid crises, raises concerns about the short- and long-term effects of prenatal exposure to opioids. The case vignette illustrates the challenge to isolate the impact of prenatal opioid exposure on any one or any set of neurodevelopmental outcomes in children. This chapter aims to broaden the focus from a narrow "cause and effect" of prenatal exposure leading to neurodevelopmental problems in children by highlighting the myriad of factors found in the literature that contribute to adverse neurodevelopmental outcomes in children.

3.1.1 Behavioral Teratology Shaped the Study of Prenatal Substance Exposure

The term behavioral teratology was introduced in 1963 by Jack Werboff whose rodent studies showed that doses of some psychotherapeutic agents could induce behavioral reactions in the offspring without creating physical malformations (Vorhees, 1986). Key concepts that comprise behavioral teratology include:

1. Developmental injuries to the nervous system have a protracted period of susceptibility. While organogenesis is most sensitive, vulnerability spans through infancy.
2. Most developing nervous system alterations are functional abnormalities, not CNS malformation. Such effects are often not detectable at birth, i.e., the organism may 'grow into its deficit.'
3. An ordinal relationship exists between the different expressions of developmental toxicity, but prenatal exposure to substances of misuse are exceptions (Vorhees, 1986).

Recognizing a wider window of vulnerability and greater sensitivity to injury over a longer developmental time led to a flurry of research to demonstrate these two themes with every drug and environmental agent that investigators could pursue. Crack cocaine and opioids were quickly examined. Developmental neurotoxicology extended the examination of prenatal exposure to substances on developmental outcomes to also recognize the importance of developmental stage at the time of exposure, the threshold of the dose required to produce effects, the development of dose–response relationships between exposure and outcomes, the potential for compensatory mechanisms, and the period of development during which outcomes are measured (Vorhees, 1986).

3.1.2 The Conceptualization of "Environment" in the Study of Prenatal Exposure to Psychoactive Substances Shapes the Questions, Study Methodology, and Result Interpretation

Of equal importance is the recognition and examination of the reciprocal roles of genetics and the "environment." The word "environment" can represent important influences such as socioeconomic and caregiving factors in child development (Sameroff & Chandler, 1975). The conceptualization of "environment" in the study of prenatal exposure to psychoactive substances has commonly been tinged with misogyny. The intrauterine environment has been weaponized against women, with pregnant individuals frequently being reduced to an incubator for the child. For example, women have been examined in research studies as vectors of disease, or as vessels, or as the "environment" for the embryo and fetus, instead of as a dyad and a separate entity unto themselves (Faden et al., 1996). Certainly, the way prenatal exposure to addictive substances, including cocaine and opioids in the past and present, has been studied, reflects both uses of the word environment (Chasnoff et al., 1988; Jones, Kaltenbach et al., 2009).

3.2 Defining Neurodevelopmental Disorders

The impact of Vorhees (1986) and colleagues on the shaping of the examination of outcomes of prenatal exposure to substances cannot be overstated. Based on such work, a body of clinical research now examines children for neurodevelopmental problems and a smaller body of work develops, tests, and implements interventions to mitigate the observed problems. Neurodevelopmental problems are a group of conditions where the integrity and function of the central and autonomic nervous systems are harmed during sensitive periods of brain development spanning from in utero to the first two years of life.

Children with neurodevelopmental disorders can experience a wide range of signs, including compromised emotional regulation, low muscle control, reduced traditional learning ability, and problems with social integration (Morris-Rosendahl & Croq, 2020). Researchers have identified several root causal categories of neurodevelopmental disorders, including: (1) genetic factors that can increase the risk of developing these disorders (e.g., Down syndrome); (2) prenatal factors such as maternal infections (e.g., rubella, toxoplasmosis), exposure to toxins or drugs (e.g., alcohol, Thalidomide), inadequate nutrition, and complications during pregnancy or birth (e.g., prematurity, low birth weight) can impact the developing brain; (3) environmental factors (e.g., lead, mercury, pollution); (4) brain injury can disrupt normal neurodevelopment and lead to neurological impairments; and (5) certain neurological conditions (e.g., epilepsy, tumors) that can affect brain development. It is likely that a combination of genetic, epigenetic, and environmental factors, as well as complex interactions between them, contribute to the development of neurodevelopmental disorders.

Disorders of early brain development are often called neurodevelopmental disorders and include attention-deficit/hyperactivity disorder (ADHD), autism spectrum disorder (ASD), learning disabilities (e.g. dyslexia), intellectual disabilities, motor disabilities (e.g., cerebral palsy), and seizures (Morris-Rosendahl & Crocq, 2020). Preterm birth and low birth weight are known high-risk factors related to infants' neurodevelopmental abnormalities (Vohr, 2013).

3.2.1 Multiple Factors Influence Neurodevelopmental Outcomes

Applying key concepts from Vorhees (1986), it is recognized that the neurodevelopment of the fetus, infant, and child is affected by multiple factors, such as genetics, epigenetics, and environment. A discussion of these factors is outside the scope of this chapter. As noted above, "environment" is a broad term that can include different factors and interpretations of who or what it is.

Figure 3.1 shows numerous examples of environmental factors that cause or are related to adverse neurodevelopmental outcomes, independent or separate from prenatal substance exposure. These "environmental" factors may be internal or external to the woman or birthing person and her child. As shown in Figure 3.1, epigenetic processes are gaining attention as an important mechanism through which the "memory" of various developmental exposures is held, with possible neurodevelopmental alternations as outcomes (Godfrey et al., 2015). There is also emerging evidence that epigenetic processes can act over several generations, including three or more generations and through the paternal line (McPherson et al., 2015). Paternal exposure to environmental stimuli (e.g., stress, diet) can result in behavioral and epigenetic changes in children. Some children of fathers using substances have shown developmental and physiological abnormalities as well as deficits in cognitive and emotional domains (Nieto & Kosten, 2019). Examining sensitivity to drugs in children of fathers who use substances is a growing area of research.

3.2.2 Typically Reported External Environmental Factors

Examples of external environmental factors reported in the literature include poverty and racial and class discrimination. Growing up in poverty has diffuse and enduring effects on children's development, such as risk of

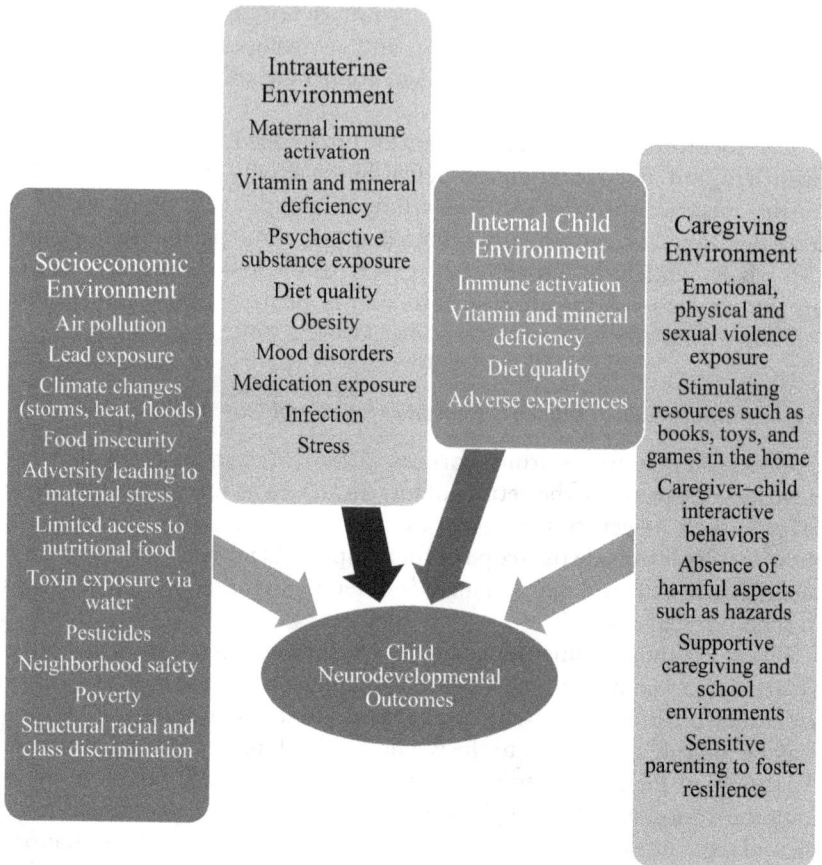

Figure 3.1 The complex relationship between internal and external environmental factors, epigenetics, and child neurodevelopmental outcomes

adverse childhood event exposure (ACEs), poor physical health, high rates of behavioral problems, and low school achievement, yet the mechanisms causing these effects have yet to be fully elucidated (Pollak & Wolfe, 2020). For race and class discrimination, neurotoxicant exposures are of particular concern in historically and currently marginalized communities.

Often a consequence of structural racism, low-income minoritized populations experience a disproportionate burden of hazardous exposures through proximity to high traffic roads, industrial facilities, and suboptimal housing. A review of 20 studies that investigated exposure disparities and neurodevelopment in children found that many studies focused on air pollution, metal exposures, and water contamination (Dickerson et al., 2023). Several of the 20 studies showed differences in exposure–outcome associations by income and education. Relatedly, macrolevel issues are manifested in exposure to environmental contaminants, such as lead in pipes and paint. Lead, even in low levels of exposure, is related to negative health, learning, and behavioral sequelae (e.g., Min et al., 2009). Greater pesticide exposure has also been associated with poorer mental development, pervasive developmental disorder, inattention, and attention-deficit/hyperactivity disorder (Roberts et al., 2012).

3.2.3 Typically Reported Internal Environmental Factors

There are numerous examples of internal maternal environmental factors outside of substance use that can alter neurodevelopment. This section provides several examples but is not intended to be an exhaustive list. Obesity, maternal stress, undernutrition, and Maternal Immune Activation (MIA), or infection during pregnancy can induce abnormal births (e.g., Pacheco, 2020). For example, maternal obesity is seen as a major determinant of early and later life health. Observational studies provide evidence for effects of maternal obesity on children's risks of asthma, coronary heart disease, obesity, stroke, and type 2 diabetes. Maternal obesity may also lead to poorer cognitive performance in children and an increased risk of neurodevelopmental disorders including cerebral palsy (Godfrey et al., 2017). A prospective study examined maternal stress during pregnancy and demonstrated a higher rate of delay in motor and mental development in children whose mothers demonstrated higher stress levels during pregnancy (Huizink et al., 2003). The relationship between maternal nutrition during pregnancy and neurodevelopment in children is highly studied. A scoping review of two decades of publications on maternal diets (e.g., high fat, ketogenic, hypercaloric), undernutrition and inadequate intake of macronutrients (e.g., fatty acids, proteins), micronutrients (e.g., choline, iron, zinc), and vitamins (e.g., B12, folate, vitamin D, vitamin A) included 84 studies. Inadequate nutrient intake during pregnancy was associated with brain defects (e.g., hypothalamic and hippocampal pathways altered, small cerebral volume, spina bifida), neuropsychiatric disorders (ASD, ADHD, schizophrenia, anxiety, depression), altered cognition, visual impairment, motor deficits, and an increased risk of abnormal behavior (Cortés-Albornoz et al., 2021).

Maternal Immune Activation (MIA), an inflammatory response triggered by pathogenic infection and autoimmune diseases, is known to be a risk factor for neurodevelopmental and psychiatric disorders (Estes & McAllister, 2016). Susceptibility to MIA may be greater in dyads where there is micronutrient deficiency (e.g., Estes & McAllister, 2016). An example of a micronutrient deficiency that creates neurodevelopmental problems (e.g., neural tube deficit) is a folic acid deficiency (Greenberg et al., 2011).

Other causes of MIAs include cytomegalovirus, herpes simplex virus, rubella, toxoplasma, and Zika viruses that are vertically transmitted to the fetus, affecting its development and resulting in severe complications such as miscarriage and malformations (Meyer, 2019). Infections with non-vertically transmitted pathogens such as influenza during pregnancy can cause neurodevelopmental disorders in children too. While these many issues have been deemed internal environmental factors of the birthing person, it is critical to understand to what extent external environmental issues (poverty, stress, ACEs, living in areas without access to healthy foods, living in areas where access to virus prevention measures are not easily accessible) prevent women and birthing people from being able to keep themselves safe from harm. Thus, we cannot examine neurodevelopmental outcomes without a full appreciation of the numerous factors that lead to behavior and internal disease states. Lessons from these studies can be applied to examining neurodevelopment of children prenatally exposed to opioids.

Another variable that has a complex relationship to neurodevelopmental outcomes in children is maternal depression. Women who experience depression during pregnancy have a higher risk of having a child with autism spectrum disorder (ASD) than women who are not affected regardless of antidepressant use (Hagberg et al., 2018). This risk was marginally higher in women with treated depression compared to those with untreated depression; however, the fact that the risk of ASD was not higher in women who were taking antidepressants for other reasons suggests that antidepressants are not responsible (Hagberg et al., 2018). It is well known that depression is common among pregnant patients treated for opioid use disorder (OUD) (Fitzsimons et al., 2007) and the cause of such depression is likely related to the stressful, toxic, and violent environment that many patients grew up in and may also live in. Relatedly, other factors such as age and maternal physical and mental health are often considered internal environmental factors and these have been shown to affect fetal growth (Miguel et al., 2019).

Maternal depression is often linked to stress and anxiety, and this combination of factors is related to adverse neurodevelopment in children. Stress, depression, and anxiety during pregnancy are related to neurodevelopmental effects on infants, including behavioral disturbances, lower cephalic circumference, and worse cognitive development than children whose mothers did not have these issues (O'Donnell et al., 2009).

Another important but often neglected factor in a discussion of maternal substance use is tobacco smoking. Intrauterine exposure to tobacco can affect expression of selected fetal brain regulatory genes responsible for brain growth, myelination, and neuronal migration, altering brain structure and function. Prenatal smoking has been associated with a greater risk for ADHD, bipolar disorder, and depression (Nakamura et al., 2021). A large body of literature has also connected disadvantaged status to nicotine use (Hiscock et al., 2012).

3.3 Prematurity and Low Birth Weight Are Related to Adverse Neurodevelopmental Outcomes

Preterm birth and low birth weight are negative outcomes in and of themselves and can be triggered by a myriad of factors. For example, potential negative effects of climate change such as air pollution, floods, food insecurity, heat, and storms can lead to maternal stress, undernutrition, and toxic exposure, eventually leading to the onset of preterm birth, low birth weight, and neurodevelopmental disorders (Singh et al., 2013). Preterm birth and low birth weight can also lead to ASD and ADHD. Preterm birth is an adverse event that contributes to poor socioemotional development. Prematurity is also associated with deficits in conversational language at 3 years old (Sanchez et al., 2020). The premature brain may present with disturbances such as alterations in myelination, changes in synaptic efficacy, loss of volume, and enlarged ventricles (Miller et al., 2004). While the effects of prematurity are seen in all gestational age subgroups, a meta-analysis showed that extremely low birth weight children have a more robust association with hyperactivity, inattention, and internalizing problems in childhood and adolescence and higher rates of anxiety, depression, and social problems in adulthood compared to their non-premature counterparts (Estes & McAllister, 2016). Advances in medical care for premature neonates may be related to the rates of some neurologic and developmental conditions being lower in recent versus historical data (Chung et al., 2020).

3.4 Examining Prenatal Opioid Exposure and Its Relationship to Neurodevelopmental Disorders

Patients who use opioids during pregnancy are comprised of unique subgroups: those who take opioids as prescribed for chronic pain, those who take opioids as prescribed for addiction, those who take prescribed opioids for both pain and addiction, those who misuse opioids but do not meet criteria for an OUD, and those with untreated OUD. While some have said that opioid exposure is all the same to the embryo or fetus, the external and internal environments that accompany such prenatal exposure may influence the child outcomes in different ways.

A discussion of groups treated for chronic pain is outside the scope of this chapter in lieu of a focus on patients with treated and untreated OUD.

During pregnancy, chronic untreated OUD is associated with many barriers to accessing care which can lead to inadequate prenatal care, increased risk of fetal growth restriction, abruptio placentae, fetal death, preterm labor, and intrauterine passage of meconium (Center for Substance Abuse Treatment, 2005). Given that most people in active addiction are pushed to the margins of society for survival, untreated addiction is associated with engagement in high-risk activities. Such behaviors leave women and birthing people vulnerable to sexually transmitted infections (STIs), violence, and legal consequences, including loss of child custody, criminal proceedings, or incarceration. As discussed in section 3.3.2 above, pregnant women with OUD often need help with co-occurring mental health conditions, particularly depression, posttraumatic stress disorder (PTSD), and anxiety. More than 30% of pregnant women enrolled in a substance use treatment program screened positive for moderate to severe depression, and more than 40% reported symptoms of postpartum depression (Holbrook & Kaltenbach, 2012).

In addition, these women are at increased risk of use of other substances, including tobacco, marijuana, and cocaine (Jones, Heil, et al., 2009). Understanding the effects of opioid-polysubstance use on the fetus is important because their additive or synergistic effects may be different from those of opioids alone. Polydrug exposure may increase the risk to the fetus or may moderate negative opioid effects, depending on the type of substances, the dosages, and the timing of exposure. When opioids are combined with alcohol or benzodiazepines, the reward effects of opioids are enhanced, but respiratory depression is exaggerated. When stimulants are used with opioids, the sedative effects are masked, sometimes resulting in extreme heart rate variability, increased blood pressure, and heart rate effects. Some drug combinations may have unique biochemical effects on the developing fetal brain and have been shown to predict poor fetal growth in some studies (Singer et al., 1994).

3.4.1 Pre-Clinical Pathophysiology of Prenatal Opioid Exposure

Animal models data suggest that in utero opioid exposure yields compromised outcomes later in life (Weller et al., 2021). Animal studies have shown a broad range of negative developmental effects on both neurons and glia after prenatal opioid exposure (Ross et al., 2015). With prenatal morphine exposure, decreased dendritic length and spine density and increased neuronal apoptosis are noted during early postnatal development (Hu et al., 2002). Prenatal heroin exposure resulted in hippocampal cholinergic alterations and may play a role in explaining spatial learning and memory deficits (Wang & Han, 2009). For prenatal exposure to buprenorphine and methadone, early myelination has been reported (Vestal-Laborde et al., 2014; Wu et al., 2014). Taken together, these results support the notion that prenatal opioid exposure in a rodent model living in a context of isolation may have a negative impact on neurodevelopment. However, the translatability of pre-clinical findings to the human fetus and neonate is complicated because of differences in neurodevelopmental trajectories, receptor expression, and central opioid pharmacokinetics (Radhakrishnan et al., 2021).

3.4.2 Brain Imaging Studies of Children Prenatally Exposed to Opioids and Other Substances

Consistent with the pre-clinical literature, imaging studies in humans report changes related to opioid exposure that have been associated with anatomical brain differences compared to other samples of children. For example, a cross-sectional magnetic resonance imaging (MRI) study of "prenatally opioid-exposed" children, of which 70 were invited and 16 completed with adequate data, were compared to 16 sex- and age-matched unexposed controls. The authors reported that opioid-exposed infants had decreased basal ganglia and cerebellar volumes (Sirnes et al., 2017). Another study of 16 infants "prenatally opioid-exposed" reported that brain volumes and basal ganglia volumes were smaller than population means (Yuan et al., 2014).

Further, Merhar et al. (2021) published outcomes from an unreported number of infants who were screened and yielded 29 infants with prenatal opioid exposure and 42 unexposed controls. Analyses controlled for a few of the many baseline differences between groups. Compared to non-prenatally substance-exposed infants, prenatally opioid-exposed infants had, with a few exceptions, significantly smaller relative volumes of brain regions (Merhar et al., 2021).

Not controlling for prenatal tobacco exposure is a concerning limitation to these findings, as there is an association between continued maternal smoking and smaller total brain volume (El Marroun et al., 2014). Given the earlier discussion of the myriad of factors that may help explain neurodevelopmental outcomes of children, the limitations of small-sample brain imaging studies to determine the extent to which prenatal opioid exposure is related to anatomical brain alterations are discussed below.

3.4.3 Long-Term Follow-Up for Children With Neonatal Abstinence Syndrome (NAS)

Five meta-analyses concluded that young children prenatally exposed to opioids, whether their birth parent used illicitly and/or was on agonist medication to treat opioid use disorder, showed worse cognitive, language, and motor skills compared to children with no prenatal substance exposure (Andersen et al., 2020; Lee, Bora, et al., 2020; Monnelly et al., 2019; Nelson et al., 2020; Yeoh et al., 2019).

However, meta-analyses are only as strong as the weakest study they include, and a commentary on these studies rightly noted that the overall literature in this area has been plagued by the same limitations since the first studies reported outcomes in the 1970s. Such design limitations include: significant heterogeneity in terms of the opioids examined, definition of opioid exposure groups, how control or comparison samples were defined and selected, small sample sizes, outcomes limited to early childhood, and an inability to account for various confounders (e.g., quality of home and child-rearing environment, socioeconomic factors, maternal mental health, inadequate nutrition, disruptions in maternal care, placement in foster, adoptive or kinship care, the presence or absence of polysubstance exposures, contribution of opioid withdrawal and possible pharmacologic treatment in the neonatal period, and genetic and epigenetic factors (e.g., Andersen et al., 2020; Lee et al., 2023; Singer et al., 2020). To address noted issues, recent studies of children with neonatal opioid withdrawal syndrome (NOWS) underscore the need for large a prospective follow-up with systematic assessments and careful evaluation of contributing factors (Benninger et al., 2020; Benninger et al., 2022).

3.4.4 Attempts to Address Complex Confounding Issues

The need to control for multiple potential confounders to understand the effects of prenatal exposure to alcohol on long-term developmental outcomes is seen in a study where 150 covariates were evaluated (Streissguth et al., 1986). For opioids, several cohort studies aimed to disentangle the effects of some of these complex confounding issues, yet their effect sizes were still too limited to control for the multiple possible factors (Kim et al., 2021; Lee, Pritchard, et al., 2020).

One large prospective cohort study found that the use of opioids in pregnant women did not affect language development or communication skills in children at 3 years of age (Skovlund et al., 2017). In a follow-up to the MOTHER study (Jones et al., 2010), a second study followed 96 infants to 36 months of age (Kaltenbach et al., 2018). The results showed no differences in outcomes between infants born to mothers who had received antenatal methadone or buprenorphine. Although a separate control group of unexposed infants was not included, infants in the MOTHER study appeared to have developed normally over this time period as compared to population norms on the outcomes measures. Finally, a large retrospective cohort study using a national database followed pregnant women without opioid use disorders or drug dependence and women prenatally exposed to prescription opioids and their infants. The authors reported no association between fetal opioid exposure and the risk of neurodevelopmental disorders in early childhood overall but reported an association within a subgroup of children born to women receiving prescription opioids for a longer duration and at higher doses during pregnancy (Wen et al., 2021). To summarize, the majority of studies in which confounders were controlled for revealed no differences in infant neurodevelopment as a function of prenatal opioid exposure (Conradt et al., 2019; Hans & Jeremy, 2001; Levine & Woodward, 2018; Messinger et al., 2004).

3.4.5 Avoiding the Single-Cause Fallacy

Prenatal opioid exposure associated with compromised neurodevelopment may incorrectly lead to the single-cause fallacy – neurodevelopmental problems are related to prenatal opioid exposure, so, implicitly, prenatal opioid exposure causes neurodevelopmental problems. Hence, when prenatal opioid exposure is found to be a marker for later developmental problems, it is argued that neonates who have experienced prenatal opioid exposure must be identified and specialized services rendered. This well-meaning attribution is inaccurate. Children experience neurodevelopmental problems for a wide variety of reasons. As noted in Figure 3.1 and above, the controlled data indicate that to the extent there are neurodevelopmental differences between children with and without prenatal opioid exposure, such differences are likely due to multiple causes. Deciding how to account for these multiple factors or causes is a challenge.

3.5 Future Recommendations for Research

Given that there are a number of studies examining the effects of prenatal exposure to opioids and other psychoactive substances launched that will follow mothers, birthing parents, and infants prenatally or at birth throughout childhood for the development of neurodevelopmental diagnoses (Lee et al., 2023), it is imperative that the mistakes of the crack cocaine era are not repeated. This section provides recommendations for future studies.

Reviews of the 1980s crack cocaine literature revealed that prenatal cocaine exposure research needed to: (1) include an appropriate comparison group, define the population of interest and exclude participants exposed in utero to other substances; (2) recruit samples prospectively during pregnancy; and (3) use masked assessment (Frank et al., 2001). This section highlights some needs and also includes: (4) statistical considerations and (5) bioethical issues.

1. *Include an appropriate comparison or contrast group, define the population of interest, and exclude participants exposed in utero to other substances*:

   Studies of prenatally cocaine-exposed infants were primarily conducted using samples of African-American women of low-socioeconomic status, exposed to violence and who received inadequate prenatal care (Coles et al., 1992). While defined contrast groups were included, social and psychological factors were often confounded with drug use and were related to child outcomes (Singer et al., 2002). Therefore, samples of convenience to investigate the impact of prenatal cocaine exposure led to the exposure being significantly confounded with the effects of structural racism and disadvantage and may have attributed effects to cocaine exposure which are actually related to other covariates. Thus, little is known about the use of cocaine by women of middle or higher socioeconomic status (SES) during pregnancy and its effects on children. For prenatal opioid exposure, choosing comparison group children prenatally exposed to illicit psychoactive substances other than opioids may be important as well as widening the SES of study participants. Moreover, comparative research should focus on multiple comparison groups. Using a variety of well-defined comparison groups that encompass SES, other substances, and race and ethnicity allows for mapping both the range and extent of the potential neurodevelopmental problems associated with prenatal opioid exposure. Relatedly, there is a need to define the population of interest and exclude participants exposed in utero to other substances. Sample selection must be based on an unambiguously defined population of interest. Care is needed to define the selection variables to optimally reflect the construct of interest (e.g., prenatal opioid exposure time, quantity, duration of use in times of gestation).

2. *Recruit samples prospectively in the perinatal period*: Samples need to be selected with a clearly defined population of interest (e.g., untreated opioid use disorder – fentanyl) and recruit during pregnancy to allow long-term follow-up of the dyad. Jones et al. (2019) describe details that can be followed in planning research.

3. *Use masked assessment*: Given the subjective nature of many child assessments (e.g., NAS measures), standardized administration policies and training are needed, as is blinding of the assessors to reduce bias and

isolate the effect of the intervention or prenatal exposure itself. Jones et al. (2019) provide a detailed description of this recommendation.

4. *Statistical analysis recommendations*: Modern statistical approaches such as propensity scores, causal inference assessment, adjustment for multiple comparisons, and changes in how statistical significance is determined should be incorporated into study design and analysis.

5. *Bioethical considerations*: It is imperative to complete a thoughtful bioethical analysis before the initiation of such studies. Mothers, birthing people, caregivers, and children with living experience must shape research priorities and design considerations. The values of potential research participants can inform and reframe research questions and bioethics debates, such as the ethics of studying prenatal exposure to substances with or without intervention and the ethics of reporting requirements and risk of harm versus real benefit to participants.

It is also important to ask how gendered norms within social structures might be shaping the research that is developed, deployed, and justified. An unanswered question in the field of prenatal exposure to opioids and other psychoactive substances is whether the same results would be obtained among upper-middle-class people. Attention must be paid to the problems with enrolling populations in research who are made vulnerable by our society.

Drawing on these debates, one possible answer as to why our studies rely on populations who are Medicaid recipients or uninsured is that only these women would enroll in such a study because they lack other options, or because they were swayed by ancillary benefits (e.g., child assessment, money, health care, transportation) that the study provided. Thus, exploitation in this clinical research deserves examination. This is also critically important as attrition remains a major threat to longitudinal cohort studies, as it is often differential, and related to lower SES and family stressors that are more likely to be prevalent in families in which a parent has a substance use disorder (Aylward et al., 1985). Sample retention is central to accurate understanding of outcomes and must be considered in research design and implementation.

Given that studies with high longitudinal cohort retention rates were notable for providing adequate financial incentives, transportation, lunch, snacks for participants, and flexibility of scheduling (Corrigan et al., 2018; Room, 2005), the point at which these "retention procedures" cross over from helpful to coercive needs careful ethical review.

The fact remains that even today, in some states, admission of use of illegal substances, during pregnancy especially, may result in mandated reports for child abuse to courts or government agencies and even lead to incarceration. Research methods are needed to remove the risk of mandated reporting of drug use during pregnancy.

Box 3.2 Case Vignette: Ways to Respond

Talking points to support patients can include praising the parent for bringing the child in and asking questions. One can say: "It's natural to wonder about the reasons for the things our children deal with. It would be impossible for me to tell you that your using opioids during your pregnancy had any specific effect on your child. What I do know is that your seeking prenatal care and bravely getting treatment for your substance use disorder would have had positive impacts on your pregnancy and on your child's health today. Let's make sure we have a plan for continuing to have your child evaluated, cared for, and getting all the support you both need to thrive."

3.6 Summary

Identifying developmental problems in children and adolescents prenatally exposed to opioids needs to focus on causal factors. To date, it remains difficult to differentiate the primary impact of prenatal opioid exposure from other associated medical, genetic, and/or internal and external environmental influences. Studies have not shown a simple linear cause-and-effect relationship between either NOWS diagnosis or prenatal opioid exposure and compromised neurodevelopmental outcomes. A focus on multiple variables is merited to recognize the complexities of interpersonal, intrapersonal, and environmental factors that contribute to long-term developmental trajectories of children.

References

Andersen, J. M., Høiseth, G., & Nygaard, E. (2020). Prenatal exposure to methadone or buprenorphine and long-term outcomes: A meta-analysis. *Early Human Development, 143*. https://doi.org/10.1016/j.earlhumdev.2020.104997

Aylward, G. P., Hatcher, R. P., Stripp, B., Gustafson, N. F., & Leavitt, L. A. (1985). Who goes and who stays: Subject loss in a multicenter, longitudinal follow-up study. *Journal of Developmental and Behavioral Pediatrics, 6*(1), 3–8. https://doi.org/10.1097/00004703-198502000-00003

Benninger, K. L., Borghese, T., Kovalcik, J. B., Moore-Clingenpeel, M., Isler, C., Bonachea, E. M., Stark, A. R., Patrick, S. W., & Maitre, N. L. (2020). Prenatal exposures are associated with worse neurodevelopmental outcomes in infants with neonatal opioid withdrawal syndrome. *Frontiers in Pediatrics, 8*, 462. https://doi.org/10.3389/fped.2020.00462

Benninger, K. L., Richard, C., Conroy, S., Newton, J., Taylor, H. G., Sayed, A., Pietruszewski, L., Nelin, M. A., Batterson, N., & Maitre, N. L. (2022). One-year neurodevelopmental outcomes after neonatal opioid withdrawal syndrome: A prospective cohort study. *Perspectives of the ASHA Special Interest Groups*, 7(4), 1019–1032. https://doi.org/10.1044/2022_PERSP-21-00270

Center for Substance Abuse Treatment. (2005). *Medication-assisted treatment for opioid addiction in opioid treatment programs: Treatment Improvement Protocol (TIP) Series, No. 43*. Substance Abuse and Mental Health Services Administration (US). http://www.ncbi.nlm.nih.gov/books/NBK64164/

Chasnoff, I. J., Chisum, G. M., & Kaplan, W. E. (1988). Maternal cocaine use and genitourinary tract malformations. *Teratology*, 37(3), 201–204. https://doi.org/10.1002/tera.1420370304

Chung, E. H., Chou, J., & Brown, K. A. (2020). Neurodevelopmental outcomes of preterm infants: A recent literature review. *Translational Pediatrics*, 9(1), 3–8. https://doi.org/10.21037/tp.2019.09.10

Coles, C. D., Platzman, K. A., Smith, I., James, M. E., & Falek, A. (1992). Effects of cocaine and alcohol use in pregnancy on neonatal growth and neurobehavioral status. *Neurotoxicology and Teratology*, 14(1), 23–33. https://doi.org/10.1016/0892-0362(92)90025-6

Conradt, E., Flannery, T., Aschner, J. L., Annett, R. D., Croen, L. A., Duarte, C. S., Friedman, A. M., Guille, C., Hedderson, M. M., Hofheimer, J. A., Jones, M. R., Ladd-Acosta, C., McGrath, M., Moreland, A., Neiderhiser, J. M., Nguyen, R. H. N., Posner, J., Ross, J. L., Savitz, D. A., ... Lester, B. M. (2019). Prenatal opioid exposure: Neurodevelopmental consequences and future research priorities. *Pediatrics*, 144(3), https://doi.org/10.1542/peds.2019-0128

Corrigan, P. W., Shah, B. B., Lara, J. L., Mitchell, K. T., Simmes, D., & Jones, K. L. (2018). Addressing the public health concerns of Fetal Alcohol Spectrum Disorder: Impact of stigma and health literacy. *Drug and Alcohol Dependence*, 185, 266–270. https://doi.org/10.1016/j.drugalcdep.2017.12.027

Cortés-Albornoz, M. C., García-Guáqueta, D. P., Velez-van-Meerbeke, A., & Talero-Gutiérrez, C. (2021). Maternal nutrition and neurodevelopment: A scoping review. *Nutrients*, 13(10), 3530. https://doi.org/10.3390/nu13103530

Dickerson, A. S., Frndak, S., DeSantiago, M., Mohan, A., & Smith, G. S. (2023). Environmental exposure disparities and neurodevelopmental risk: A review. *Current Environmental Health Reports*, 10(2), 73–83. https://doi.org/10.1007/s40572-023-00396-6

El Marroun, H., Schmidt, M. N., Franken, I. H., Jaddoe, V. W., Hofman, A., van der Lugt, A., Verhulst, F. C., Tiemeier, H., & White, T. (2014). Prenatal tobacco exposure and brain morphology: A prospective study in young children. *Neuropsychopharmacology*, 39(4), 792–800. https://doi.org/10.1038/npp.2013.273

Estes, M. L., & McAllister, A. K. (2016). Maternal immune activation: Implications for neuropsychiatric disorders. *Science*, 353(6301), 772–777. https://doi.org/10.1126/science.aag3194

Faden, R., Kass, N., & McGraw, D. (1996). Women as vessels and vectors: Lessons from the HIV epidemic. In S. Wolf (Ed.), *Feminism and bioethics: Beyond reproduction* (pp. 252–281). Oxford University Press.

Fitzsimons, H. E., Tuten, M., Vaidya, V., & Jones, H. E. (2007). Mood disorders affect drug treatment success of drug-dependent pregnant women. *Journal*

of Substance Abuse Treatment, *32*(1), 19–25. https://doi.org/10.1016/
j.jsat.2006.06.015

Frank, D. A., Augustyn, M., Knight, W. G., Pell, T., & Zuckerman, B. (2001).
Growth, development, and behavior in early childhood following prenatal
cocaine exposure: A systematic review. *JAMA, 285*(12), 1613–1625. https://doi.
org/10.1001/jama.285.12.1613

Godfrey, K. M., Costello, P. M., & Lillycrop, K. A. (2015). The developmental environment, epigenetic biomarkers and long-term health. *Journal of
Developmental Origins of Health and Disease, 6*(5), 399–406. https://doi.org/
10.1017/S204017441500121X

Godfrey, K. M., Reynolds, R. M., Prescott, S. L., Nyirenda, M., Jaddoe, V. W.,
Eriksson, J. G., & Broekman, B. F. (2017). Influence of maternal obesity on
the long-term health of offspring. *The Lancet. Diabetes & Endocrinology, 5*(1),
53–64. https://doi.org/10.1016/S2213-8587(16)30107-3

Greenberg, J. A., Bell, S. J., Guan, Y., & Yu, Y. H. (2011). Folic acid supplementation and pregnancy: More than just neural tube defect prevention. *Reviews in
Obstetrics & Gynecology, 4*(2), 52–59.

Hagberg, K. W., Robijn, A. L., & Jick, S. (2018). Maternal depression and
antidepressant use during pregnancy and the risk of autism spectrum disorder
in offspring. *Clinical Epidemiology, 10,* 1599–1612. https://doi.org/10.2147/
CLEP.S180618

Hans, S. L., & Jeremy, R. J. (2001). Postneonatal mental and motor development
of infants exposed in utero to opioid drugs. *Infant Mental Health Journal, 22*(3),
300–315. https://doi.org/10.1002/imhj.1003

Hiscock, R., Bauld, L., Amos, A., Fidler, J. A., & Munafò, M. (2012). Socioeconomic
status and smoking: A review. *Annals of the New York Academy of Sciences,
1248,* 107–123. https://doi.org/10.1111/j.1749-6632.2011.06202.x

Holbrook, A., & Kaltenbach, K. (2012). Co-occurring psychiatric symptoms in
opioid-dependent women: The prevalence of antenatal and postnatal depression.
The American Journal of Drug and Alcohol Abuse, 38(6), 575–579. https://doi.
org/10.3109/00952990.2012.696168

Hu, S., Sheng, W. S., Lokensgard, J. R., & Peterson, P. K. (2002). Morphine
induces apoptosis of human microglia and neurons. *Neuropharmacology, 42*(6),
829–836. https://doi.org/10.1016/s0028-3908(02)00030-8

Huizink, A. C., Robles de Medina, P. G., Mulder, E. J., Visser, G. H., & Buitelaar,
J. K. (2003). Stress during pregnancy is associated with developmental outcome
in infancy. *Journal of Child Psychology and Psychiatry, and Allied Disciplines,
44*(6), 810–818. https://doi.org/10.1111/1469-7610.00166

Jones, H. E., Heil, S. H., O'Grady, K. E., Martin, P. R., Kaltenbach, K., Coyle,
M. G., Stine, S. M., Selby, P., Arria, A. M., & Fischer, G. (2009). Smoking in
pregnant women screened for an opioid agonist medication study compared to
related pregnant and non-pregnant patient samples. *The American Journal of
Drug and Alcohol Abuse, 35*(5), 375–380. https://doi.org/10.1080/0095299090
3125235

Jones, H. E., Kaltenbach, K., Benjamin, T., Wachman, E. M., & O'Grady, K. E.
(2019). Prenatal opioid exposure, neonatal abstinence syndrome/neonatal opioid

withdrawal syndrome, and later child development research: Shortcomings and solutions. *Journal of Addiction Medicine, 13*(2), 90–92. https://doi.org/10.1097/ADM.0000000000000463

Jones, H. E., Kaltenbach, K., Heil, S. H., Stine, S. M., Coyle, M. G., Arria, A. M., O'Grady, K. E., Selby, P., Martin, P. R., & Fischer, G. (2010). Neonatal abstinence syndrome after methadone or buprenorphine exposure. *The New England Journal of Medicine, 363*(24), 2320–2331. https://doi.org/10.1056/NEJMoa1005359

Jones, H. E., Kaltenbach, K., & O'Grady, K. E. (2009). The complexity of examining developmental outcomes of children prenatally exposed to opiates. A response to the Hunt et al. Adverse neurodevelopmental outcome of infants exposed to opiates in-utero. *Early Human Development, 85*(4), 271–272. https://doi.org/10.1016/j.earlhumdev.2008.10.001

Kaltenbach, K., O'Grady, K. E., Heil, S. H., Salisbury, A. L., Coyle, M. G., Fischer, G., Martin, P. R., Stine, S., & Jones, H. E. (2018). Prenatal exposure to methadone or buprenorphine: Early childhood developmental outcomes. *Drug and Alcohol Dependence, 185*, 40–49. https://doi.org/10.1016/j.drugalcdep.2017.11.030

Kim, H. M., Bone, R. M., McNeill, B., Lee, S. J., Gillon, G., & Woodward, L. J. (2021). Preschool language development of children born to women with an opioid use disorder. *Children (Basel, Switzerland), 8*(4), 268. https://doi.org/10.3390/children8040268

Lee, S. J., Bora, S., Austin, N. C., Westerman, A., & Henderson, J. M. T. (2020). Neurodevelopmental outcomes of children born to opioid-dependent mothers: A systematic review and meta-analysis. *Academic Pediatrics, 20*(3), 308–318. https://doi.org/10.1016/j.acap.2019.11.005

Lee, S. J., Pritchard, V. E., Austin, N. C., Henderson, J. M. T., & Woodward, L. J. (2020). Health and neurodevelopment of children born to opioid-dependent mothers at school entry. *Journal of Developmental and Behavioral Pediatrics, 41*(1), 48–57. https://doi.org/10.1097/DBP.0000000000000711

Lee, J. J., Saraiya, N., & Kuzniewicz, M. W. (2023). Prenatal opioid exposure and neurodevelopmental outcomes. *Journal of Neurosurgical Anesthesiology, 35*(1), 142–146. https://doi.org/10.1097/ANA.0000000000000876

Levine, T. A., & Woodward, L. J. (2018). Early inhibitory control and working memory abilities of children prenatally exposed to methadone. *Early Human Development, 116*, 68–75. https://doi.org/10.1016/j.earlhumdev.2017.11.010

McPherson, N. O., Owens, J. A., Fullston, T., & Lane, M. (2015). Preconception diet or exercise intervention in obese fathers normalizes sperm microRNA profile and metabolic syndrome in female offspring. *American Journal of Physiology. Endocrinology and Metabolism, 308*(9), 805–821. https://doi.org/10.1152/ajpendo.00013.2015

Merhar, S. L., Kline, J. E., Braimah, A., Kline-Fath, B. M., Tkach, J. A., Altaye, M., He, L., & Parikh, N. A. (2021). Prenatal opioid exposure is associated with smaller brain volumes in multiple regions. *Pediatric Research, 90*(2), 397–402. https://doi.org/10.1038/s41390-020-01265-w

Messinger, D. S., Bauer, C. R., Das, A., Seifer, R., Lester, B. M., Lagasse, L. L., Wright, L. L., Shankaran, S., Bada, H. S., Smeriglio, V. L., Langer, J. C., Beeghly, M., & Poole, W. K. (2004). The maternal lifestyle study: Cognitive, motor, and behavioral outcomes of cocaine-exposed and opiate-exposed infants through three years of age. *Pediatrics, 113*(6), 1677–1685. https://doi.org/10.1542/peds.113.6.1677

Meyer, U. (2019). Neurodevelopmental resilience and susceptibility to maternal immune activation. *Trends in Neurosciences, 42*(11), 793–806. https://doi.org/10.1016/j.tins.2019.08.001

Miguel, P. M., Pereira, L. O., Silveira, P. P., & Meaney, M. J. (2019). Early environmental influences on the development of children's brain structure and function. *Developmental Medicine and Child Neurology, 61*(10), 1127–1133. https://doi.org/10.1111/dmcn.14182

Miller, M. T., Strömland, K., Ventura, L., Johansson, M., Bandim, J. M., & Gillberg, C. (2004). Autism with ophthalmologic malformations: The plot thickens. *Transactions of the American Ophthalmological Society, 102*, 107–121.

Min, M. O., Singer, L. T., Kirchner, H. L., Minnes, S., Short, E., Hussain, Z., & Nelson, S. (2009). Cognitive development and low-level lead exposure in poly-drug exposed children. *Neurotoxicology and Teratology, 31*(4), 225–231. https://doi.org/10.1016/j.ntt.2009.03.002

Monnelly, V. J., Hamilton, R., Chappell, F. M., Mactier, H., & Boardman, J. P. (2019). Childhood neurodevelopment after prescription of maintenance methadone for opioid dependency in pregnancy: A systematic review and meta-analysis. *Developmental Medicine and Child Neurology, 61*(7), 750–760. https://doi.org/10.1111/dmcn.14117

Morris-Rosendahl, D. J., & Crocq, M. A. (2020). Neurodevelopmental disorders – the history and future of a diagnostic concept. *Dialogues in Clinical Neuroscience, 22*(1), 65–72. https://doi.org/10.31887/DCNS.2020.22.1/macrocq

Nakamura, A., François, O., & Lepeule, J. (2021). Epigenetic alterations of maternal tobacco smoking during pregnancy: A narrative review. *International Journal of Environmental Research and Public Health, 18*(10), 5083. https://doi.org/10.3390/ijerph18105083

Nelson, L. F., Yocum, V. K., Patel, K. D., Qeadan, F., Hsi, A., & Weitzen, S. (2020). Cognitive outcomes of young children after prenatal exposure to medications for opioid use disorder: A systematic review and meta-analysis. *JAMA Network Open, 3*(3). https://doi.org/10.1001/jamanetworkopen.2020.1195

Nieto, S. J., & Kosten, T. A. (2019). Who's your daddy? Behavioral and epigenetic consequences of paternal drug exposure. *International Journal of Developmental Neuroscience, 78*, 109–121. https://doi.org/10.1016/j.ijdevneu.2019.07.002

O'Donnell, K., O'Connor, T. G., & Glover, V. (2009). Prenatal stress and neurodevelopment of the child: Focus on the HPA axis and role of the placenta. *Developmental Neuroscience, 31*(4), 285–292. https://doi.org/10.1159/000216539

Pacheco, S. E. (2020). Catastrophic effects of climate change on children's health start before birth. *The Journal of Clinical Investigation, 130*(2), 562–564. https://doi.org/10.1172/JCI135005

Pollak, S. D., & Wolfe, B. L. (2020). Maximizing research on the adverse effects of child poverty through consensus measures. *Developmental Science, 23*(6). https://doi.org/10.1111/desc.12946

Radhakrishnan, R., Grecco, G., Stolze, K., Atwood, B., Jennings, S. G., Lien, I. Z., Saykin, A. J., & Sadhasivam, S. (2021). Neuroimaging in infants with prenatal opioid exposure: Current evidence, recent developments and targets for future research. *Journal of Neuroradiology, 48*(2), 112–120. https://doi.org/10.1016/j.neurad.2020.09.009

Roberts, J. R., Karr, C. J., Council on Environmental Health, Paulson, J. A., Brock-Utne, A. C., Brumberg, H. L., Campbell, C. C., Lanphear, B. P., Osterhoudt, K. C., Sandel, M. T., Trasande, L., & Wright, R. O. (2012). Pesticide exposure in children. *Pediatrics, 130*(6), 1765–1788. https://doi.org/10.1542/peds.2012-2758

Room, R. (2005). Stigma, social inequality and alcohol and drug use. *Drug and Alcohol Review, 24*(2), 143–155. https://doi.org/10.1080/09595230500102434

Ross, E. J., Graham, D. L., Money, K. M., & Stanwood, G. D. (2015). Developmental consequences of fetal exposure to drugs: What we know and what we still must learn. *Neuropsychopharmacology, 40*(1), 61–87. https://doi.org/10.1038/npp.2014.147

Sameroff, A. J., & Chandler, M. J. (1975). Reproductive risk and the continuum of caretaking casualty. In F. D. Horowitz, M. Hetherington, S. Scarr-Salapatek, & G. Siegel (Eds.), *Review of child development research* (pp. 187–244). University of Chicago Press.

Sanchez, K., Spittle, A. J., Boyce, J. O., Leembruggen, L., Mantelos, A., Mills, S., Mitchell, N., Neil, E., John, M. S., Treloar, J., & Morgan, A. T. (2020). Conversational language in 3-year-old children born very preterm and at term. *Journal of Speech, Language, and Hearing Research, 63*(1), 206–215. https://doi.org/10.1044/2019_JSLHR-19-00153

Singer, L. T., Arendt, R., Minnes, S., Farkas, K., Salvator, A., Kirchner, H. L., & Kliegman, R. (2002). Cognitive and motor outcomes of cocaine-exposed infants. *JAMA, 287*(15), 1952–1960. https://doi.org/10.1001/jama.287.15.1952

Singer, L., Arendt, R., Song, L. Y., Warshawsky, E., & Kliegman, R. (1994). Direct and indirect interactions of cocaine with childbirth outcomes. *Archives of Pediatrics & Adolescent Medicine, 148*(9), 959–964. https://doi.org/10.1001/archpedi.1994.02170090073014

Singer, L. T., Chambers, C., Coles, C., & Kable, J. (2020). Fifty years of research on prenatal substances: Lessons learned for the opioid epidemic. *Adversity and Resilience Science, 1*, 223–234. https://doi.org/10.1007/s42844-020-00021-7

Singh, G. K., Kenney, M. K., Ghandour, R. M., Kogan, M. D., & Lu, M. C. (2013). Mental health outcomes in US children and adolescents born prematurely or with low birthweight. *Depression Research and Treatment, 2013*. https://doi.org/10.1155/2013/570743

Sirnes, E., Oltedal, L., Bartsch, H., Eide, G. E., Elgen, I. B., & Aukland, S. M. (2017). Brain morphology in school-aged children with prenatal opioid exposure: A structural MRI study. *Early Human Development, 106–107*, 33–39. https://doi.org/10.1016/j.earlhumdev.2017.01.009

Skovlund, E., Handal, M., Selmer, R., Brandlistuen, R. E., & Skurtveit, S. (2017). Language competence and communication skills in 3-year-old children after prenatal exposure to analgesic opioids. *Pharmacoepidemiology and Drug Safety*, 26(6), 625–634. https://doi.org/10.1002/pds.4170

Streissguth, A. P., Sampson, P. D., Barr, H. M., Clarren, S. K., & Martin, D. C. (1986). Studying alcohol teratogenesis from the perspective of the fetal alcohol syndrome: Methodological and statistical issues. *Annals of the New York Academy of Sciences*, 477, 63–86. https://doi.org/10.1111/j.1749-6632.1986.tb40322.x

Vestal-Laborde, A. A., Eschenroeder, A. C., Bigbee, J. W., Robinson, S. E., & Sato-Bigbee, C. (2014). The opioid system and brain development: Effects of methadone on the oligodendrocyte lineage and the early stages of myelination. *Developmental Neuroscience*, 36(5), 409–421. https://doi.org/10.1159/000365074

Vohr, B. (2013). Long-term outcomes of moderately preterm, late preterm, and early term infants. *Clinics in Perinatology*, 40(4), 739–751. https://doi.org/10.1016/j.clp.2013.07.006

Vorhees, C.V. (1986). Origins of behavioral teratology. In E. P. Riley & C. V. Vorhees (Eds.), *Handbook of behavioral teratology* (pp. 3–22). Plenum Press.

Wang, Y., & Han, T. Z. (2009). Prenatal exposure to heroin in mice elicits memory deficits that can be attributed to neuronal apoptosis. *Neuroscience*, 160(2), 330–338. https://doi.org/10.1016/j.neuroscience.2009.02.058

Weller, A. E., Crist, R. C., Reiner, B. C., Doyle, G. A., & Berrettini, W. H. (2021). Neonatal opioid withdrawal syndrome (NOWS): A transgenerational echo of the opioid crisis. *Cold Spring Harbor Perspectives in Medicine*, 11(3). https://doi.org/10.1101/cshperspect.a039669

Wen, X., Lawal, O. D., Belviso, N., Matson, K. L., Wang, S., Quilliam, B. J., & Meador, K. J. (2021). Association between prenatal opioid exposure and neurodevelopmental outcomes in early childhood: A retrospective cohort study. *Drug Safety*, 44(8), 863–875. https://doi.org/10.1007/s40264-021-01080-0

Wu, C. C., Hung, C. J., Shen, C. H., Chen, W. Y., Chang, C. Y., Pan, H. C., Liao, S. L., & Chen, C. J. (2014). Prenatal buprenorphine exposure decreases neurogenesis in rats. *Toxicology Letters*, 225(1), 92–101. https://doi.org/10.1016/j.toxlet.2013.12.001

Yeoh, S. L., Eastwood, J., Wright, I. M., Morton, R., Melhuish, E., Ward, M., & Oei, J. L. (2019). Cognitive and motor outcomes of children with prenatal opioid exposure: A systematic review and meta-analysis. *JAMA Network Open*, 2(7). https://doi.org/10.1001/jamanetworkopen.2019.7025

Yuan, Q., Rubic, M., Seah, J., Rae, C., Wright, I. M., Kaltenbach, K., Feller, J. M., Abdel-Latif, M. E., Chu, C., Oei, J. L., & BOB (Brains, Opioids and Babies) Collaborative group (2014). Do maternal opioids reduce neonatal regional brain volumes? A pilot study. *Journal of Perinatology*, 34(12), 909–913.

4 Maximizing Outcomes for Infants With Neonatal Opioid Withdrawal Syndrome Through a Multidisciplinary Collaborative Approach

Lori A. Devlin

4.1 Introduction

No individual healthcare provider has the expertise to deliver the comprehensive care that is needed to optimize both short-term outcomes during the newborn hospitalization and behavioral and developmental outcomes for infants with neonatal opioid withdrawal syndrome (NOWS). Thus, the importance of a collaborative multidisciplinary team cannot be understated. Healthcare systems that effectively care for infants with NOWS support the development and education of a team of physicians, advanced practice providers, nurses, therapists, nutritionists, lactation consultants, and social workers to provide consistent evidence-based care for opioid-dependent mothers and their infants. This multidisciplinary team should: 1) be trained in a trauma informed approach to care, 2) empower parents to care advocate for their infants, and 3) integrate high-quality evidence into clinical care.

A previous history of personal trauma such as childhood abuse (Kors et al., 2022) and intimate partner violence (Henninger et al., 2022) has been associated with opioid dependency during pregnancy. Repeat trauma may be triggered by stigmatizing verbal and nonverbal communication with healthcare providers (Weber et al., 2021). Internalized stigma may promote disengagement from the healthcare team and suboptimal outcomes for the mother–infant dyad (Weber et al., 2021; Yanos et al., 2015). Integration of trauma-informed practices into clinical care can minimize stigma and empower parenting women with opioid dependency to advocate for and actively engage in caring for their infants (Marcellus, 2014).

The term neonatal abstinence syndrome (NAS) was originally used to describe the signs of opioid withdrawal after birth after recurrent antenatal exposure to opioids (Finnegan, Kron, et al., 1975). Since the 1970s,

DOI: 10.4324/9781003397267-4

the definition of NAS has subsequently been expanded to include neonatal withdrawal after antenatal exposure to other psychotropic substances. To accurately identify infants with antenatal opioid exposure, a more specific term was needed, and neonatal opioid withdrawal syndrome (NOWS) was coined by the Food and Drug Administration between 2013 and 2016 (Food and Drug Administration [FDA], 2013; FDA, 2016). Throughout this chapter the term NOWS will be used to preferentially describe opioid withdrawal in the neonatal period, but the term NAS may be used when referring directly to works in which NAS was the authors' chosen terminology.

NOWS presents as placentally transferred opioids are cleared from the infant's system, and is characterized by dysfunction in three primary areas: the central nervous system, the autonomic nervous system, and the gastrointestinal system (Finnegan, Kron, et al., 1975). Clinical signs of NOWS include, but are not limited to, irritability, tremors, increased tone, poor sleep, and poor feeding tolerance (Finnegan, Kron, et al., 1975). Although neonatal opioid withdrawal has been treated for over 50 years, a standardized definition has not been widely accepted across the field. Lack of a clear definition may lead to misdiagnosis and suboptimal treatment. In 2020 researchers used a modified Delphi approach to develop consensus across panels of experts in the field. Expert panels concluded that the following were needed for the diagnosis of neonatal opioid withdrawal: in utero exposure (known by history, not necessarily by toxicology testing) to opioids with or without the presence of other psychotropic substances, and the presence of at least two of the most common clinical signs characteristic of withdrawal (excessive crying, fragmented sleep, tremors, increased muscle tone, gastrointestinal dysfunction) (Jilani et al., 2022).

A gold standard for the clinical care of infants with NOWS has not yet been established and as a consequence clinical care varies substantially between hospitals (Young et al., 2021). Variation in care has been correlated with differences in healthcare outcomes (Goodman et al., 2019). The development of a standard evidence-based approach to care will optimize outcomes for infants with NOWS. To be generalizable, this approach must be based on high-quality research conducted via large studies that include a diverse sample of infants from multiple geographically diverse care settings. The Advancing Clinical Trials in Neonatal Opioid Withdrawal (ACT NOW) Collaborative, which is supported by the National Institutes of Health Helping to End Addiction Long Term (National Institutes of Health HEAL Initiative, 2023a) is conducting research that is designed to inform clinical care and ultimately improve outcomes for this vulnerable population.

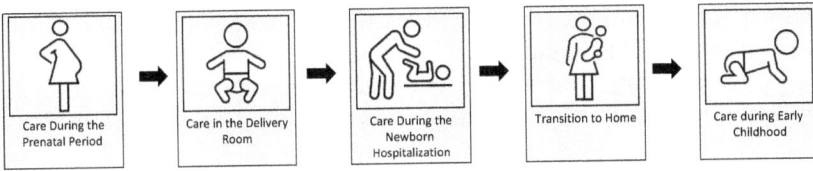

Figure 4.1 Periods of collaborative care for opioid-exposed infants and children through early childhood

This chapter will focus on how a trauma-informed, multidisciplinary team can use an evidence-based approach to further improve expectations for the pregnant woman with opioid use during pregnancy and outcomes for her infant prior to birth, during the newborn period, and into early childhood (see Figure 4.1).

4.2 Prenatal Counseling

Consultation with newborn specialists during the third trimester of pregnancy will prepare women with opioid dependency for their infants' clinical course after delivery. Collaboration between maternal health, addiction medicine, and newborn specialists provides consistent messaging and sets realistic expectations for potential infant outcomes during the newborn period. Discussions with the pregnant woman and her family should be informed by evidence-based research and include: 1) the definition of NOWS, 2) the incidence of neonatal opioid withdrawal after birth, 3) the benefits of both nonpharmacologic and pharmacologic care, and 4) the overall structure and daily function of the unit in which the infant will be cared for. Perceived barriers to care for both the mother and her infant should also be discussed and addressed to maximize bonding and attachment for the dyad after delivery.

Educational materials for families that mirror key discussion points in the prenatal consult should be developed by each hospital that cares for infants with NOWS. These materials should be vetted with women who have lived experience to decrease stigmatizing language (Pivovarova & Stein, 2019). Sharing educational materials with all hospital and community care providers will standardize and reinforce consistent messaging for parents and other caregivers. A unified approach will help to set realistic expectations, facilitate open dialogue, and improve knowledge.

Engagement with a peer mentor with lived experience is another way to support pregnant women with opioid dependency as they learn to parent their infants. A recent qualitative survey of ten postpartum women with opioid use disorder who were attending outpatient substance use treatment programs found that nine of the ten women reported a perception of being treated differently by the medical team once a substance use history was disclosed and admitted to fear of being reported to child services and losing custody of their child. This fear guided all aspects of the new mother's decision making (Proulx & Fantasia, 2021). Early engagement with a peer mentor may improve care for the infant by improving maternal expectations and identifying and resolving implicit bias across the medical team.

4.3 Optimizing Care After Delivery

A collaborative trauma-informed approach to care in the delivery room and during the newborn stay decreases maternal and family stress and maximizes satisfaction with and the quality of medical care. The medical team supporting women with opioid use during pregnancy and their infants should avoid punitive and exclusionary practices. When asked, these women report receiving judgmental verbal and nonverbal reactions from healthcare workers which made them feel powerless and discouraged active participation in the care of themselves and their infants (Cleveland & Bonugli, 2014; Howard, 2016; Recto et al., 2020).

In the delivery room birthing women should be given the opportunity to place their infant skin-to-skin after birth if the mother and infant are clinically stable. This practice has been shown to improve bonding and attachment and encourage early breastfeeding if desired (Bogen & Whalen, 2019; Bremer & Knippen, 2023). Infants with antenatal opioid exposure are at increased risk for disorganized attachment (Kondili & Duryea, 2019), which makes the implementation of early measures to develop and strengthen the maternal–infant bond essential. Maintaining the mother and infant together, through practices such as rooming-in, will enhance a mother's ability to learn her infant's cues and develop her responses (Lawlor et al., 2020; Singh et al., 2021). The medical stability and safety of the mother and infant must be taken into consideration prior to establishing rooming-in.

During the newborn hospital stay opioid-exposed infants and their families benefit from consistency in healthcare providers and treatment by a multidisciplinary medical team who are knowledgeable and skilled in recognizing and appropriately treating the signs of opioid withdrawal. Although some transition is inevitable, face-to-face handoffs that include the parent(s)/primary caregiver(s) can promote trust and enhance collaboration.

4.4 Assessment and Management Approaches for Neonatal Opioid Withdrawal Syndrome (NOWS)

The traditional approach to the assessment and management for infants with NOWS is based on a tool developed by Dr. Loretta Finnegan in 1975 (Finnegan, Kron, et al., 1975). The Finnegan Neonatal Abstinence Scoring Tool (FNAST) has been used in the clinical care of infants with NOWS since that time. This tool is composed of a comprehensive weighted list of the signs of neonatal opioid withdrawal and is accompanied by a threshold for the initiation of pharmacologic treatment (Finnegan, Connaughton, et al., 1975). This threshold is also used to determine escalation and weaning of opioid therapy. The traditional treatment approach used with the FNAST consists of a tapered opioid dosing regimen that is slowly weaned over a period of weeks while the infant is monitored in the hospital for worsening signs of withdrawal. Active collaboration across the medical team was implied with the use of the FNAST, but not measured. Parents/primary caregivers were not integrated into the care of their infants and often relegated to bystanders by the healthcare team. In addition, the complexity of the FNAST and the subjectivity inherent in the assessment of the clinical signs of withdrawal led to discontent with the tool among both medical and nursing providers and resulted in multiple attempts to modify the original FNAST (Chervoneva et al., 2020; Devlin et al., 2020; Gomez Pomar et al., 2017).

One such attempt, the Eating, Sleeping and Consoling (ESC) approach developed by Dr. Matthew Grossman and colleagues at Yale University, challenged the status quo (Grossman et al., 2017). The ESC approach was implemented as part of a single center quality improvement (QI) initiative and embraced a focus on the functional components of withdrawal, if an infant could eat, sleep, and be consoled. This approach also advocated for early and consistent individualized nonpharmacologic care provided by parents/primary caregivers who roomed-in with their infants. The results of this initiative showed a marked decrease in the proportion of infants who were initiated on pharmacologic treatment and a substantial reduction in the length of hospital stay for infants who were assessed and managed with ESC versus the FNAST (Grossman et al., 2017). A subsequent single center QI initiative, designed to enhance generalizability and demonstrate the reproducibility of the primary findings, was conducted by Dr. Elisha Wachman and colleagues at Boston Medical Center. This QI initiative included infants whose parents/primary caregivers were unable to room-in and introduced the ESC Care Tool which provides a structured approach to the ESC assessment (Wachman et al., 2018). The ESC Care Tool includes "caregiver huddles" which enhance collaborative practice. Huddles offered an opportunity for all members of the medical team (e.g., nurses, therapists, physicians, etc.) to meet with the parent(s)/ primary caregiver(s) to review the infant's ability to conduct the activities of daily living (i.e., eating, sleeping, and consoling) and to determine the next step in treatment. The ESC care approach moved collaborative care to the center of the treatment paradigm and empowered parents to advocate for their infants.

Other single center and regional quality improvement initiatives conducted at hospitals across the US continued to show improvement in short-term outcomes for infants assessed and managed with the ESC care approach when compared to the FNAST (Blount et al., 2019; Hwang et al., 2020; Wachman et al., 2020). QI initiatives are limited by a reliance on the QI bundle which includes implementation of the ESC care approach in conjunction with other interventions over time. Thus, QI work cannot fully speak to the efficacy, safety, and generalizability of the ESC care approach (Schiff & Grossman, 2019). In addition, hospital-based QI initiatives do not assess neurodevelopmental outcomes in the first two years of life which are necessary to recommend treatment approaches in the newborn period.

A large, randomized, controlled clinical trial was needed to determine if the ESC care approach is efficacious, safe, and generalizable. The Eating, Sleeping, Consoling for Neonatal Opioid Withdrawal (ESC-NOW): a Function-Based Assessment and Management Approach trial (Clinical Trials Number, CT04057820) was developed through the collaboration of two established clinical trial networks – the NIH Environmental Influence on Child Health Outcomes (ECHO) IDeA States Pediatric Clinical Trials Network (ISPCTN) clinical trials network and the Eunice Kennedy Shriver NICHD Neonatal Research Network – with support from the National Institutes of Health Helping to End Addiction Long-Term (NIH-HEAL) initiative (Young et al., 2022). This trial enrolled over 1,300 infants from 26 hospitals across the United States and found that when compared to usual care with the FNAST, infants assessed and managed with the ESC care approach had an almost seven-day reduction in the time until they were medically ready for discharge and a 32.5 percentage point decrease in the initiation of pharmacologic treatment. In hospital and post-hospital safety was measured and there were no substantial differences in three-month safety outcomes between groups (Young et al., 2023). A subset of infants enrolled in the ESC trial are completing measures of family and infant wellness through the first two years and neurodevelopmental and behavioral assessments at 2 years of age. The results of this long-term follow-up are anticipated in 2025. These results will not only further inform the use of the ESC care approach for the assessment and management of infants with NOWS, but they will also provide a more definitive understanding of the impact of opioid use during pregnancy on the overall well-being of the maternal–infant dyad.

Development of strong evidence to support the best practice for the assessment and management of infants with NOWS further supports best practice for the treatment of infants with NOWS.

4.5 Nonpharmacologic Treatment

The American Academy of Pediatrics (AAP) recommends nonpharmacologic care as the foundation of treatment for infants with antenatal opioid exposure (Patrick et al., 2020). Nonpharmacologic interventions should ideally begin after birth, continue during the newborn hospitalization, and extend through the first few months of age (Jansson & Patrick, 2019). Nonpharmacologic care should be tailored to the physiologic needs of each infant (Velez & Jansson, 2008) and supported through a trauma-informed multidisciplinary team. Although there is evidence to support some components of nonpharmacologic care, evidence is emerging for other components of care. This section will briefly review several of the components of nonpharmacologic care through the lens of the multidisciplinary team.

4.5.1 Rooming-In

Traditionally infants with moderate to severe withdrawal who require increased monitoring and/or pharmacologic treatment were transferred to hospital care settings that limit direct parental involvement. Separating infants from their parents decreases support for nonpharmacologic interventions such as holding, swaddling, on-demand feeding, and breastfeeding. Studies focused on parental rooming-in, although limited either by the retrospective nature of the study design and/or small sample size, have shown that family-centered care reduces the initiation of pharmacologic therapy, the length of hospital stay, and healthcare costs (Abrahams et al., 2007; Grossman et al., 2017; Holmes et al., 2016; Hunseler et al., 2013; Lawlor et al., 2020; MacMillan et al., 2018; McKnight et al., 2016; Singh et al., 2021). Perinatal nurses report three primary barriers to the implementation of rooming-in: 1) inadequate physical spaces to accommodate parents as they care for their infants, 2) poor inter- and intradisciplinary communication, and 3) a lack of care coordination (Shuman et al., 2021).

Developing a physical space that meets the clinical needs of the infant while accommodating the parent(s)/primary caregiver(s)will enhance engagement in nonpharmacologic care. Such a space would facilitate 24/7 visitation (MacMillan, 2019), include environmental controls for light and sound (McQueen & Murphy-Oikonen, 2016), and provide a space where both the nursing staff and the parents could comfortably care for the infant. The provision of other accommodations for parents, such as a restroom and a comfortable sleeping space in the room with the infants, in addition to in-room meals and on-site opioid use disorder (OUD) treatment, while the infant is in the hospital will allow parents to focus on the needs of their infant. If responsibilities outside of the hospital do not allow for parents/primary caregivers to room-in, additional support to ensure the families have transportation to the hospital and policies that allow for other vetted care providers (e.g., other family members, friends, and volunteer cuddlers) should be strongly considered.

Use of a single integrated approach to care for infants with NOWS across different care settings within a hospital can minimize incongruencies in care and optimize outcomes. Such an approach should facilitate high-quality handoffs between healthcare providers and encourage cross-disciplinary conferences that engage infants' parents/primary caregivers in the decision making for their child. An integrated approach to care requires flexibility in staffing models that enhance provider continuity and account for the heightened requirements on providers' time as they work to meet the physiologic needs of the infant and address the psychosocial and educational needs of the parenting women (Shuman et al., 2021). Development of mechanisms to support the emotional health of providers as they care for this, and all other high-risk populations, will decrease provider burnout.

4.5.2 Breastfeeding

Receipt of maternal breastmilk is generally considered safe and has been associated with a decrease in the severity of NOWS and improved hospital outcomes for infants whose mothers are compliant with their prescribed methadone and buprenorphine therapy (Abdel-Latif et al., 2006; Isemann et al., 2011; Liu et al., 2015; McQueen et al., 2011; Pritham et al., 2012; Short et al., 2016; Wachman et al., 2010; Welle-Strand et al., 2013). Breastfeeding is less prevalent among infants with NOWS (Tolia et al., 2015), but the rates of breastfeeding may be improved through the use of integrated models of care.

Breastfeeding education for mothers in substance dependency treatment has been associated with the higher rates of breastfeeding after delivery (McQueen et al., 2011). Mothers who are receiving treatment for opioid dependency and have abstained from illicit substance use should consult with lactation specialists prior to delivery and breastfeeding and/or the provision of breastmilk should be encouraged by newborn specialists during prenatal consultation. After delivery the medical team should promote practices such as skin-to-skin care and on-demand breastfeeding, and support from dedicated lactation specialists should continue throughout the hospital stay. All members of the healthcare team should be versed in the benefits of maternal breastmilk and breastfeeding. They should encourage opioid-dependent women who have the desire to breastfeed and who are stable in their opioid treatment to provide breastmilk for their infants.

Past trauma may influence the decision to breastfeed. Women who were sexually abused commonly cited their breastfeeding experiences as uniquely challenging and noted that at times they felt the focus on breastfeeding was overwhelming and guilt-inducing, but women who were successful in breastfeeding their infants reported it as an empowering experience (Sobel et al., 2018).

4.5.3 Emerging Nonpharmacologic Practices

Whole-body massage for infants with antenatal opioid exposure has been evaluated to date in a single prospective observational pilot study of 30 term infants. Researchers noted improvement in heart rate, respiratory rate, and blood pressure after a 30-minute whole-body massage administered by a single certified massage therapist when compared to baseline vital signs. This improvement was more pronounced for infants who received pharmacologic therapy for NOWS (Rana et al., 2022). Additional research is needed to determine the safety and efficacy of this adjunctive nonpharmacologic therapy for infants with NOWS.

A small single-site randomized pilot study found that aromatherapy with lavender or chamomile in addition to standard treatment decreased the duration of opioid treatment and the length of stay when compared to standard care alone (Daniel et al., 2020). Additional studies are also needed to validate these findings in a large and diverse population of infants with NOWS.

Laser acupuncture has been evaluated for the treatment of NOWS in a single randomized controlled clinical trial of 28 infants and was found to decrease the duration of opioid treatment and the length of hospital stay when compared to infants who received opioids alone (Raith et al., 2015). In addition, a single randomized controlled clinical trial of 31 study participants evaluated influence of foot reflexology and auricular seed acupressure on NOWS severity and found that both interventions decreased opioid withdrawal symptoms as measured by the FNAST (Sajadi et al., 2019). Additional multi-center clinical trials are needed to determine the efficacy and safety of all approaches. If they are proven to be safe and effective, emerging nonpharmacologic practices may enhance collaborative care for infants with NOWS.

Nonpharmacologic care has been identified as the preferred primary approach to treatment for infants with NOWS (Patrick et al., 2020) and as such hospitals that care for infants with NOWS should develop physical spaces that facilitate rooming-in for mother–infant dyads, and utilize staffing ratios to support the goal of integrated care. Nurses, physicians, therapists, nutritionists, lactation specialists, and social workers must all individually and as a team develop a trusting relationship with the parents/primary caregivers. This is facilitated by: 1) a single consistent and unified approach to medical care that has been developed and refined with input from the entire healthcare team, 2) a trauma-informed approach to care, and 3) open communication with the parents/primary caregivers on changes in clinical care for their infants, including the criteria for hospital discharge. It is essential that parents/caregivers are seen as important members of the team caring for their infant and are educated on the important role that they play in improving short- and long-term outcomes.

4.6 Pharmacologic Treatment

While nonpharmacologic care has been shown to be an effective approach to the treatment of infants with NOWS and is recommended as the first line of treatment (Patrick et al., 2020; Young et al., 2023), pharmacologic therapy remains an important component of care for infants whose signs of withdrawal are not well controlled by nonpharmacologic care alone. The optimal approach to pharmacologic treatment, including the ideal opioid, dosing, and treatment duration, remains unknown and the impact of postnatal pharmacologic treatment on developmental and behavioral outcomes for infants with NOWS during childhood has not been well studied.

A regional quality improvement initiative in Ohio demonstrated improvement in hospital outcomes when a treatment algorithm guides pharmacologic treatment for infants with NOWS (Walsh et al., 2018). This improvement was noted to be independent from the type of opioid used to treat NOWS. Collaboration with a multidisciplinary team of pharmacists, physicians, nurses, and therapists in the development of a treatment algorithm will help to maintain a global perspective on the use of pharmacologic treatment, enhance compliance with the treatment algorithm, and optimize hospital outcomes.

Prolonged hospital stays are primarily driven by the management of pharmacologic treatment. Extended time in the hospital may negatively impact bonding and attachment, increase parental stress, and result in high healthcare utilization. To address the potential negative outcomes associated with prolonged hospital stays, some institutions have advocated for discharging infants from the hospital while still receiving medications to treat NOWS. Greater than 25% of infants treated in one of 200 centers participating in the Vermont Oxford Network were discharged home on pharmacologic treatment over the two-year collaborative (Patrick et al., 2016). Retrospective single center studies have shown a reduction in length of hospital stay when infants are stabilized in the hospital and then discharged to home to complete the weaning process (Backes et al., 2012; Lee et al., 2015; Oei et al., 2001; Smirk et al., 2014). Yet, infants who are weaned at home typically had a prolonged duration of pharmacologic treatment (Backes et al., 2012; Maalouf et al., 2018). As little is known about the implications of prolonged pharmacologic treatment on neurodevelopmental outcomes, further studies are needed to evaluate the safety and efficacy of home weaning. This practice is not currently recommended by the AAP (Patrick et al., 2020).

Additional research is needed to identify the best approach to pharmacologic treatment and the best opioid medication for the treatment of infants with moderate to severe withdrawal that does not adequately respond to nonpharmacologic care alone. The HEAL Evaluation of Limited Pharmacotherapies for Neonatal Opioid Withdrawal Syndrome (HELP for NOWS) Consortium is a multi-center initiative that is designing and conducting two comparative effectiveness, randomized controlled trials focused on pharmacologic treatment for NOWS. The results of these trials will provide evidence to support a standard approach to the pharmacologic treatment provided for infants with NOWS (National Institutes of Health HEAL Initiative, 2023b).

4.7 Optimizing Care With the Transition to Home

Infants treated for acute withdrawal after antenatal opioid exposure are at risk for suboptimal outcomes after hospital discharge (Uebel et al., 2015). Coordinated verbal handoffs between the inpatient to the outpatient teams may mitigate the risk of poor outcomes soon after hospital discharge. Development of a plan of safe care for the maternal–infant dyad that is informed by multidisciplinary inpatient and outpatient teams and vetted by the parenting woman is essential to bridge the transition from inpatient to outpatient care.

The postpartum period is a vulnerable time for women with opioid dependency. Physical recovery, breastfeeding, and the adaptation to parenting a new child is often further complicated by mental health diagnoses such as anxiety or depression (Corr et al., 2020), social adversity such as poverty and food insecurity, intimate partner violence (Cizmeli et al., 2018; Pallatino et al., 2021), and relapse into substance misuse (Gopman, 2014; Proulx & Fantasia, 2021). Women with OUD overdose more frequently in the postpartum period than during pregnancy, with the highest rates occurring 7–12 months after delivery (Schiff et al., 2018). Treatment after delivery should be designed to decrease stigma, break down barriers to care, and empower women in their role as parents (Proulx & Fantasia, 2021). The well-being of a parenting woman is key to the wellness of her infant.

After the acute phase of withdrawal, infants with NOWS remain at risk for suboptimal growth and development during early childhood which necessitates close medical and social follow-up (Favara et al., 2022; Lee et al., 2020). Engagement shortly after discharge with a medical provider who is versed on the infant's hospital course, educated on the potential short- and longer-term complications of NOWS, trauma-informed, and able to provide consistent and if needed flexible access to care will optimize outcomes. This medical provider should be supported by a multidisciplinary team that can address feeding and nutritional, developmental, and social concerns that arise during the first few years of life. In addition, close attention should be paid to the bond between the infant's primary caregiver and the infant. Infants with NOWS have an increased risk for disorganized attachment with their caregivers which, when coupled with a chaotic home environment, may compromise the caregiver–infant bond and lead to suboptimal caregiving experiences (Kondili & Duryea, 2019; Martin et al., 2022) which increases the risk of neglect and maltreatment for the infant (Deutsch et al., 2020; Uebel et al., 2015).

Opioid-dependent women who are parenting and receiving substance treatment in the postpartum period identify the health and welfare of their children as a priority (Proulx & Fantasia, 2021); although they often have physiologic, psychological, and social stressors that may interfere with quality parenting. Hospital-based attachment-informed interventions (e.g., skin-to-skin care, rooming-in) provide the foundation for the relationship between the parenting mother and her infant. After discharge, special care should be taken to support the mother–infant dyad and additional methods to improve attachment and bonding and enhance quality caregiving may be needed (Kondili & Duryea, 2019; Martin et al., 2022). The Attachment and Biobehavioral Catch-up (ABC), a preventative program which promotes sensitive parenting, has been extensively studied in multiple vulnerable populations and has been found to enhance parental sensitivity and decrease infant stress, promote autonomic nervous system regulation, improve emotional expression and language development, and enhance executive functioning in childhood (Martin et al., 2022). A randomized controlled trial of a modified ABC program is ongoing in this population (Modified ABC Clinical Trial Number NCT03891628). This trial will provide generalizable evidence on sensitive parenting which may mitigate risk and improve behavioral and development outcomes for infants with NOWS (Martin et al., 2022).

During the transition to home after the initial newborn hospital stay, pediatric medical providers should partner with a social and developmental team who have or are willing to develop expertise in the care of the opioid-affected mother–infant dyad. As maternal health and wellness directly impacts the health of the infant, pediatric care providers should also establish open lines of communication with providers who care for women during the postpartum period, and together they can work to improve outcomes for the dyad during the transition from hospital to home and into early childhood.

4.8 The Role of the Multidisciplinary Team in Developmental Follow-Up

Families impacted by substance use often have co-occurring morbidities such as psychological trauma, mental health conditions, economic insecurity, and domestic violence that may complicate the developmental trajectory for opioid-exposed infants and children (Deutsch et al., 2020). The diagnosis of NOWS in the newborn period has been associated with an increased risk for rehospitalization due to nonaccidental trauma and neglect and this risk has been shown to persist throughout childhood (Uebel et al., 2015). These associations emphasize the critical need for multidisciplinary collaborative programs which support opioid-affected families and optimize outcomes for exposed children.

A better understanding of the behavioral and neurodevelopmental outcomes commonly seen during the first two years of age in children with antenatal opioid exposure is needed to identify the focus of developmental intervention programs for this population. A recent meta-analysis of studies designed to evaluate neurodevelopmental outcomes for children who were born to mothers with opioid use during pregnancy found that opioid-exposed infants had worse behavioral and neurodevelopmental outcomes than their non-opioid-exposed counterparts (Lee et al., 2020). Careful interpretation of these results is needed as the diverse and small studies included in this meta-analysis have substantial limitations, which include incomplete and inadequate confirmation of antenatal drug exposure, variability in assessor blinding, and variability in the statistical approach across studies. In addition, comparison groups in some studies were not well defined or well matched (Devlin et al., 2022). Large-scale studies that account for confounding factors are needed to better define neurodevelopmental outcomes during early childhood and thus guide the multidisciplinary team best suited to improve outcomes. The ESC-NOW trial is currently collecting data on behavioral and neurodevelopmental outcomes and infant and family well-being during the first two years of life in a large, consented group of maternal–infant dyads with opioid exposure during pregnancy (Young et al., 2022). The results will begin to address this knowledge gap and will further inform developmental care for children with a history of NOWS.

Outcomes for children with NOWS are influenced by multiple socioeconomic, home, and environmental factors that may not be easily controlled for. Large-scale studies will allow researchers to begin to differentiate behavioral and neurodevelopmental outcomes while controlling for confounding factors. This knowledge will inform best practices in developmental care for infants with NOWS.

4.9 Summary

A multidisciplinary healthcare team is needed to enhance the safety and well-being of infants with NOWS and to support parenting women with opioid dependency. With a focus on optimizing short- and longer-term outcomes, this team can use high-quality evidence to develop a unified approach to clinical care. If generalizable evidence has not been established, the team can support the research necessary to build the evidence. If medical and social service providers work with hospital leadership and families, they can: 1) enhance the delivery of nonpharmacologic care, 2) empower parents/caregivers in caring for their infants and mitigate stigma, 3) promote the judicious use of pharmacologic therapy, and 4) advocate for the resource and support needed to enhance the optimal growth and development for infants and children with antenatal opioid exposure.

References

Abdel-Latif, M. E., Pinner, J., Clews, S., Cooke, F., Lui, K., & Oei, J. (2006). Effects of breast milk on the severity and outcome of neonatal abstinence syndrome among infants of drug-dependent mothers. *Pediatrics, 117*(6), 1163–1169. https://doi.org/10.1542/peds.2005-1561

Abrahams, R. R., Kelly, S. A., Payne, S., Thiessen, P. N., Mackintosh, J., & Janssen, P. A. (2007). Rooming-in compared with standard care for newborns of mothers using methadone or heroin. *Can Fam Physician, 53*(10), 1722–1730. https://www.ncbi.nlm.nih.gov/pubmed/17934036

Backes, C. H., Backes, C. R., Gardner, D., Nankervis, C. A., Giannone, P. J., & Cordero, L. (2012). Neonatal abstinence syndrome: Transitioning methadone-treated infants from an inpatient to an outpatient setting. *J Perinatol, 32*(6), 425–430. https://doi.org/10.1038/jp.2011.114

Blount, T., Painter, A., Freeman, E., Grossman, M., & Sutton, A. G. (2019). Reduction in length of stay and morphine use for NAS with the "Eat, Sleep, Console" method. *Hosp Pediatr, 9*(8), 615–623. https://doi.org/10.1542/hpeds.2018-0238

Bogen, D. L., & Whalen, B. L. (2019). Breastmilk feeding for mothers and infants with opioid exposure: What is best? *Semin Fetal Neonatal Med, 24*(2), 95–104. https://doi.org/10.1016/j.siny.2019.01.001

Bremer, M. J., & Knippen, K. L. (2023). Breastfeeding experiences in women from ten states reporting opioid use before or during pregnancy: PRAMS, Phase 8. *Matern Child Health J, 27*(4), 747–756. https://doi.org/10.1007/s10 995-022-03497-0

Chervoneva, I., Adeniyi-Jones, S. C., Blanco, F., & Kraft, W. K. (2020). Development of an abbreviated symptom score for the neonatal abstinence syndrome. *J Perinatol, 40*(7), 1031–1040. https://doi.org/10.1038/s41372-020-0606-4

Cizmeli, C., Lobel, M., Harland, K. K., & Saftlas, A. (2018). Stability and change in types of intimate partner violence across pre-pregnancy, pregnancy, and the postpartum period. *Women's Reprod Health (Phila), 5*(3), 153–169. https://doi.org/10.1080/23293691.2018.1490084

Cleveland, L. M., & Bonugli, R. (2014). Experiences of mothers of infants with neonatal abstinence syndrome in the neonatal intensive care unit. *J Obstet Gynecol Neonatal Nurs, 43*(3), 318–329. https://doi.org/10.1111/1552-6909.12306

Corr, T. E., Schaefer, E. W., Hollenbeak, C. S., & Leslie, D. L. (2020). One-year postpartum mental health outcomes of mothers of infants with neonatal abstinence syndrome. *Matern Child Health J, 24*(3), 283–290. https://doi.org/10.1007/s10995-019-02839-9

Daniel, J. M., Davidson, L. N., Havens, J. R., Bauer, J. A., & Shook, L. A. (2020). Aromatherapy as an adjunctive therapy for neonatal abstinence syndrome: A pilot study. *J Opioid Manag, 16*(2), 119–125. https://doi.org/10.5055/jom.2020.0558

Deutsch, S. A., Donahue, J., Parker, T., Hossain, J., & De Jong, A. (2020). Factors associated with child-welfare involvement among prenatally substance-exposed infants. *J Pediatr, 222*, 35–44. https://doi.org/10.1016/j.jpeds.2020.03.036

Devlin, L. A., Breeze, J. L., Terrin, N., Gomez Pomar, E., Bada, H., Finnegan, L. P., O'Grady, K. E., Jones, H. E., Lester, B., & Davis, J. M. (2020). Association of a simplified Finnegan neonatal abstinence scoring tool with the need for pharmacologic treatment for neonatal abstinence syndrome. *JAMA Netw Open, 3*(4). https://doi.org/10.1001/jamanetworkopen.2020.2275

Devlin, L. A., Young, L. W., Kraft, W. K., Wachman, E. M., Czynski, A., Merhar, S. L., Winhusen, T., Jones, H. E., Poindexter, B. B., Wakschlag, L. S., Salisbury, A. L., Matthews, A. G., & Davis, J. M. (2022). Neonatal opioid withdrawal syndrome: A review of the science and a look toward the use of buprenorphine for affected infants. *J Perinatol, 42*(3), 300–306. https://doi.org/10.1038/s41 372-021-01206-3

Favara, M. T., Smith, J., Friedman, D., Lafferty, M., Carola, D., Adeniyi-Jones, S., Greenspan, J., & Aghai, Z. H. (2022). Growth failure in infants with neonatal abstinence syndrome in the neonatal intensive care unit. *J Perinatol, 42*(3), 313–318. https://doi.org/10.1038/s41372-021-01183-7

Finnegan, L. P., Connaughton, J. F., Jr., Kron, R. E., & Emich, J. P. (1975). Neonatal abstinence syndrome: Assessment and management. *Addict Dis, 2*(1–2), 141–158. https://www.ncbi.nlm.nih.gov/pubmed/1163358

Finnegan, L. P., Kron, R. E., Connaughton, J. F., & Emich, J. P. (1975). Assessment and treatment of abstinence in the infant of the drug-dependent mother. *Int J Clin Pharmacol Biopharm*, 12(1–2), 19–32. https://www.ncbi.nlm.nih.gov/pub med/1100537

Food and Drug Administration. (2013, September 10). *FDA announces safety labeling changes and postmarket study requirements for extended-release and long-acting opioid analgesics* [News release]. https://wayback.archive-it.org/ 7993/20170112130229/http:/www.fda.gov/NewsEvents/Newsroom/PressAn nouncements/ucm367726.htm

Food and Drug Administration. (2016, March 22). *FDA announces enhanced warnings for immediate-release opioid pain medications related to risks of misuse, abuse, addiction, overdose and death* [News release]. https://www. fda.gov/news-events/press-announcements/fda-announces-enhanced-warnings-immediate-release-opioid-pain-medications-related-risks-misuse-abuse

Gomez Pomar, E., Finnegan, L. P., Devlin, L., Bada, H., Concina, V. A., Ibonia, K. T., & Westgate, P. M. (2017). Simplification of the Finnegan Neonatal Abstinence Scoring System: Retrospective study of two institutions in the USA. *BMJ Open*, 7(9). https://doi.org/10.1136/bmjopen-2017-016176

Goodman, D. C., Little, G. A., Harrison, W. N., Moen, A., Mowitz, M. E., & Ganduglia-Cazaban, C. (2019). In *The Dartmouth atlas of neonatal intensive care: A report of the Dartmouth Atlas Project*. https://www.ncbi.nlm.nih.gov/ pubmed/36264871

Gopman, S. (2014). Prenatal and postpartum care of women with substance use disorders. *Obstet Gynecol Clin North Am*, 41(2), 213–228. https://doi.org/ 10.1016/j.ogc.2014.02.004

Grossman, M. R., Berkwitt, A. K., Osborn, R. R., Xu, Y., Esserman, D. A., Shapiro, E. D., & Bizzarro, M. J. (2017). An initiative to improve the quality of care of infants with neonatal abstinence syndrome. *Pediatrics*, 139(6). https://doi.org/ 10.1542/peds.2016-3360

Henninger, M. W., Clements, A. D., Kim, S., Rothman, E. F., & Bailey, B. A. (2022). Prevalence of opioid use and intimate partner violence among pregnant women in South-Central Appalachia, USA. *Subst Use Misuse*, 57(8), 1220–1228. https://doi.org/10.1080/10826084.2022.2076872

Holmes, A. V., Atwood, E. C., Whalen, B., Beliveau, J., Jarvis, J. D., Matulis, J. C., & Ralston, S. L. (2016). Rooming-in to treat neonatal abstinence syndrome: Improved family-centered care at lower cost. *Pediatrics*, 137(6). https://doi.org/10.1542/peds.2015-2929

Howard, H. (2016). Experiences of opioid-dependent women in their prenatal and postpartum care: Implications for social workers in health care. *Soc Work Health Care*, 55(1), 61–85. https://doi.org/10.1080/00981389.2015.1078427

Hunseler, C., Bruckle, M., Roth, B., & Kribs, A. (2013). Neonatal opiate withdrawal and rooming-in: A retrospective analysis of a single center experience. *Klin Padiatr*, 225(5), 247–251. https://doi.org/10.1055/s-0033-1347190

Hwang, S. S., Weikel, B., Adams, J., Bourque, S. L., Cabrera, J., Griffith, N., Hall, A. M., Scott, J., Smith, D., Wheeler, C., Woodard, J., & Wymore, E. (2020). The Colorado hospitals substance exposed newborn quality improvement collaborative: Standardization of care for opioid-exposed newborns shortens length of stay and reduces number of infants requiring opiate therapy. *Hosp Pediatr, 10*(9), 783–791. https://doi.org/10.1542/hpeds.2020-0032

Isemann, B., Meinzen-Derr, J., & Akinbi, H. (2011). Maternal and neonatal factors impacting response to methadone therapy in infants treated for neonatal abstinence syndrome. *J Perinatol, 31*(1), 25–29. https://doi.org/10.1038/jp.2010.66

Jansson, L. M., & Patrick, S. W. (2019). Neonatal abstinence syndrome. *Pediatr Clin North Am, 66*(2), 353–367. https://doi.org/10.1016/j.pcl.2018.12.006

Jilani, S. M., Jones, H. E., Grossman, M., Jansson, L. M., Terplan, M., Faherty, L. J., Khodyakov, D., Patrick, S. W., & Davis, J. M. (2022). Standardizing the clinical definition of opioid withdrawal in the neonate. *J Pediatr, 243*, 33–39. https://doi.org/10.1016/j.jpeds.2021.12.021

Kondili, E., & Duryea, D. G. (2019). The role of mother-infant bond in neonatal abstinence syndrome (NAS) management. *Arch Psychiatr Nurs, 33*(3), 267–274. https://doi.org/10.1016/j.apnu.2019.02.003

Kors, S., Kurdziel-Adams, G., Towers, C., Fortner, K., & Macfie, J. (2022). Sexual abuse as a risk factor for opioid misuse in pregnancy. *J Child Sex Abus, 31*(5), 538–549. https://doi.org/10.1080/10538712.2022.2056104

Lawlor, M. L., Shook, L. A., McQuerry, K., Srinivasan, A., Johnson, Q. B., Chavan, N. R., & Critchfield, A. S. (2020). Care-by-parent model as a tool for reduction of neonatal opioid withdrawal syndrome in neonates exposed to buprenorphine maintenance therapy in-utero. *J Matern Fetal Neonatal Med, 33*(16), 2718–2722. https://doi.org/10.1080/14767058.2018.1558201

Lee, J., Hulman, S., Musci, M., Jr., & Stang, E. (2015). Neonatal abstinence syndrome: Influence of a combined inpatient/outpatient methadone treatment regimen on the average length of stay of a Medicaid NICU population. *Popul Health Manag, 18*(5), 392–397. https://doi.org/10.1089/pop.2014.0134

Lee, S. J., Bora, S., Austin, N. C., Westerman, A., & Henderson, J. M. T. (2020). Neurodevelopmental outcomes of children born to opioid-dependent mothers: A systematic review and meta-analysis. *Acad Pediatr, 20*(3), 308–318. https://doi.org/10.1016/j.acap.2019.11.005

Liu, A., Juarez, J., Nair, A., & Nanan, R. (2015). Feeding modalities and the onset of the neonatal abstinence syndrome. *Front Pediatr, 3*, 14. https://doi.org/10.3389/fped.2015.00014

Maalouf, F. I., Cooper, W. O., Slaughter, J. C., Dudley, J., & Patrick, S. W. (2018). Outpatient pharmacotherapy for neonatal abstinence syndrome. *J Pediatr, 199*, 151–157. https://doi.org/10.1016/j.jpeds.2018.03.048

MacMillan, K. D. L. (2019). Neonatal abstinence syndrome: Review of epidemiology, care models, and current understanding of outcomes. *Clin Perinatol, 46*(4), 817–832. https://doi.org/10.1016/j.clp.2019.08.012

MacMillan, K. D. L., Rendon, C. P., Verma, K., Riblet, N., Washer, D. B., & Volpe Holmes, A. (2018). Association of rooming-in with outcomes for neonatal abstinence syndrome: A systematic review and meta-analysis. *JAMA Pediatr, 172*(4), 345–351. https://doi.org/10.1001/jamapediatrics.2017.5195

Marcellus, L. (2014). Supporting women with substance use issues: Trauma-informed care as a foundation for practice in the NICU. *Neonatal Netw, 33*(6), 307–314. https://doi.org/10.1891/0730-0832.33.6.307

Martin, C., Chen, H. B., & Dozier, M. (2022). Intervening with opioid-exposed newborns: Modifying an evidence-based parenting intervention. *Dela J Public Health, 8*(2), 94–98. https://doi.org/10.32481/djph.2022.05.014

McKnight, S., Coo, H., Davies, G., Holmes, B., Newman, A., Newton, L., & Dow, K. (2016). Rooming-in for infants at risk of neonatal abstinence syndrome. *Am J Perinatol, 33*(5), 495–501. https://doi.org/10.1055/s-0035-1566295

McQueen, K., & Murphy-Oikonen, J. (2016). Neonatal abstinence syndrome. *N Engl J Med, 375*(25), 2468–2479. https://doi.org/10.1056/NEJMra1600879

McQueen, K. A., Murphy-Oikonen, J., Gerlach, K., & Montelpare, W. (2011). The impact of infant feeding method on neonatal abstinence scores of methadone-exposed infants. *Adv Neonatal Care, 11*(4), 282–290. https://doi.org/10.1097/ANC.0b013e318225a30c

National Institutes of Health Heal Initiative. (2023a) Advancing clinical trials in neonatal opioid withdrawal (ACT NOW). Retrieved September 16, 2023, from https://heal.nih.gov/research/infants-and-children/act-now

National Institutes of Health Heal Initiative. (2023b) The HEAL Evaluation of Limited Pharmacotherapies for Neonatal Opioid Withdrawal Syndrome (HELP for NOWS). Retrieved September 16, 2023, from https://helpfornows.rti.org

Oei, J., Feller, J. M., & Lui, K. (2001). Coordinated outpatient care of the narcotic-dependent infant. *J Paediatr Child Health, 37*(3), 266–270. https://doi.org/10.1046/j.1440-1754.2001.00657.x

Pallatino, C., Chang, J. C., & Krans, E. E. (2021). The intersection of intimate partner violence and substance use among women with opioid use disorder. *Subst Abus, 42*(2), 197–204. https://doi.org/10.1080/08897077.2019.1671296

Patrick, S. W., Barfield, W. D., Poindexter, B. B., Committee on Fetus and Newborn, Committee on Substance Use and Prevention, Cummings, J., Hand, I., Adams-Chapman, I., Aucott, S. W., Puopolo, K. M., Goldsmith, J. P., Kaufman, D., Martin, C., Mowitz, M., Gonzalez, L., Camenga, D. R., Quigley, J., Ryan, S. A., & Walker-Harding, L. (2020). Neonatal opioid withdrawal syndrome. *Pediatrics, 146*(5). https://doi.org/10.1542/peds.2020-029074

Patrick, S. W., Schumacher, R. E., Horbar, J. D., Buus-Frank, M. E., Edwards, E. M., Morrow, K. A., Ferrelli, K. R., Picarillo, A. P., Gupta, M., & Soll, R. F. (2016). Improving care for neonatal abstinence syndrome. *Pediatrics, 137*(5). https://doi.org/10.1542/peds.2015-3835

Pivovarova, E., & Stein, M. D. (2019). In their own words: Language preferences of individuals who use heroin. *Addiction, 114*(10), 1785–1790. https://doi.org/10.1111/add.14699

Pritham, U. A., Paul, J. A., & Hayes, M. J. (2012). Opioid dependency in pregnancy and length of stay for neonatal abstinence syndrome. *J Obstet Gynecol Neonatal Nurs, 41*(2), 180–190. https://doi.org/10.1111/j.1552-6909.2011.01330.x

Proulx, D., & Fantasia, H. C. (2021). The lived experience of postpartum women attending outpatient substance treatment for opioid or heroin use. *J Midwifery Womens Health, 66*(2), 211–217. https://doi.org/10.1111/jmwh.13165

Raith, W., Schmolzer, G. M., Resch, B., Reiterer, F., Avian, A., Koestenberger, M., & Urlesberger, B. (2015). Laser acupuncture for neonatal abstinence syndrome: A randomized controlled trial. *Pediatrics*, *136*(5), 876–884. https://doi.org/10.1542/peds.2015-0676

Rana, D., Garde, K., Elabiad, M. T., & Pourcyrous, M. (2022). Whole body massage for newborns: A report on non-invasive methodology for neonatal opioid withdrawal syndrome. *J Neonatal Perinatal Med*, *15*(3), 559–565. https://doi.org/10.3233/NPM-220989

Recto, P., McGlothen-Bell, K., McGrath, J., Brownell, E., & Cleveland, L. M. (2020). The role of stigma in the nursing care of families impacted by neonatal abstinence syndrome. *Adv Neonatal Care*, *20*(5), 354–363. https://doi.org/10.1097/ANC.0000000000000778

Sajadi, S., Kazemi, M., Bakhtar, B., & Ostadebrahimi, H. (2019). Comparing the effects of auricular seed acupressure and foot reflexology on neonatal abstinence syndrome: A modified double blind clinical trial. *Complement Ther Clin Pract*, *36*, 72–76. https://doi.org/10.1016/j.ctcp.2019.06.002

Schiff, D. M., & Grossman, M. R. (2019). Beyond the Finnegan scoring system: Novel assessment and diagnostic techniques for the opioid-exposed infant. *Semin Fetal Neonatal Med*, *24*(2), 115–120. https://doi.org/10.1016/j.siny.2019.01.003

Schiff, D. M., Nielsen, T., Terplan, M., Hood, M., Bernson, D., Diop, H., Bharel, M., Wilens, T. E., LaRochelle, M., Walley, A. Y., & Land, T. (2018). Fatal and nonfatal overdose among pregnant and postpartum women in Massachusetts. *Obstet Gynecol*, *132*(2), 466–474. https://doi.org/10.1097/AOG.0000000000002734

Short, V. L., Gannon, M., & Abatemarco, D. J. (2016). The association between breastfeeding and length of hospital stay among infants diagnosed with neonatal abstinence syndrome: A population-based study of in-hospital births. *Breastfeed Med*, *11*, 343–349. https://doi.org/10.1089/bfm.2016.0084

Shuman, C. J., Wilson, R., VanAntwerp, K., Morgan, M., & Weber, A. (2021). Elucidating the context for implementing nonpharmacologic care for neonatal opioid withdrawal syndrome: A qualitative study of perinatal nurses. *BMC Pediatr*, *21*(1), 489. https://doi.org/10.1186/s12887-021-02955-y

Singh, R., Houghton, M., Melvin, P., Wachman, E. M., Diop, H., Iverson, R., Jr., Picarillo, A., Rhein, L., & Gupta, M. (2021). Predictors of pharmacologic therapy for neonatal opioid withdrawal syndrome: A retrospective analysis of a statewide database. *J Perinatol*, *41*(6), 1381–1388. https://doi.org/10.1038/s41372-021-00969-z

Smirk, C. L., Bowman, E., Doyle, L. W., & Kamlin, O. (2014). Home-based detoxification for neonatal abstinence syndrome reduces length of hospital admission without prolonging treatment. *Acta Paediatr*, *103*(6), 601–604. https://doi.org/10.1111/apa.12603

Sobel, L., O'Rourke-Suchoff, D., Holland, E., Remis, K., Resnick, K., Perkins, R., & Bell, S. (2018). Pregnancy and childbirth after sexual trauma: Patient perspectives and care preferences *Obstet Gynecol*, *132*(6), 1461–1468. https://doi.org/10.1097/AOG.0000000000002956

Tolia, V. N., Patrick, S. W., Bennett, M. M., Murthy, K., Sousa, J., Smith, P. B., Clark, R. H., & Spitzer, A. R. (2015). Increasing incidence of the neonatal abstinence syndrome in U.S. neonatal ICUs. *N Engl J Med*, *372*(22), 2118–2126. https://doi.org/10.1056/NEJMsa1500439

Uebel, H., Wright, I. M., Burns, L., Hilder, L., Bajuk, B., Breen, C., Abdel-Latif, M. E., Feller, J. M., Falconer, J., Clews, S., Eastwood, J., & Oei, J. L. (2015). Reasons for rehospitalization in children who had neonatal abstinence syndrome. *Pediatrics*, *136*(4), 811–820. https://doi.org/10.1542/peds.2014-2767

Velez, M., & Jansson, L. M. (2008). The opioid dependent mother and newborn dyad: Non-pharmacologic care. *J Addict Med*, *2*(3), 113–120. https://doi.org/10.1097/ADM.0b013e31817e6105

Wachman, E. M., Byun, J., & Philipp, B. L. (2010). Breastfeeding rates among mothers of infants with neonatal abstinence syndrome. *Breastfeed Med*, *5*(4), 159–164. https://doi.org/10.1089/bfm.2009.0079

Wachman, E. M., Grossman, M., Schiff, D. M., Philipp, B. L., Minear, S., Hutton, E., Saia, K., Nikita, F., Khattab, A., Nolin, A., Alvarez, C., Barry, K., Combs, G., Stickney, D., Driscoll, J., Humphreys, R., Burke, J., Farrell, C., Shrestha, H., & Whalen, B. L. (2018). Quality improvement initiative to improve inpatient outcomes for neonatal abstinence syndrome. *J Perinatol*, *38*, 1114–1122. https://doi.org/10.1038/s41372-018-0109-8

Walsh, M. C., Crowley, M., Wexelblatt, S., Ford, S., Kuhnell, P., Kaplan, H. C., McClead, R., Macaluso, M., & Lannon, C. (2018). Ohio perinatal quality collaborative improves care of neonatal narcotic abstinence syndrome. *Pediatrics*, *141*(4). https://doi.org/10.1542/peds.2017-0900

Weber, A., Miskle, B., Lynch, A., Arndt, S., & Acion, L. (2021). Substance use in pregnancy: Identifying stigma and improving care. *Subst Abuse Rehabil*, *12*, 105–121. https://doi.org/10.2147/SAR.S319180

Welle-Strand, G. K., Skurtveit, S., Jansson, L. M., Bakstad, B., Bjarko, L., & Ravndal, E. (2013). Breastfeeding reduces the need for withdrawal treatment in opioid-exposed infants. *Acta Paediatr*, *102*(11), 1060–1066. https://doi.org/10.1111/apa.12378

Yanos, P. T., Lucksted, A., Drapalski, A. L., Roe, D., & Lysaker, P. (2015). Interventions targeting mental health self-stigma: A review and comparison. *Psychiatr Rehabil J*, *38*(2), 171–178. https://doi.org/10.1037/prj0000100

Young, L. W., Hu, Z., Annett, R. D., Das, A., Fuller, J. F., Higgins, R. D., Lester, B. M., Merhar, S. L., Simon, A. E., Ounpraseuth, S., Smith, P. B., Crawford, M. M., Atz, A. M., Cottrell, L. E., Czynski, A. J., Newman, S., Paul, D. A., Sanchez, P. J., Semmens, E. O., ... Devlin, L. A. (2021). Site-level variation in the characteristics and care of infants with neonatal opioid withdrawal. *Pediatrics*, *147*(1). https://doi.org/10.1542/peds.2020-008839

Young, L. W., Ounpraseuth, S. T., Merhar, S. L., Hu, Z., Simon, A. E., Bremer, A. A., Lee, J. Y., Das, A., Crawford, M. M., Greenberg, R. G., Smith, P. B., Poindexter, B. B., Higgins, R. D., Walsh, M. C., Rice, W., Paul, D. A., Maxwell, J. R., Telang, S., Fung, C. M., ... Devlin, L. A. (2023). Eat, sleep, console approach or usual care for neonatal opioid withdrawal. *New England Journal of Medicine*. https://doi.org/10.1056/NEJMoa2214470

Young, L. W., Ounpraseuth, S. T., Merhar, S. L., Simon, A. E., Das, A., Greenberg, R. G., Higgins, R. D., Lee, J., Poindexter, B. B., Smith, P. B., Walsh, M., Snowden, J., Devlin, L. A., & Eunice Kennedy Shriver National Institute of Child Health and Human Development Neonatal Research Network and the NIH Environmental Influences on Child Health Outcomes (ECHO) Program Institutional Development Awards States Pediatric Clinical Trials Network. (2022). Eating, sleeping, consoling for neonatal opioid withdrawal (ESC-NOW): A function-based assessment and management approach study protocol for a multi-center, stepped-wedge randomized controlled trial. *Trials*, 23(1), 638. https://doi.org/10.1186/s13063-022-06445-z

5 Trauma-Informed Care as a Foundational Approach to Supporting Children and Families

Lenora Marcellus and Catherine Ringham

5.1 Introduction

The use of opioids and their related health impacts continue to rise globally (United Nations Office on Drugs and Crime, 2022). Women now represent almost half of consumers of pharmaceutical opioids. In the United States, the number of women with opioid-related diagnoses reported at birth more than quadrupled between 1999 and 2014 (Haight et al., 2018). Women with substance use disorders who are pregnant and parenting face many complex challenges. They have a greater physiological response than men to opioids, less access to supportive treatments, violence and trauma in their personal lives, risk of criminalization and separation from children, and exposure to stigma in their communities, including when they access health care services (Faherty et al., 2019, Hand et al., 2021; Meinhofer & Anglero-Diaz, 2019).

Infants who are exposed to opioids prenatally may develop Neonatal Opioid Withdrawal Syndrome (NOWS, previously commonly known as Neonatal Abstinence Syndrome, or NAS). NOWS is a cluster of signs that develop after birth, predominantly within the central nervous system and gastrointestinal tract (Patrick et al., 2020). Infants may require non-pharmacological and pharmacological treatment and support during the withdrawal period, with subacute signs of opioid withdrawal lasting for up to six months. The presence of NOWS has been noted to be significantly associated with future child maltreatment, mental health diagnoses, visual problems, speech and language impairment, and poor school performance. However, there is a paucity of high-quality longitudinal outcome research available and causation cannot be suggested (Oei et al., 2017; Rees et al., 2020). Overall, researchers suggest that prenatal opioid exposure may be associated with a range of potential future morbidities (Andersen et al., 2020; Oei, 2018; Rees et al., 2020; Yeoh et al., 2019). These morbidities are also greatly influenced by the presence of cumulative social adversities

DOI: 10.4324/9781003397267-5

and disparities, intergenerationally within families and across communities (Meulewaeter et al., 2019; Schoon & Melis, 2019; Zhang et al., 2022). These adversities are not limited to families within the context of substance use. Halfon et al. (2014), in their review of contemporary children's health trends, note that the epidemiology and social context of American childhood is rapidly changing. They identify trauma and violence as one of the "new epidemiologies of childhood," along with family substance use, chronic mental health challenges, chronic health issues, and persistent health and social disparities from gender, racial, ethnic, geographic, and economic perspectives (Halfon et al., 2014, p. 2116).

Within the context of substance use, infants, children, parents, and families are more likely to face stressful and constrained circumstances of daily living. Studies of women with substance use disorder (SUD) report greater incidences of poverty, lower levels of education and employment, insecure and unsafe housing, a history of child abuse and/or neglect, and child removal (Goodman et al., 2020; Seng & Taylor, 2015). There is now compelling evidence that these circumstances are often linked to individual and intergenerational experiences of trauma and violence (Meulewaeter et al., 2019; Zhang et al., 2022).

Many trauma-informed care (TIC) resources have been targeted toward providers who work in settings where they are most likely to encounter individuals with substance use disorders, such as shelters, child protection services, psychiatric programs, counseling services, and recovery programs. This knowledge is also helpful for health and social care providers practicing across diverse infant, child, and family health settings. Many state, national, and international organizations are beginning to integrate trauma-informed care as an organizational priority and professional standard of practice. For example, the American Medical Association (2021) recently recognized the importance of fully integrating knowledge about trauma-informed care into practice.

Awareness of trauma is important in speech-language pathology (SLP) services, as children with a history of prenatal substance exposure or those who have experienced trauma may present with difficulties in language development (Robertson & Lund, 2022). Robertson and Lund (2022) conducted a survey of school-based SLPs' attitudes and knowledge about TIC. They found variation in responses, with a small number of participants having completed trauma-informed training. Those who completed training did not necessarily feel confident in their ability to provide TIC or felt that implementation was unsupported by their organization. Robertson and Lund (2022) noted that, currently, accreditation standards for SLP education programs do not yet require instruction related to trauma and its effects. Similarly, medical, nursing, social work, and public health curricula do not yet generally incorporate education in trauma-informed principles (Menschner & Maul, 2016).

TIC is an approach and organizational framework that recognizes the prevalence and significance of trauma experienced by individuals, families, and communities (Substance Abuse and Mental Health Services Administration [SAMHSA], 2014). Addressing trauma is increasingly viewed as a required component of effective health services delivery. TIC is becoming a standard of practice and fundamental obligation for care in human-serving sectors, including health, education, and criminal justice. In this chapter, the concept of TIC will be reviewed. An overview of the NEAR science framework is provided, illustrating understandings of neurobiology, epigenetics, adverse childhood experiences (ACEs), and resilience in relation to the impact of stress and trauma. Strategies for integrating trauma-informed principles into interdisciplinary practice settings will be identified. Within the context of NOWS, these strategies are applicable to both the child and the family.

5.2 Trauma-Informed Care

In her landmark book, *Trauma and recovery*, Judith Herman (1997) highlighted the essential connections between the biological, psychological, social, and political dimensions of trauma. Exemplars of later works focus on trauma-informed services for survivors of violent victimization (Harris & Fallot, 2001), principles for designing trauma-informed services (Elliot et al., 2005), trauma-informed and gender-sensitive addiction and recovery programs (Covington, 2008), TIC in the perinatal period (Seng & Taylor, 2015), and trauma-informed care in the Neonatal Intensive Care Unit (Coughlin, 2021; Marcellus & Cross, 2016). The American Academy of Pediatrics recently published a policy statement on trauma-informed care in child health systems (Duffee et al., 2021). This statement is notable for integrating a life course perspective and moving from associating trauma only with specific groups to acknowledging its widespread nature, including the cross-cutting impact of racism. The accompanying clinical report (Forkey et al., 2021) provides guidance on implementing trauma-informed care, related to awareness, readiness, detection and assessment, and management. Beyond professional literature and practices, trauma has also become a popularized cultural concept with substantial general literature and resources available (Birnbaum, 2019).

The US SAMHSA defines trauma as the response that happens when an *event*, series of events, or set of circumstances (such as the death of a significant parent or child, experiencing significant injury or illness, neglect, abuse, witnessing violence, chronic stressors such as poverty and racism) is *experienced* by an individual as physically or emotionally harmful or threatening (SAMHSA, 2014). Experiences can have lasting adverse *effects* on the individual's functioning and physical, social, emotional, or spiritual well-being, depending on contextual factors like developmental stage, social supports, and access to resources. There are many forms of trauma (simple, complex, developmental, and intergenerational) and many variations in how trauma is experienced by individuals (Marcellus & Cross, 2016). SAMHSA has framed trauma with a "three E" approach (taking into account the *event* itself, the *experience* of the individual, and the *effect* on the individual) to capture the diversity of these variations. It is important to note that some of the harm experienced by people is caused by, or made worse by the structures, organizations, and systems in which they live or access care. For example, state policies that treat substance use during pregnancy as a criminal act versus a health concern, create harms with children often removed from families and mothers incarcerated (Faherty et al., 2019).

Child and family service delivery is typically grounded in a family-centered care approach (Institute for Patient- and Family-Centered Care, n.d.). Family-centered care (FCC) is a philosophical foundation that provides a mechanism for collaboration and recognizing families as the experts in the care of their child. Within the context of family histories of perinatal substance use disorders, there are some limitations to the clinical direction that an FCC philosophy can provide and additional approaches to care are required. TIC approach provides a complementary way to address the unique support needs of this group of infants, parents, and families (Duffee et al., 2021; SAMHSA, 2014). The principles of FCC align closely with the principles of TIC (see Table 5.1). A trauma-informed, person- and family-centered care approach is fundamental in health care, particularly in the care of vulnerable children and families in high-stress situations.

5.3 The Science Behind Trauma-Informed Care: The NEAR Framework

A TIC approach is based on growing bodies of evidence in the fields of clinical psychology, genetics, and neuroscience. New theoretical models or frameworks are being developed to represent this evidence in an integrated way, many building on Bronfenbrenner's (2005) ecological systems theory, which views child development as a complex system of relationships affected by multiple levels of the surrounding environment. One example is the American Academy of Pediatrics Basic Science of Pediatrics Model (Shonkoff et al., 2012), These models all share a focus on understanding and responding to root causes of adversity, intentions to break cycles of disadvantage, and build strength in children, families, and communities.

Table 5.1 Comparison of family-centered care principles and trauma-informed care principles (Institute for Patient-and Family-Centered (IPFCC)[1], SAMHSA, and Trauma Informed Oregon[2])

Family-centered care	Trauma-informed care
	Safety Throughout the organization, staff and the people they serve feel physically and psychologically safe.[2]
Respect and dignity Health care practitioners listen to and honor patient and family perspectives and choices. Patient and family knowledge, values, beliefs, and cultural backgrounds are incorporated into the planning and delivery of care.[1]	*Empowerment, voice, and choice* Organization aims to strengthen the staff, client, and family members' experience of choice and recognizes that every person's experience is unique and requires an individualized approach. This builds on what clients, staff, and communities have to offer, rather than responding to perceived deficits.[2]
Information sharing Health care practitioners communicate and share complete and unbiased information with patients and families in ways that are affirming and useful. Patients and families receive timely, complete and accurate information in order to effectively participate in care and decision-making.[1]	*Trustworthiness and transparency* Organizational operations and decisions are conducted with transparency and the goal of building and maintaining trust among staff, clients, and family members of those receiving services.[2]
Participation Patients and families are encouraged and supported in participating in care and decision-making at the level they choose.[1]	*Peer support and mutual self-help* These are integral to the organizational and service delivery approach and are understood as a key vehicle for building trust, establishing safety, and empowerment.[2]
Collaboration Patients, families, health care practitioners, and health care leaders collaborate in policy and program development, implementation, and evaluation; in facility design; in professional education; and in research; as well as in the delivery of care.[1]	*Collaboration and mutuality* There is recognition that healing happens in relationships and in the meaningful sharing of power and decision-making. The organization recognizes that everyone has a role to play in a trauma-informed approach. One does not have to be a therapist to be therapeutic.[2]
	Cultural, historical, and gender issues The organization actively moves past cultural stereotypes and biases, offers culturally responsive services, leverages the healing value of traditional cultural connections, and recognizes and addresses historical trauma.[2]

Anda and Porter, members of the landmark Adverse Childhood Event (ACE) study research team, developed the NEAR framework to integrate these fields of evidence (Lile & Ryser, 2020). The framework provides a more holistic and integrated understanding of how a person's experiences of trauma can impact health outcomes over their life course. In this framework the concepts of neurobiology, epigenetics, adverse childhood events, and resilience are considered.

It is important to note that the manner in which these concepts are incorporated into standards of practice has been critiqued by various authors. One risk of science-based approaches is that they can obscure the fact that many of the causes of trauma and health inequities in childhood and society are social-structural and political in nature (Birnbaum, 2019; Legrenzi & Umilta, 2011; Wastell & White, 2017). A second risk is that responsibility for child development primarily falls on the shoulders of individual women, as typical primary caregivers during the early years, with blame and stigma when there are child health challenges (Reimer & Sahagian, 2015). There can be unintended consequences associated with development of social policy based on neuroscientific evidence, such as increased involvement of child protection and child removal (Featherstone et al., 2014). A third critique is that the science continues to evolve. Limitations in some of the foundational studies and concerns with rapid or uncritical uptake and adaptation have been noted (Karatekin et al., 2022; Kelly-Irving & Delpierre, 2019). These critiques may help health care providers see the broader socio-political effects on people experiencing trauma and consider effective, practical approaches to supporting vulnerable families.

5.3.1 The Neurobiology of Stress

The concept of stress was developed in the field of physics to describe various types of physical pressures or forces. Selye, an endocrinologist considered the early leader in stress research in the 1930s, noted in his clinical practice that patients with chronic illnesses shared symptoms that he attributed to what is now commonly called stress, further impacting their health (Robinson, 2018). In Selye's general adaptation syndrome, he suggested that disruptions in homeostasis led to a stress response, including phase of alarm reaction, stage of resistance, and stage of exhaustion, mediated by the release of neurotransmitters and hormones. Stress was not adapted as an accepted scientific term until the 1950s, building on attention on the psychological experiences of soldiers in world wars. Further research moved beyond the behavioral to consider how individuals interpreted or made meaning of stressors. In the 1980s, the concept of coping as a mediator of stress was introduced by Lazarus, a cognitive scientist (Robinson, 2018).

The past three decades are considered the era of brain science, a time of rapid advances in the understanding of neurobiology, molecular science, genetics, epigenetics, and transgenerational transmission of stress. The landmark National Research Council (US) and Institute of Medicine (US) Committee on Integrating the Science of Early Childhood Development (2020) report "From neurons to neighborhoods: The science of early childhood development" presented evidence establishing that brain development is heavily influenced by relationships and life experiences, including social and economic circumstances. Key brain development occurs rapidly during the prenatal and early childhood periods, featuring neuronal proliferation, differentiation and migration, synaptic formation, systematic pruning, programmed cell death, and myelination. These processes are supported by enriching experiences and disrupted by exposure to a range of negative influences, including diet, infection, environment, adversity, and stress. These adverse early experiences can be biologically embedded in the stress response systems of the child's brain, with specific effects depending on the timing, intensity, and duration of exposure to these influences (Hunter et al., 2018; Shonkoff et al., 2012).

The neurobiology of stress is complex, but this science provides an understanding of how toxic stress, adverse experiences, and trauma affect brain development and function over time. Human biological systems are acutely responsive to stress (McEwan, 2017). The autonomic nervous system responds with "rest and digest" on the parasympathetic side and on the sympathetic side, with "fight or flight." Perceived threats elicit a response from the amygdala, often resulting in instinctual, outward reaction like anger, fear, and anxiety. The hypothalamic–pituitary–adrenal (HPA) axis response is a longer-term physiological response, with activation resulting in cortisol, the primary stress hormone, secretion from the adrenal gland. Together, these two systems exert important effects on biological systems that prepare the individual for stress or challenge (Hunter et al., 2018).

The concept of allostasis addresses how well these multiple complex biological systems work together to support adaptation of the body to threat. Allostasis refers to the process that maintains homeostatic systems in balance, enabling an individual to respond to its physical state and cope with various stressors or external stimuli (McEwan, 2017). Allostatic load is the burden carried by the body in response to continued and repeated exposure to stressors, and is associated with increased risk for disease and poor health across the lifespan. Chronic "wear and tear" (high allostatic load) results from prolonged activation and overburdening of biological systems that are designed primarily for short-term activation (McEwan,

2017). Excessive, persistent, or uncontrollable levels of stress, without sufficient protective factors, can contribute to negative effects on multiple organ systems, including the brain, leading to illness throughout the life course (Herrman et al., 2011).

Researchers have also identified other important biomarkers in the stress response affecting immune functioning, cellular aging, epigenetics, and changes to brain structure (Bush & Roubinov, 2021). As early as conception, the cellular impact of toxic stress, malnutrition, and environmental toxicity can be imprinted. Adverse experiences in early childhood can have a scaffolding effect, particularly at highly sensitive periods of development and with exposure to potential toxic situations. The result is the development of physiological deficits affecting neuroendocrine, metabolic, cardiovascular, immune systems, and the brain (Shonkoff et al., 2012). These effects have impacts across the life course.

5.3.2 Beyond Nature Versus Nurture: An Introduction to Epigenetics

The term epigenetics was first conceptualized in the 1940s and 1950s by Conrad Waddington, an embryologist, and David Nanney, a geneticist (Deichmann, 2016). Framed as a paradigm shift from Darwin's theory of biological evolution and the nature versus nurture debate, the concept and known mechanisms of epigenetics have evolved over time. The term originally referred to the complex interactions that occur between the genotype (the DNA sequence in the genome, or initial blueprint) and the phenotype (specific characteristic attributed to the gene's protein product, or the final outcome) (Garner & Saul, 2018). Its meaning has broadened and diversified over time to emphasize the importance of both genetic and nongenetic factors in controlling gene expression. Although there remains ambiguity in terminology, the National Human Genome Research Institute (2023) currently defines epigenetics as the field of study focused on changes in DNA that do not involve alterations to the underlying sequence. Finally, the Centers for Disease Control and Prevention (2022) define epigenetics as the study of how behaviors and environment can cause changes that affect the way genes work.

Factors that regulate the progression from DNA to RNA to protein are now known to be influenced by the environment. Epigenetic changes are evidence that "genes are not destiny, that the early childhood ecology can be biologically embedded within the epigenome, and that subsequent events can also alter the way that the genetic blueprint is used (Garner & Saul, 2018, p. 29). Epigenetic changes and health outcomes influenced by these changes are attributed to circumstances such as altered food availability, stress, pain exposure, parental nurturing, maternal chronic disease, and maternal substance use (Tiffon, 2018; Yen et al., 2023). For example, recent research found that epigenetic variation in the opioid receptor mu 1 (OPRM1) gene is associated with differences in severity of NOWS and hospitalization outcomes (Wachman & Farrer, 2019). In relation to trauma, if women are exposed to stress during pregnancy, or infants are exposed to stress after birth, epigenetic changes that control cortisol can be produced and may determine the body's response to the threat. This epigenomic modification can persist through to adulthood, influencing how individuals respond to stress and potentially increasing risk of adult disease. Alternatively, supportive environments and learning experiences can generate positive epigenetic signatures that activate, rather than suppress, genetic potential (Shonkoff et al., 2012).

5.3.3 The Impact of Adverse Childhood Experiences on Child Development and Well-Being

Many research studies have measured the long-term health and social impacts of exposure to early childhood adversity, with the intent of designing interventions that may reduce these adversities and their nega-tive impacts on the mental and physical health of children and adults (Asmundson & Afifi, 2020). One influential study has raised the profile of the pervasive, intergenerational impact of trauma on children, families, and communities.

The Kaiser Permanente *Adverse Childhood Experiences (ACE) Study* was conducted in the United States from 1998 to 2010 (Felitti et al., 1998). Researchers looked at the life histories of 17,000 individuals to determine the connections between adverse childhood events (related to abuse and living in dysfunctional households) and health in adulthood. Seven cat-egories of events were considered, including psychological, physical, or sexual abuse, violence against mother, or living with household members who were substance abusers, mentally ill or suicidal, or ever imprisoned. They reported that more than 60% of their participants had experienced at least one category of childhood trauma, and, of this group, 20% had experienced three or more categories of trauma. This study found a strong correlation between exposure to stress and abuse during childhood and the subsequent development of multiple risk factors (i.e. smoking, obesity, physical inactivity, and mental illness) leading to chronic disease (i.e. ischemic heart disease, cancer, and lung disease) in later life. A conceptual model of the long-term effects of early stress was developed through this research. It illustrates the life course of early stress, from disruption of neurodevelopment leading to impairments in social, emotional, and cogni-tive capacity, through the adoption of risk behaviors, resulting in chronic diseases and disabilities (see Figure 5.1).

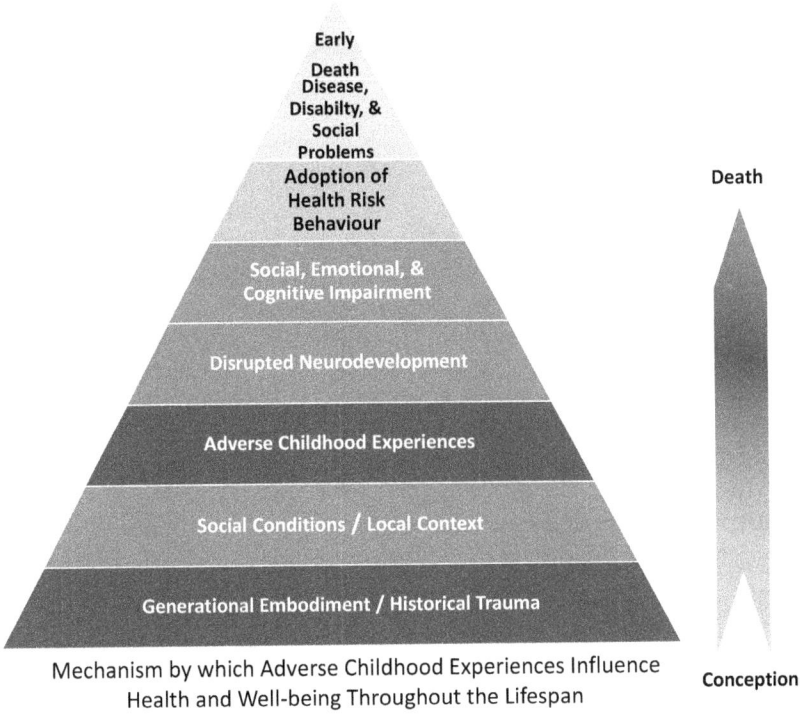

Mechanism by which Adverse Childhood Experiences Influence
Health and Well-being Throughout the Lifespan

Figure 5.1 A pyramid describing the impacts adverse childhood experiences can have on an individual throughout the lifespan (Figure developed by the CDC. The use of this figure does not imply endorsement of this chapter by the CDC. This figure is available on the CDC website: https://www. cdc.gov/violenceprevention/aces/about.html.)

Adverse childhood events (ACEs) are considered a collection of potentially negative, stressful, traumatic exposures that individuals may experience during childhood and confer health risk across the life course (Anda et al., 2006; Asmundson & Afifi, 2020; Goddard, 2021). The best studied ACEs are divided into umbrellas of abuse, neglect, and dysfunction; however, they are interrelated and have cumulative impact (Hays-Grudo & Sheffield Morris, 2020). These exposures create toxic stress, beyond that considered positive or tolerable, biologically embedding stress and leading to a wide range of health risk behaviors, chronic physical and mental health conditions, and all-cause mortality (Karatekin et al., 2022).

ACEs are common globally and are now prioritized in the United Nations' 2030 Sustainable Development Goals to end abuse and all forms of violence against children (Rutter, 2021). The scope and depth of the long-term consequences of ACEs on physical, mental, cognitive, and social health warrant recognition as a public health issue (Tonmyr et al., 2020).

It is estimated that up to 90% of the population will experience at least one traumatic event during their lives (Norris & Slone, 2007) and that over half of children and adolescents (51.2%) in the US have experienced at least one type of adverse childhood experience (Crouch et al., 2019). Most commonly for children, this includes experiencing economic hardship or parental/guardian divorce. Women with substance use disorders who are pregnant typically have experienced multiple adverse events, including a history of abuse and household dysfunction, across socio-economic gradients (Currie & Tough, 2021; Osofsky et al., 2021). There is a dose–response association between the number of ACEs and the risk for substance use during pregnancy: women with four or more ACEs had almost a four-fold increase in the odds of illicit drug use in pregnancy (Currie & Tough, 2021). Dr. Robert Block, the former President of the American Academy of Pediatrics, has noted that adverse childhood experiences are the single greatest unaddressed public health threat facing the United States (Burke-Harris, 2014).

5.3.4 Resilience: Positive Adaption in the Face of Adversity

The roots of the term resilience are thought to have emerged in the field of physics and engineering to capture the elastic ability of materials to spring back after pressures or shocks. As a concept, resilience has been explored and applied in diverse disciplinary fields such as psychology, social work, systems ecology, economic policy, urban planning, and more recently, genetics and neuroscience. It has been examined at multiple levels, from the molecular to the global (Masten, 2007). Resilience, as a counterpoint to dominant problem or deficit models used in health care, is typically framed as the "ability of the individual to cope, adapt, or mobilize protective resources in the face of adversity" (Hutcheon & Lashewicz, 2014, p. 1383). In the fields of psychology and child development, the term refers to positive adaptation during or following exposure to adversities that have the potential to harm development. Despite many decades of research, resilience continues to be defined in a variety of ways, with a shared element of having the ability to weather adversity (Southwick et al., 2014).

Building on Bronfenbrenner's (2005) ecological approach to child development, research on the concept of resilience emerged from studies exploring the impact of childhood adversity on adult health and well-being. Research on "the invulnerable child" began in the 1970s by psychiatrists who, building on previous decades of study on the impact of trauma and stress, were intrigued by how some children could adapt positively when living under conditions of extreme vulnerability and hardship (Anthony, 1974). Later research moved beyond the individual to families and communities. Most recently, research is addressing how resilience is shaped by dynamic interactions across multiple levels and integrated pathways, including gene-environment, and social networks (Masten & Barnes, 2018). As resilience science shifts more to a systems perspective, there is now much greater recognition that much of what promotes resilience originates outside the individual.

Resiliency theory describes how promotive/protective factors may counteract the negative effects of risks. Sources of resilience include personal, biological, environmental, and systemic factors, and dynamic interaction between these factors (Herrman et al., 2011). The most significant determinant of resilience – noted in nearly every review or study of resilience in the last 50 years – is the quality of close personal relationships, especially with parents and primary caregivers (Gartland et al., 2019). Risk factors include adverse childhood experiences, adverse community environments, and for families with substance use disorders, socio-political factors (Ellis & Dietz, 2017). For example, there has been a recent proliferation of punitive state policies for people who are pregnant or parenting with substance use disorders. They are less likely to be able to access recovery treatment and more likely to be confronted with the potential of being charged with child abuse or another criminal act (Faherty et al., 2019).

Many interventions have been developed to promote resiliency, by increasing protective factors and lessening the impact of cumulative negative effects, at individual, family, and community levels. One framework, related to ACEs, called the PACEs (Protective and Compensatory Experiences) approach, integrates strategies to enhance resilience (Hays-Grudo and Sheffield Morris, 2020). Hays-Grudo and Sheffield Morris (2020) developed the PACE scale to assess experiences that are known from research to promote resilience in the face of adversity, for children as well as adults. These experiences are relationship-based (e.g. unconditional love, being part of a social group) and resource-dependent (e.g. living in a safe and clean home with enough food, having resources to learn).

5.4 Integrating Trauma-Informed Care Approaches Into Practice

A *trauma-informed approach* refers to how people within organizations think about and respond to those who have experienced or may be at risk for experiencing trauma (Marcellus, 2014). SAMHSA (2014) outlines a "four R" perspective for the elements that are required to create this shift in organizational culture: (1) *realizing* the prevalence of trauma, (2) *recognizing* how trauma affects all individuals involved with the organization (clients, families, and team members), (3) *responding* by putting this knowledge into practice, and (4) actively *resisting* retraumatization. In this next section, this "four R" perspective is applied to SLP practice and interdisciplinary clinical settings. Specific activities for each element are summarized in Table 5.2.

Table 5.2 Examples of activities for integrating a trauma-informed approach, based on the SAMHSA elements (adapted from: Duffee et al., 2021; Forkey et al., 2021; Marcellus & Cross, 2016; Marcellus, 2014; SAMHSA, 2014)

Element	*Activities*
Realizing	• Gather data for your state on mental health and trauma/violence in infants, young children, women, and families • Collaborate with partners such as local child welfare agencies, infant development programs, women's recovery and support programs, schools, and public health to learn about the scope of the issue in your community
Recognizing	• Learn more about the concepts of infant, early childhood and family stress, trauma and trauma-informed care; for example, review current resources, share information in team meetings, and attend workshops • Conduct trauma-informed care self-assessments for individual team members and your unit/organization • Develop opportunities for clinicians to be supported through consultation, role support, and supervision • Recognize that any client and their family members could have experienced past or ongoing adverse events
Responding	• Establish a welcoming, non-stigmatizing and non-judgmental environment, with an integrated and consistent approach from all program team members. Emphasize physical and emotional safety • Interpret behaviors, which may be "fight or flight" responses, with a trauma-informed lens • Use clear communication and strengths-focused approaches to providing diagnostic and treatment information. Provide choices as much as possible and ensure informed consent • Use strengths-based, person-first language (change language away from "manipulative, uncooperative, drug-seeking" to "they have survived trauma, they have developed these survival skills to help them make it this far, recovery takes time") • Shift from "what is wrong" to "what is happening" and integrate this knowledge into every aspect of service design and delivery

Table 5.2 (Continued)

Element	Activities
Resisting retraumatization	• Reassess routine procedures from perspective of trauma and stigma, including intake processes and testing procedures. Talk people through the testing processes and ask if there are modifications that would make them more comfortable. • Employ emotional regulation techniques – environmental (i.e. light, sound, activity, pacing of activities, complexity of instructions), sensory motor (i.e. swinging or fidgeting to increase or decrease arousal, improve attentiveness, and self-soothe), language (i.e. labeling emotions, validating emotions, providing visuals to support language, modeling self-talk to cope with a difficulty) • Be mindful of potential triggers in your practice environment and routine practices • Ensure program policies and procedures support parent–child relationships. Be careful to not position parents as the primary risk factor for children. Women who have infants/children with NOWS or FASD (Fetal Alcohol Spectrum Disorder) already feel shamed and stigmatized (Stone, 2015)

5.4.1 Realizing the Prevalence of Trauma

In a trauma-informed approach, all people at all levels of the organization have a basic realization about trauma and understand how trauma can affect families, groups, organizations, and communities as well as individuals (SAMHSA, 2014). Developing an awareness of the pervasiveness of the issue of trauma in the lives of the families in our communities creates an opportunity to view how service delivery can be improved (Marcellus, 2014). There are a growing number of resources and tools available through many different organizations to support teams in examining their practices from a trauma-informed perspective, including individual and organizational checklists, team self-assessment activities, and program planning guidelines. Examples of organizations with available resources include the Centers for Disease Control and Prevention, National Child Traumatic Stress Network, the Trauma-Informed Care Implementation Resource Center, and Zero to Three.

5.4.2 Recognizing How Trauma Affects People

People in the organization or system are also able to recognize the signs of trauma (SAMHSA, 2014). Survivors of trauma and abuse often live in environments where they constantly face the threat of danger and fear, which then becomes the lens through which they see the world (Marcellus, 2014). A biopsychosocial approach is an effective way to understand the effects of trauma. From a physiologic perspective, experiences of trauma have been linked to a range of physical symptoms (i.e. eating and sleeping disturbances, sensitivity to noise and being touched), emotional concerns (i.e. anxiety, fearfulness, anger), behavioral issues (i.e. self-harm, substance use, hypervigilance), cognitive challenges (i.e. memory lapses, difficulty making decisions), and spiritual concerns (i.e. guilt, shame) (Haskell, 2013). It is also important to be aware of the effects on cognitive, behavioral, and emotional systems. Without an understanding of trauma, symptoms that are seen in practice, such as anger, acting out, or not coming to appointments, may be attributed solely to the substance use or judgmentally to the people themselves (Marcellus, 2014). Many of the adaptations that people who have experienced trauma develop to survive may be seen as pathologic (including using drugs and alcohol) unless they are interpreted through a trauma lens (Haskell, 2013; Stone, 2015).

5.4.3 Responding by Putting Knowledge Into Action

The program, organization, or system responds by applying the principles of a trauma-informed approach to all areas of functioning and by all health care providers (SAMHSA, 2014). After learning about the prevalence of trauma in their community and how to recognize signs of trauma in infants, children, and families, there are several initial steps that teams can take to respond to this knowledge and begin to incorporate a trauma-informed approach into their care (Marcellus & Cross, 2016). Two key preliminary steps foundational to this work are developing new interdisciplinary partnerships and incorporating the voices of families into service delivery design. One key approach is to embed this understanding of trauma into all aspects of service delivery – a *universal precautions* approach, operating as if everyone who comes into care has experienced a traumatic event (Owens et al., 2022; Racine et al., 2019). It is important to note that providers who work from a trauma-informed approach do not have to be specialists in providing treatment for trauma; instead, they need to be able to recognize the effects of trauma and alter their practices to provide appropriate safe support. A trauma-informed approach should therefore not be an "add-on" practice but should be a *fundamental shift* in the way health care services are organized and delivered.

5.4.4 Actively Resisting Retraumatization

A trauma-informed approach seeks to resist retraumatization of clients as well as staff (SAMHSA, 2014). Health care environments and the routine practices and policies that are in place may be experienced by people as traumatizing, and can trigger stress and trauma responses. By understanding this relationship, teams can proactively examine these practices and policies to develop an environment that will be more likely to be experienced as safe (Marcellus & Cross, 2016).

In addition to trauma-informed strategies, there are actions that health care teams can take to ensure that their services are accessible and welcoming for families who may be coping with cumulative stressors and disadvantages:

- Learn about the context of each family's own daily life (that could include adversities such as poverty, mental health challenges, substance use issues, violence, and trauma). Partner with other community agencies and services to address issues.
- Reduce and/or remove barriers that prevent families from attending services, such as transportation, childcare for other children, and flexible appointment scheduling and reminders.

5.5 Summary

Many of today's families are facing increasing challenges, including substance use, violence, and trauma. Inequities develop in life opportunities and resources, creating stress and adversity. Early intervention and support, a foundation of child health services, is even more critical for families living within the context of cumulative disadvantage. Every child health encounter provides an opportunity for promoting family resilience and relational health (Duffee et al., 2021). Integration of TIC principles into all aspect of practice is an important protective factor for those experiencing adversity.

References

American Medical Association. (2021). *Adverse childhood experiences and trauma-informed care.* https://policysearch.ama-assn.org/policyfinder/det ail/Adverse%20Childhood%20Experiences%20and%20Trauma-Infor med%20Care%C2%A0%20H-515.952?uri=%2FAMADoc%2FHOD.xml-H-%09515.952.xml

Anda, R. F., Felitti, V. J., Bremner, J. D., Walker, J. D., Whitfield, C. H., Perry, B., Dube, S. R., & Giles, W. H. (2006). The enduring effects of abuse and related adverse experiences in childhood. *European Archives of Psychiatry and Clinical Neuroscience, 256*(3), 174–186. https://doi.org/10.1007/s00406-005-0624-4

Andersen, J., Hoiseth, G., & Nygaard, E. (2020). Prenatal exposure to methadone or buprenorphine and long-term outcomes: A meta-analysis. *Early Human Development, 143.* https://doi.org/10.1016/j.earlhumdev.2020.104997

Anthony, E. (1974). The syndrome of the psychologically invulnerable child. In E. Anthony & C. Koupernik (Eds.), *The child in his family: Children at psychiatric risk* (pp. 529–545). Wiley.

Asmundson, G., & Afifi, T. (2020). *Adverse childhood experiences: Using evidence to advance research, practice, policy, and prevention.* Academic Press. https://doi.org/10.1016/C2017-0-03827-2

Birnbaum, S. (2019). Confronting the social determinants of health: Has the language of trauma informed care become a defence mechanism? *Issues in Mental Health Nursing, 40*(6), 476–481. https://doi:10.1080/01612840.2018.1563256

Bronfenbrenner, U. (2005). *Making human beings human: Bioecological perspectives on human development.* Sage Publications.

Burke-Harris, N. (2014). *How childhood trauma affects health across a lifetime* [Video]. TED. https://www.ted.com/talks/nadine_burke_harris_how_childhood_trauma_affects_health_across_a_lifetime

Bush, N., & Roubinov, D. (2021). Bringing a neurobiological perspective to resilience. In M. Ungar (Ed.), *Multisystemic resilience: Adaptation and transformation in contexts of change* (pp. 35–56). Oxford. https://doi.org/10.1093/oso/9780190095888.003.0003

Centers for Disease Control and Prevention. (2022). *What is epigenetics?* https://www.cdc.gov/genomics/disease/epigenetics.htm

Coughlin, M. (2021). *Trauma-informed care in the NICU: Evidence-based practice guidelines for neonatal clinicians.* Springer.

Covington, S. (2008). Women and addiction: A trauma-informed approach. *Journal of Psychoactive Drugs, SARC Supplement 5*, 377–385. https://doi.org/10.1080/02791072.2008.10400665

Crouch, E., Radcliff, E., & Hung, P. (2019). Challenges to school success and the role of adverse childhood experiences. *Academic Pediatrics, 19*, 899–907. https://doi:10.1016/j.acap.2019.08.006

Currie, C., & Tough, S. (2021). Adverse childhood experiences are associated with drug use among pregnant women with middle to high socioeconomic status: Findings from the All Our Families cohort. *BMC Pregnancy and Childbirth, 21*(133). https://doi:10.1186/s12884-021-03591-1

Deichmann, U. (2016). Epigenetics: The origins and evolution of a fashionable topic. *Developmental Biology, 416*(1), 249–254. https://doi:10.1016/j.ydbio.2016.06.005

Duffee, J., Szilagyi, M., Forkey, H., Kelly, E., & Council on Community Pediatrics, Council on Foster Care, Adoption and Kinship Care, Council on Child Abuse and Neglect, Committee on Psychosocial Aspects of Child and Family Health. (2021). Trauma-informed care in child health systems. *Pediatrics, 148*(2). https://doi.org/10.1542/peds.2021-052579

Elliot, D., Bjelajac, P., Fallot, R., Markoff, L., & Reed, B. (2005). Trauma-informed or trauma-denied: Principles and implementation of trauma-informed services for women. *Journal of Community Psychology, 33*(4), 461–477. https://doi.org/10.1002/jcop.20063

Ellis, W., & Dietz, W. (2017). A new framework for addressing adverse childhood and community experiences: The building community resilience model. *Academic Pediatrics, 17*(7), S86–S93. https://doi:10.1016/j.acap.2016.12.011

Faherty, L., Kranz, A., Russell-Fritch, J., Patrick, S., Cantor, J., & Stein, B. (2019). Association of punitive and reporting state policies related to substance use in pregnancy with rates of neonatal opioid withdrawal. *JAMA Network Open*, 2(11). https://doi.org/10.1001/jamanetworkopen.2019.14078

Featherstone, B., Morris, K., & White, S. (2014). A marriage made in hell: Early intervention meets child protection. *British Journal of Social Work*, 44(7), 1735–1749. https://doi.org/10.1093/bjsw/bct052

Felitti, V. J., Anda, R. F., Nordenberg, D., Williamson, D. F., Spitz, A. M., Edwards, V., Koss, M. P., & Marks, J. S. (1998). Relationship of childhood abuse and household dysfunction to many of the leading causes of death in adults. The Adverse Childhood Experiences (ACE) study. *American Journal of Prevention Medicine, 14*, 245–258. http://doi:org/10.1016/S0749-3797(98)00017-8

Forkey, H., Szilagyi, M., Kelly, E., American Academy of Pediatrics Council on Foster Care, Adoption, and Kinship Care, Council on Community Pediatrics, Council on Child Abuse and Neglect, Committee on Psychosocial Aspects of Child and Family Health. (2021). Trauma-informed care. *Pediatrics, 148(2)*. https://doi.org/10.1542/peds.2021-052580

Garner, A., & Saul, R. (2018). *Thinking developmentally: Nurturing wellness in childhood to promote lifelong health*. American Academy of Pediatrics. https://doi.org/10.1542/9781610021531

Gartland, D., Riggs, E., Muyeen, S., Giallo, R., Afifi, T. O., MacMillan, H., Herrman, H., Bulford, E., & Brown, S. J. (2019). What factors are associated with resilient outcomes in children exposed to social adversity? A systematic review. *BMJ Open, 9*(4). http://dx.doi.org/10.1136/bmjopen-2018-024870

Goddard, A. (2021). Adverse childhood experiences and trauma-informed care. *Journal of Pediatric Health Care, 35*(2), 145–155. https://doi.org/10.1016/j.pedhc.2020.09.001

Goodman, D., Saunders, E., & Wolff, K. (2020). In their own words: A qualitative study of factors promoting resilience and recovery among postpartum women with opioid use disorders. *BMC Pregnancy and Childbirth, 20*, 178.

Haight, S., Ko, J., Tong, V., Bohm, M., & Callaghan, W. (2018). Opioid use disorder documented at delivery hospitalization – United States, 1999–2014. *Morbidity and Mortality Weekly Report, 67*, 845–849. https://doi.org/10.15585/mmwr.mm673a1

Halfon, N., Wise, P., & Forrest, C. (2014). The changing nature of children's health development: New challenges require different policy solutions. *Health Affairs, 33*(12), 2116–2124. https://doi.org/10.1377/hlthaff.2014.0944

Hand, D. J., Fischer, A. C., Gannon, M. L., McLaughlin, K. A., Short, V. L., & Abatemarco, D. J. (2021). Comprehensive and compassionate responses for opioid use disorder among pregnant and parenting women. *International Review of Psychiatry, 33*(6), 514–527. https://doi.org/10.1080/09540261.2021.1908966

Harris, M., & Fallot, R. D. (Eds.). (2001). *Using trauma theory to design service systems*. Jossey-Bass/Wiley.

Haskell, L. (2013). A developmental understanding of complex trauma. In N. Poole & L. Greaves (Eds.), *Becoming trauma-informed* (pp. 9–27). Centre for Addiction and Mental Health.

Hays-Grudo, J., & Sheffield Morris, A. (2020). *Adverse and protective childhood experiences: A developmental perspective.* American Psychological Association.

Herman, J. (1997). *Trauma and recovery.* Basic Books.

Herrman, H., Stewart, D., Diaz-Granados, N., Berger, E., Jackson, B., & Yuen, T. (2011). What is resilience? *Canadian Journal of Psychiatry, 56*(5), 258–265. https://doi.org/10.1177/070674371105600504

Hunter, R., Gray, J., & McEwan, B. (2018). The neuroscience of resilience. *Journal of the Society for Social Work and Research, 9*(2), 305–339. https://doi.org/10.1086/697956

Hutcheon, E., & Lashewicz, B. (2014). Theorizing resilience: Critiquing and unbounding a marginalizing concept. *Disability & Society, 29,* 1383–1397. https://doi.org/10.1080/09687599.2014.934954

Institute for Patient- and Family-Centered Care (n.d.). *What is patient- and family-centered care?* https://www.ipfcc.org/about/pfcc.html

Karatekin, C., Mason, S., Riegelman, A., Bakker, C., Hunt, S., Gresham, B., Corcoran, F., & Barnes, A. (2022). Adverse childhood experiences: A scoping review of measures and methods. *Children and Youth Services Review, 136.* https://doi.org/10.1016/j.childyouth.2022.106425

Kelly-Irving, M., & Delpierre, C. (2019). A critique of the Adverse Childhood Experience Framework in epidemiology and public health: Uses and misuses. *Social Policy and Society, 18*(3), 445–456. https://doi.org/10.1017/S1474746419000101

Legrenzi, P., & Umilta, C. (2011). *Neuromania: On the limits of brain science.* Oxford Scholarship. https://doi.org/10.1093/acprof:oso/9780199591343.001.0001

Lile, J., & Ryser, L. (2020). *Using NEAR sciences to address community health: A primer.* Washington State University Extension. https://rex.libraries.wsu.edu/esploro/outputs/report/Using-NEAR-sciences-to-address-community/99900501624401842#file-0

Marcellus, L. (2014). Supporting women with substance use issues: Trauma-informed care as a foundation for practice in the NICU (Part 1). *Neonatal Network, 33*(6), 307–314. https://doi.org/10.1891/0730-0832.33.6.307

Marcellus, L., & Cross, S. (2016). Trauma-informed care in the NICU: Implications for early childhood development (Part II). *Neonatal Network, 35*(6), 359–366. https://doi.org/10.1038/jp.2017.124

Masten, A. (2007). Resilience in developing systems: Progress and promise as the fourth wave rises. *Development and Psychopathology, 19,* 921–930. https://doi.org/10.1017/S0954579407000442

Masten, A., & Barnes, A. (2018). Resilience in children: Developmental perspectives. *Children, 5*(7), 98. https://doi.org/10.3390/children5070098

McEwan, B. (2017). Stress: Homeostasis, rheostasis, reactive scope, allostasis and allostatic load. *Reference Module in Neuroscience and Behavioral Psychology.* Elsevier. https://doi.org/10.1016/B978-0-12-809324-5.02867-4

Meinhofer, A., & Anglero-Diaz, Y. (2019). Trends in foster care entry among children removed from their homes because of parental drug use, 2000–2017. *JAMA Pediatrics, 173*(9), 881–883. https://doi.org/10.1001/jamapediatrics.2019.1738

Menschner, C., & Maul, A. (2016). *Key ingredients for successful trauma-informed care implementation.* https://www.samhsa.gov/sites/default/files/programs_ca mpaigns/childrens_mental_health/atc-whitepaper-040616.pdf

Meulewaeter, F., De Pauw, S., & Vanderplasschen, W. (2019). Mothering, substance use disorders and intergenerational trauma transmission: An attachment-based perspective. *Frontiers in Psychiatry, 10,* 728. https://doi.org/10.3389/fpsyt.2019.00728

National Human Genome Research Institute. (2023). *Definition of epigenetics.* https://www.genome.gov/genetics-glossary/Epigenetics

National Research Council (US) and Institute of Medicine (US) Committee on Integrating the Science of Early Childhood Development. (2000). *From neurons to neighborhoods: The science of early childhood development* (J. Shonkoff & D. Phillips, Eds.). National Academies Press. PMID: 25077268.

Norris, F., & Slone, L. (2007). The epidemiology of trauma and PTSD. In M Friedman, T. Keane, & P. Reswick (Eds.), *Handbook of PTSD: Science and practice* (pp. 78–98). Guilford Press.

Oei, J. (2018). Adult consequences of prenatal drug exposure. *Internal Medicine Journal, 48,* 25–31. https://doi.org/10.1111/imj.13658

Oei, J. L., Melhuish, E., Uebel, H., Azzam, N., Breen, C., Burns, L., Hilder, L., Bajuk, B., Abdel-Latif, M., Ward, M., Feller, J., Falconer, J., Clews, S., Eastwood, J., Li, A., & Wright, I. (2017). Neonatal Abstinence Syndrome and high school performance. *Pediatrics, 139*(2). https://doi.org/10.1542/peds.2016-2651

Osofsky, J. D., Osofsky, H. J., Frazer, A. L., Fields-Olivieri, M. A., Many, M., Selby, M., Holman, S., & Conrad, E. (2021). The importance of adverse childhood experiences during the perinatal period. *American Psychologist, 76*(2), 350–363. https://doi.org/10.1037/amp0000770

Owens, L., Terrell, S., Kane Low, L., Loder, C., Rhizal, D., Scheiman, L., & Seng, J. (2022). Universal precautions: The case for consistently trauma-informed reproductive healthcare. *American Journal of Obstetrics and Gynecology, 226*(5), 671–677. https://doi.org/10.1016/j.ajog.2021.08.012

Patrick, S. W., Barfield, W. D., Poindexter, B. B., Committee on Fetus and Newborn, & Committee on Substance Use and Prevention. (2020). Neonatal Opioid Withdrawal Syndrome. *Pediatrics, 146*(5). https://doi.org/10.1542/peds.2020-029074

Racine, N., Killam, T., & Madigan, S. (2019). Trauma-informed care as a universal precaution: Beyond the adverse childhood experiences questionnaire. *JAMA Pediatrics, 174*(1), 5–6. https://doi.org/10.1001/jamapediatrics.2019.3866

Rees, P., Stilwell, P., Bolton, C., Akillioglu, M., Carter, B., Gale, C., & Sutcliffe, A. (2020). Childhood health and educational outcomes after Neonatal Abstinence Syndrome: A systematic review and meta-analysis. *Journal of Pediatrics, 226,* 149–156. https://doi.org/10.1016/j.jpeds.2020.07.013

Reimer, V., & Sahagian, S. (2015). *The mother-blame game.* Demeter.

Robertson, M., & Lund, E. (2022). School-based speech-language pathologists' attitudes and knowledge about trauma-informed care. *Language, Speech and Hearing Services in Schools, 53*(4), 1117–1128. https://doi.org/10.1044/2022_LSHSS-21-00172

Robinson, A. (2018). Let's talk about stress: History of stress research. *Review of General Psychology, 22*(3), 334–342. https://doi.org/10.1037/gpr0000137

Rutter, A. (2021). The relevance of the adverse childhood experience international questionnaire to working children: Knowledge gaps and implications for policy makers. *Children, 8*(10), 897. https://doi.org/10.3390/children8100897

Schoon, I., & Melis, G. (2019). Intergenerational transmission of family adversity: Examining constellations of risk factors. *PLoS ONE, 14*(4). https://doi.org/10.1371/journal.pone.0214801

Seng, J., & Taylor, J. (2015). *Trauma-informed care in the perinatal period.* Dunedin Academic Press.

Shonkoff, J. P., Garner, A. S., Committee on Psychosocial Aspects of Child and Family Health, Committee on Early Childhood, Adoption, and Dependent Care, & Section on Developmental and Behavioral Pediatrics. (2012). The lifelong effects of early childhood adversity and toxic stress. *Pediatrics, 129*(1), 232–246. https://doi.org/10.1542/peds.2011-2663

Southwick, S., Bonanno, G., Masten, A., Panter-Brick, C., & Yehuda, R. (2014). Resilience definitions, theory, and challenges: Interdisciplinary perspectives. *European Journal of Psychotraumatology, 5.* https://doi.org/10.3402/ejpt.v5.25338

Stone, R. (2015). Pregnant women and substance use: Fear, stigma, and barriers to care. *Health & Justice, 3*(2), 1– 15. https://doi.org/10.1186/s40352-015-0015-5

Substance Abuse and Mental Health Services Administration (2014). *SAMHSA's concept of trauma and guidance for a trauma-informed approach.* HHS Publication No. (SMA) 14-4884. https://store.samhsa.gov/sites/default/files/d7/priv/sma14-4884.pdf

Tiffon, C. (2018). Nutrition and environmental epigenetics on human health and disease. *International Journal of Molecular Science, 19*(11), 3425. https://doi.org/10.3390/ijms19113425

Tonmyr, L., Lacroix, J., & Herbert, M. (2020). The public health issue of ACEs in Canada. In G. Asmundson & T. Afifi (Eds.), *Adverse childhood experiences: Using evidence to advance research, practice, policy, and prevention* (pp. 185–207). Academic Press.

Trauma Informed Oregon. (2023). *Six principles of trauma informed care.* https://traumainformedoregon.org/resources/new-to-trauma-informed-care/trauma-informed-care-principles/

United Nations Office on Drugs and Crime (2022). *World drug report.* https://www.unodc.org/unodc/data-and-analysis/world-drug-report-2022.html

Wachman, E., & Farrer, L. (2019). The genetics and epigenetics of Neonatal Abstinence Syndrome. *Seminars in Fetal and Neonatal Medicine, 24*(2), 105–110. https://doi.org/10.1016/j.siny.2019.01.002

Wastell, S., & White, D. (2017). *Blinded by science: The social implications of epigenetics and neuroscience.* Policy Press. https://doi.org/10.1177/0308575919867239

Yen, E., Gaddis, N., Jantzie, L., & Davis, J. M. (2023). A review of the genomics of Neonatal Abstinence Syndrome. *Frontiers in Genetics, 14,* 208. https://doi.10.3389/fgene.2023.1140400

Yeoh, S., Eastwood, J., Wright, I., Morton, R., Melhuish, E., Ward, M., & Oei, J. (2019). Cognitive and motor outcomes of children with prenatal opioid exposure. *JAMA Network Open*, 2(7). https://doi.org/10.1001/jamanetworko pen.2019.7025

Zhang, L., Mersky, J., Gruber, A., & Kim, J. (2022). Intergenerational transmission of parental adverse childhood experiences and children's outcomes: A scoping review. *Trauma, Violence and Abuse*, 24(5), 1–14. https://doi.org/10.1177/15248380221126186

6 Neonatal Opioid Withdrawal Syndrome

Feeding Recommendations for Infants and Children

Karen McQueen and Alison Thompson

6.1 Introduction

Adequate nutrition is imperative for the growth and development of newborns, infants, and children. For infants exposed to opioids during pregnancy, obtaining adequate nutrition can be challenging as infants may develop Neonatal Opioid Withdrawal Syndrome (NOWS), also referred to as Neonatal Abstinence Syndrome (NAS). As neonatal withdrawal typically affects the central nervous system, autonomic, respiratory, and gastrointestinal systems (Cheng et al., 2021), infants with NOWS are at increased risk for nutritional deficits due to feeding difficulties, diarrhea, dehydration, and weight loss (Favara et al., 2022; Nagy et al., 2023). Thus, the nutritional needs of opioid-exposed infants are of paramount importance in the newborn period. For infants and children post-NOWS, the promotion of optimal nutrition remains important for growth and development as opioid-exposed infants and children may be at risk for altered feeding behaviours. Thus, the aim of this chapter is to summarize the current evidence on infant feeding for infants with NOWS and for infants/children post-NOWS. Readers should note that we use the term NOWS to refer to infants who have been exposed to opioids in utero and are symptomatic of withdrawal; however, we also use the term NAS when referencing the works of authors who used the term NAS.

6.2 General Recommendations for Infant Nutrition

Human milk is recognized as the optimal source of nutrition for infants. National and international organizations recommend that healthy, term newborns are exclusively breastfed for the first 6 months of life (Meek et al., 2022; World Health Organization & United Nations Children's Fund [UNICEF], 2018). Nutrient-rich complementary foods, with particular attention to iron, should be introduced around 6 months of age,

DOI: 10.4324/9781003397267-6

with continued breastfeeding for up to 2 years and beyond. If an infant is not breastfed or weaned before 12 months of age, they should receive iron-fortified formula until one year. These recommendations are endorsed by health authorities nationally and internationally.

Breastfeeding is typically described by the quantity of breastmilk provided to the infant (e.g., any, partial, or exclusive) and the mode of feeding (e.g., breast, expressed milk, or both). "Breastfeeding" is defined as the transfer of human milk from the breast directly to the infant. Whereas, when infants are fed expressed breastmilk from the mother by bottle, cup, syringe, tube (or other methods), or through human milk banking, it is often referred to as human milk feeding or mother's milk feeding. Exclusive breastfeeding is defined as giving no other foods or fluids, including water, except vitamins and medicines; whereas partial breastfeeding or any breastfeeding refers to a combination of breastmilk feedings and additional fluids, and/or solids (Bogen & Whalen, 2019).

6.3 Benefits of Breastfeeding

Breastfeeding is a complex biological process that uniquely supports infant growth and development through the provision of nutrients and bioactive compounds between the mother and infant (Victora et al., 2016). There is strong evidence highlighting the benefits for infants, mothers, and society. Breastmilk is the ideal food for infants as it is safe, clean, and contains antibodies to protect against many common illnesses (World Health Organization & United Nations Children's Fund [UNICEF], 2018). Breastmilk is uniquely adapted to support infant growth, health, and maturation (Victora et al., 2016) as it provides all the energy and nutrients that infants require for the first 6 months of life.

6.3.1 Benefits of Breastfeeding for Infants With NOWS/NAS

There are additional compelling advantages for breastfeeding for mother–infant dyads impacted by opioid use during pregnancy (Bogen & Whalen, 2019). Various studies have evaluated the relationship between infant feeding methods and NAS outcomes with consistent findings supporting the benefits of breastfeeding for infants with NAS (Chu et al., 2022; McQueen et al., 2019). In a systematic review of 8 studies, the researchers found that among newborns exposed to methadone in utero (n = 5 studies), breastfeeding was associated with a decreased incidence and duration of pharmacologic treatment, shorter hospital length of stay, and decreased severity of NAS symptoms (McQueen et al., 2019). They also found the onset of withdrawal symptoms also delayed in infants who received breastmilk. Similarly, in a review by Chu and colleagues (2022), which included a meta-analysis, breastfeeding reduced initiation of pharmacologic treatment, duration of pharmacologic treatment, and length of stay.

From a clinical perspective these findings are important as breastfeeding provides infants with NOWS optimal nutrition while simultaneously decreasing the severity of NOWS symptomatology. Reduced severity of symptoms decreases distress in newborns, the need for pharmacologic treatment, length of pharmacologic treatment, and length of hospital stay (Chu et al., 2022). Given that infants with NAS have one of the longest lengths of stay of any pediatric disorder, breastfeeding may also assist to decrease healthcare expenditures (Grossman & Berkwitt, 2019). Of additional importance in mitigating symptoms of NOWS is the potential benefits to mothers. From a psychosocial perspective, breastfeeding may help to facilitate mother–infant attachment, which has sometimes been difficult for mothers who have an infant with NOWS (Short et al., 2021).

6.4 Mechanism of Action of Breastfeeding and NOWS

The process by which breastfeeding leads to reduced NOWS symptomology is not fully understood. However, there are a few plausible explanations that support the relationship between breastfeeding and reduced NOWS symptoms, including the composition of breastmilk and the act of breastfeeding.

6.4.1 Composition of Breastmilk

It is widely accepted that medications ingested by the mother pass into the breastmilk of the mother via passive diffusion. Evidence has identified that both methadone and buprenorphine are secreted into the breastmilk in small amounts (Patrick et al., 2020). While the amounts of the medication in breastmilk are small, it may be sufficient to decrease the severity of NOWS symptoms, but not completely prevent NOWS symptoms. A dose–response has also been identified with a reduction in NAS symptoms among infants who were exclusively/highly breastfed compared to those who were partially breastfed (McQueen et al., 2019). Furthermore, breastmilk is more easily digested and is emptied by the stomach and intestines more quickly than formula (Bogen & Whalen, 2019). The increased digestion of breastmilk may reduce some of the gastrointestinal symptoms of NAS such as vomiting and diarrhea that are included in NAS scoring tools.

6.4.2 The Act of Breastfeeding

The act of breastfeeding with skin-to-skin contact, frequent feedings, and maternal presence may also help to comfort and soothe infants, which helps to reduce the severity of NOWS symptoms.

While this has been a plausible explanation for several years, there has been a more recent emphasis on nonpharmacological interventions, such as breastfeeding, as a first-line treatment for opioid-exposed infants (Grossman & Berkwitt, 2019; MacVicar et al., 2018).

6.5 Infant Feeding Recommendation and NOWS

The Academy of Breastfeeding Medicine (ABM) (Reece-Stremtan & Marinelli, 2015) and the American Academy of Pediatrics (AAP) (Meek et al., 2022) strongly endorse breastfeeding and the use of a mother's own milk for infants with NAS and/or at risk for NAS, whose mothers are stable on opioid substitution treatment (e.g., methadone or buprenorphine), provided they do not have any contraindications to breastfeeding (see below for contraindications). For mothers who do not want to feed their infant directly from the breast, breastmilk expression should be encouraged to offer the infant their mother's milk via a bottle or alternate feeding method (Taylor & Maguire, 2020). When breastfeeding is contraindicated or is not the preferred method of feeding, iron-rich infant formula should be provided until 1 year of age (Canadian Paediatric Society, 2023; Fewtrell et al., 2017).

6.5.1 Infant Feeding Decision

The decision regarding the infant feeding method should be made by the mother and the multi-disciplinary care team, based on a comprehensive assessment. The Academy of Breastfeeding Medicine (ABM) has a protocol to guide clinicians in deciding which mothers should be encouraged to breastfeed and when breastfeeding is contraindicated (Reece-Stremtan & Marinelli, 2015), as breastfeeding is not universally recommended for all substance-exposed infants. Breastfeeding is recommended for mothers who are stable on opioid agonists, who are not using illicit drugs, and who have no contraindications to breastfeeding.

While evidence indicates that opioid-exposed infants and their mothers with substance use disorders can benefit from breastfeeding, caution should be encouraged in promoting breastfeeding if the risks outweigh the benefits. Caution regarding breastfeeding should be considered for individuals who are not engaged in prenatal care, not engaged in treatment, or have no plans for treatment; have a positive urine toxicology screen for substances other than marijuana; have relapsed; exhibit behaviors or indicators of active use; and have chronic alcohol use (Reece-Stremtan & Marinelli, 2015). Education and ongoing assessment of the risks versus benefits of breastfeeding should be considered in situations such as relapse, use of other prescription medications not compatible with lactation, and lack of support systems (Holmes et al., 2017).

6.5.2 Contraindications to Breastfeeding

According to the Centers for Disease Control and Prevention (CDC), there are exceptions when breastfeeding or providing human milk is contraindicated (CDC, 2023). Mothers should be counselled *not* to breastfeed or feed expressed breastmilk to their infants in the following situations:

- Infant is diagnosed with galactosemia
- Mother has HIV, is not on antiretroviral therapy, and/or does not have a suppressed viral load during pregnancy, delivery, and postpartum
- Mother is infected with human T-cell lymphotropic virus
- Mother is using an illicit drug(s), such as opioids, phencyclidine (PCP), or cocaine (Note: For mothers who discontinue illicit opioids or other substances and are on stable methadone or buprenorphine maintenance therapy, breastfeeding should be encouraged.)
- Mother has suspected or confirmed Ebola virus disease

In certain situations, mothers may have to temporarily stop breastfeeding (e.g., active herpes lesion of the breast, hepatitis C positive with cracked or bleeding nipples) and/or providing expressed breastmilk to their infants (CDC, 2023; Patrick et al., 2020). If in doubt, consultation with a physician about the safety of breastfeeding should be obtained. Additional sources of information regarding the safety of breastfeeding may be found on various reputable websites, such as the United States National Library of Health, National Institute of Child Health and Human Development (LactMedR®) (https://www.ncbi.nlm.nih.gov/books/NBK501922/) and the Association for the Promotion of and Scientific and Cultural Research into Breastfeeding: E-lactancia (http://e-lactancia.org/).

6.6 Barriers to Breastfeeding

While breastfeeding has been associated with positive outcomes for infants with NOWS, breastfeeding rates among this population are low compared to the rates of breastfeeding among the general population (e.g., non-substance users) (Ryan et al., 2019). Attention to the barriers affecting breastfeeding is required to better support mothers who want to breast-feed and potentially decrease and/or mitigate the symptoms of NOWS.

6.6.1 NOWS Symptomatology

The signs of NOWS can present numerous barriers to establishing and maintaining breastfeeding. Excessive sucking, hyperirritability, and vomiting have been associated with poor feeding, which can put the infant at risk for increased weight loss (Nagy et al., 2023). Similarly, many infants with NAS have difficulty with the coordination of sucking, swallowing, and breathing (McGlothen-Bell et al., 2020), which can create challenges with positioning, latching, and feeding.

6.6.2 Separation of Mother and Infant

Neonates with NOWS are more likely to be separated from their mothers during their hospital stay and after discharge, which can affect breastfeeding, maternal–infant bonding, family dynamics, and long-term child health and safety (Patrick et al., 2020). Most treatment guidelines recommend nonpharmacologic care as the first line of treatment; however, most Neonatal Intensive Care Units (NICUs) do not have the physical capacity to allow parents to room-in with their newborns and often struggle to provide effective nonpharmacologic care (Cheng et al., 2021).

6.6.3 Attitudes and Stigma

Mothers who have an infant with NAS often report feelings of guilt and distress due to their infants in utero exposures and symptomatology (Cleveland et al., 2016). Many also report feeling stigmatized by healthcare providers, which can have a profound impact on the ability of mothers and healthcare providers to establish collaborative relationships (MacVicar et al., 2018). Mothers with a substance use history may have more difficulty interacting with nurses and asking for assistance in healthcare settings as some nurses are judgmental towards women who have used opiates during pregnancy.

6.6.4 Lack of Information/Breastfeeding Promotion

Lack of information or inconsistent promotion of breastfeeding by healthcare professionals has been frequently identified as a barrier to breastfeeding (Holmes et al., 2017). Historically breastfeeding among mothers on opioid replacement treatment was not encouraged and many were told they should not breastfeed by family, friends, and healthcare providers. Thus, a lack of encouragement to breastfeed from healthcare providers may be found among those who are unaware of the benefits of breastfeeding for mothers on opioid replacement therapy and have concerns about neonatal sedation or adverse effects (MacVicar et al., 2018).

6.6.5 Lack of Knowledge/Resources

Many mothers report a lack of knowledge regarding the benefits and recommendations for breastfeeding opioid-exposed infants (Short et al., 2021). Physical and mental health, lack of confidence, and social influence may also impact the decision to breastfeed (Crook & Brandon, 2017). Many opioid-dependent pregnant women are socioeconomically disadvantaged (MacVicar et al., 2018) and may lack resources to go to and from the hospital to breastfeed and pay for parking and childcare if the length of stay is prolonged. Additionally, women with an opioid use disorder often have higher rates of trauma, including sexual trauma, which affect breastfeeding decisions (Patrick et al., 2020)

6.7 Infant Feeding of Opioid-Exposed Infants

Feeding is a complex task for young infants and even more so among infants who have been exposed to opioids in utero. Findings from an integrative review identified feeding as a major challenge that requires targeted and individualized interventions (McGlothen-Bell et al., 2020). Furthermore, the ability of the infant to feed independently to achieve adequate nutrition is paramount as it is typically a criterion for discharge (Nagy et al., 2023). However, despite the evidence regarding infant feeding challenges among this population, there is relatively little information regarding best practices for feeding opioid-exposed infants. More research on this topic is needed. Thus, the strategies to support infant feeding in this section are primarily from the general infant feeding literature, with some information from the NOWS and/or NICU literature incorporated. The following strategies serve as information for practitioners and families. However, institutional guidelines and recommendations from the multi-disciplinary care team should be followed.

6.7.1 Prenatal Strategies to Support Mothers/Parents

6.7.1.1 Prenatal Education

As the choice of infant feeding method for a pregnant woman with a history of past or current substance use can be challenging, the discussion regarding infant feeding should be initiated in the prenatal period (Short et al., 2021). Prenatal encounters provide an opportunity for healthcare providers to assess, educate, and address concerns about NOWS and infant feeding. The prenatal visits can provide an opportunity for healthcare providers to provide much-needed support to the family before the birth of the infant (Patrick et al., 2020).

6.7.1.2 Anticipatory Guidance for Families

Parents should be provided with anticipatory guidance regarding the treatment for NAS and potential challenges with infant feeding (Maguire et al., 2015). Parents should be aware that poor feeding is common among infants with NOWS, which can put infants at risk for poor weight gain and lengthier hospital stays. This anticipatory guidance may in turn help develop realistic expectations regarding the newborn transition.

6.7.2 Infant Feeding In Hospital and Beyond

6.7.2.1 Provision of Skin-to-Skin Contact

Direct skin-to-skin contact is encouraged for healthy newborns at birth and beyond as it has positive effects on mothers and infants. Benefits include increased rates of breastfeeding initiation and exclusivity, more rapid mother–infant interaction, improved thermoregulation, reduced maternal and newborn stress reactivity/salivary cortisol levels, and reduced pain response in newborns (Cleveland et al., 2017).

Box 6.1

When newborns are placed skin-to-skin at birth, regular assessments of the infant should be performed for skin color, breathing effort and rate, oxygen saturation, and temperature.

6.7.2.2 Responsive Feeding

Parents intrinsically understand the importance of feeding their infant, but the stress of caregiving can undermine parents' confidence in this important task. Parents may experience worry or uncertainty about how often and how much they are feeding their infant (DiTomasso et al., 2022). As a result, parents often crave objective indicators that their infants' nutritional needs are being adequately met. In addition, parenting books have historically recommended feeding babies on a predetermined and consistent schedule – including controlling the frequency, duration, and time between feedings. Therefore, scheduled feedings, measured amounts of formula, or specific durations of feeding may be misconstrued as markers of successful feeding and infant care (Harries & Brown, 2019). In contrast, responsive feeding is based on supporting parents to recognize and respond appropriately to infant cues for hunger and satiety. Responsive feeding is very similar to cue-based feeding (Shaker, 2013) and enables parents to ensure they are feeding their infant when they are hungry and providing enough nutrition to satisfy them.

Parents should be taught signs of infant readiness such as: making sucking movements or opening of mouth, rooting (turning head towards contact with cheek or face and opening mouth), bringing hands towards mouth, making fists or having clenched hands over stomach or chest, and increased physical movements like bending of arms or legs (American Academy of Pediatrics, 2023). General recommendations for responsive infant feeding suggest a baby should be offered the breast or bottle when they begin to demonstrate readiness cues. This is particularly important for infants with NOWS as best practice for affected infants is to not disrupt the infant who is calm and at rest unless medically indicated – meaning a sleeping infant should not be awakened for scheduled feedings (Grossman & Berkwitt, 2019). Infant crying is a late sign of hunger and should be avoided if possible as infants can become frantic, making latching more difficult. Infants who display late signs of hunger and are distressed may need to be consoled before initiating a feed. All parents need support to recognize and understand the specific cues their infant demonstrates.

Parents of infants with NOWS may need additional support because cues can be more difficult to distinguish with infants who can be restless and difficult to console. For example, common NAS signs such as yawning, increased muscle tone, high-pitched crying, and excessive sucking (Grossman & Berkwitt, 2019) may be misinterpreted as readiness cues, which can be confusing for parents. Some evidence suggests that feeding patterns are most disrupted and symptomatology most problematic for infants with prenatal opioid exposure during the first month of life and may thereafter start to improve (McGlothen-Bell et al., 2020; Taylor & Maguire, 2020).

Parents need reassurance that learning their babies' cues will take time. Physical contact within the mother–infant dyad should be encouraged as it has been associated with increased responsiveness to early feeding cues, meaning that promoting skin-to skin contact and other forms of physical contact such as babywearing may help parents become attuned to their infants' cues (Little et al., 2018). In addition, paying attention to and adjusting the physical environment of feeding infants may help minimize distress and allow parents to recognize their infant's cues more easily. For example, creating a calm, quiet, and slightly darkened physical space, and implementing strategies to decrease overstimulation, such as swaddling or feeding the infant facing away from the parent, may be helpful for infants with NOWS (Maguire et al., 2018). Conversely, maternal preoccupation during feeds and a history of maternal trauma were identified as barriers to dyadic reciprocity and responsive feeding (Messina et al., 2020). Hospital feeding regimens with a focus on feeding frequency and milk volume are further barriers to the development of responsive feeding patterns (Redsell et al., 2021).

6.7.2.3 Frequency of Feeding

Infant feeding patterns vary as each mother–infant dyad is unique. Typically, newborn infants will feed between 8 and 12 times in 24 hours. Patterns of infant feeding for the first weeks of life are similar between infants taking formula or human milk and those fed by bottle or at the breast. Some infants will feed every 2 to 3 hours, whereas others will cluster feed (several feedings in a row) and then sleep for a longer period of time. Healthcare providers should be cautious to not implicitly or explicitly endorse scheduled feedings since adhering to rigid scheduling will likely result in worsening withdrawal for infants with NOWS, particularly for those fed their mother's milk.

6.7.2.4 Duration of Feeding

The duration of feedings can be highly variable. Some infants can be very efficient at the breast or bottle and get sufficient nutrition in a short time. Other infants who are sleepy at the breast may take much longer to feed. The average time for breastfeeding in the newborn period is 30 to 40 minutes per feeding. Bottle-feeding sessions may be a similar duration. It is important to teach mothers signs when the infant is actively feeding versus finished feedings so that the feeding is guided by the infant and not the clock (e.g., time). Some infants with NOWS may exhibit a strong (although potentially dis-coordinated) suck reflex and benefit from a slow-flow nipple during bottle-feeding to minimize the risk of vomiting or regurgitation associated with rapid feeding (Maguire et al., 2018). Smaller, more frequent feeding sessions may help infants develop a circadian rhythm and are typically better tolerated by infants with NAS-related gastrointestinal symptoms (Ryan et al., 2019). The amount of time the infant spends at the breast is not a reliable indicator of the amount of milk the infant receives as some feeding can be non-nutritive sucking. Similarly, parents feeding their infant with a bottle should observe infant cues indicating satiety, rather than the amount of formula consumed.

6.7.2.5 Satiety Cues

Similar to the need for parents to understand and respond to readiness and hunger cues, parents should also learn satiety cues to recognize when an infant is finished feeding. Satiety signs for infants include turning the head away from the breast or bottle, allowing the nipple to fall from the mouth, stopping sucking, closing the mouth, and relaxing of hands. Signs of sufficient milk intake can also include the infant's output (urine and stool) and weight loss/gain. Careful attention to satiety cues may help prevent overfeeding and the development of maladaptive feeding behaviours that can persist beyond infancy and may predispose children to obesity (Redsell et al., 2021). Although the process of learning infant cues may be more complex for parents of infants with NOWS, the responsive approach to soothing, feeding, and nutrition can build useful skills and perspectives for parents past infancy as their child begins complementary feeding, and beyond (Redsell et al., 2021).

6.7.2.6 Parental Presence/Rooming-In

Parental presence/rooming-in should be encouraged for infants with NOWS as parents who are continuously present are more attentive to the needs of their infants, better able to identify feeding cues early, and initiate nonpharmacologic care such as swaddling and cue-based feedings (MacMillan et al., 2018). Several advantages have also been associated with rooming-in and improved rates of breastfeeding among opioid-exposed infants (Grossman & Berkwitt, 2019). When parents room-in they are able to provide frequent skin-to-skin contact and breastfeed on demand, which helps establish milk supply (Meek et al., 2022). Parents who are involved in their infant's plan of care have also been found to experience improved health outcomes including decreased parental stress and increased attachment and relationships with healthcare providers (MacVicar et al., 2018). In cases where parental presence is not possible, an alternative caregiver may be designated to fulfill the caregiver role (e.g., family member, adoptive or foster parent) to ensure continuous newborn-centered care.

6.7.2.7 Pacifiers

Pacifier use is often part of standard care for infants with NOWS (Ryan et al., 2019) as non-nutritive sucking is beneficial in decreasing agitation (Taylor & Maguire, 2020). However, pacifier use among breastfeeding newborns has often been discouraged due to concerns regarding its association with decreased rates of breastfeeding. Healthcare providers should be knowledgeable about the benefits of pacifier use for infants with NOWS and strategies to avoid interruption of exclusive breastfeeding unless medically indicated.

6.7.2.8 Infant Weight

In-hospital weight monitoring is usually done daily until a stable pattern of weight gain has been established. After discharge, most infants can be weighed weekly or less often as they demonstrate continued growth with no new or worsening symptoms such as diarrhea, vomiting, inconsolability, or feeding difficulties.

6.7.2.9 Newborn Follow-Up

Early follow-up is recommended after discharge to assess infant growth and weight (Grossman & Berkwitt, 2019). Where available, home-based support (Patrick et al., 2020) may be provided to monitor weight and infant feeding as part of comprehensive care of infants with NOWS.

6.8 Strategies to Support Breastfeeding

Breastfeeding support (e.g., education, counseling, hands-on assistance) in the early days and weeks postpartum can be influential in improving breastfeeding duration and exclusivity (McFadden et al., 2017). As breastfeeding can be challenging, new mothers require support to initiate, maintain, and manage common breastfeeding difficulties. This also includes recognizing cues of effective milk transfer, infant satiety, and when additional support may be warranted. Access to timely, skilled breastfeeding support can assist mothers to overcome breastfeeding difficulties, increases confidence in the ability to breastfeed, and dispels myths about the need to add more foods to meet the newborn's nutritional needs (Brockway et al., 2017; McFadden et al., 2017).

6.8.1 Early Initiation of Infant Feeding

Breastfeeding initiation is recommended within the first hour of birth for healthy, term newborns. Early breastfeeding provides immunological benefits from the colostrum, assists with thermoregulation, passage of meconium, and stimulation of milk supply, and prevents hypoglycemia. For infants who have been exposed to opioids, early initiation of breastfeeding is important to potentially mitigate the signs of NOWS. It also provides an opportunity for infants and mothers to learn how to establish infant feeding (e.g., breastfeeding or bottle-feeding) before the development of

NOWS symptoms. Signs of NOWS from opioids with longer half-lives, such as methadone and buprenorphine, typically don't develop until 36 to 48 hours after birth, which provides an opportunity for infant feeding to become established.

When feeding at the breast is not possible, feeding expressed breastmilk from the infant's mother may be the next best alternative (Bogen & Whalen, 2019). For mothers who want to feed their infants expressed breastmilk, pumping should be initiated early (preferably within 6 hours of birth) to stimulate milk production (Enger & Hurst, 2023). Expression by hand or pump should occur at least 8–10 times per 24 hours, including overnight. The use of a hospital-grade double pump may assist in establishing and maintaining the milk supply. The safe storage and handling of mother's milk is important and should follow recommended guidelines.

6.8.2 Positioning and Latching

New mothers often need assistance to establish breastfeeding in the early postpartum period. Various positions are encouraged for breastfeeding (cradle hold, football hold, cross-cradle hold) based on mother and infant preferences. For infants with NAS, multiple techniques can be used in an attempt to calm the infant for feeding (Taylor & Maguire, 2020). As infants respond differently, it is important to determine what techniques work best for each infant.

6.8.3 Indicators of Effective Breastfeeding

One of the biggest concerns new mothers have regarding breastfeeding is whether the infant is receiving sufficient breastmilk. This may be enhanced among mothers with an infant with NOWS as the infant may not appear to be satisfied after feeding. Careful evaluation of the infant's breastfeeding (e.g., latch, audible swallowing) and output is required. The Best Start Resource "Signs that Feeding Is Going Well" (Best Start Health Nexus, 2020) is often used as an example of intake and output for healthy, term newborns. While this can be a helpful resource to guide families, NOWS signs such as loose, watery stools may make the assessment of urine output difficult. Likewise, assessment of satiety after a feed can be difficult to determine.

6.8.4 Referral to Lactation Consultant

Lactation consultants should be offered (if available) to assist in establishing breastfeeding (Grossman & Berkwitt, 2019) and continue after discharge (Patrick et al., 2020). Breastfeeding support is important for mothers who want to breastfeed their infant and are at high risk for feeding difficulties due to NOWS (Nagy et al., 2023).

6.8.5 Supplementing Breastfeeding

Supplementing is generally not recommended for healthy, term infants unless medically indicated. However, for infants with NOWS, supplementation to maintain weight/caloric intake may be required. Early supplementation with high-calorie formula or human milk fortifiers should be considered if there are concerns regarding the infant's weight loss (Grossman & Berkwitt, 2019). Infants losing a substantial amount of weight and/or having feeding difficulties (e.g., dis-coordinated suck, difficulty latching) may benefit from supplemental feedings with expressed breastmilk, formula, or human milk fortifier (Bogen et al., 2018).

6.8.6 Human Milk Fortification

Human milk fortifiers (HMFs) are liquid or powder products that are mixed with expressed human milk to increase the nutritional composition. HMFs are typically made from either cow's milk–based protein or from concentrated donated human milk. HMFs are often used for preterm and very-low-birth-weight infants who need additional nutrients to support growth. Similarly, some infants with NOWS may also benefit from HMFs to mitigate weight loss. Parents who are using expressed or donated human milk for infant feeding may be advised by the medical team to begin adding HMFs if weight gain is slow or the infant displays concerning weight loss. HMFs are primarily used while the infant remains in hospital and weight can be closely monitored. HMFs may be continued for a period of time when infants require higher nutritional intake to maintain their weight progression. Once the infant has shown evidence of weight and feeding stabilization, HMFs are often discontinued for home discharge.

6.9 Strategies to Support Formula Feeding

Feeding support in the postpartum period is equally important for families who are unable or elect not to breastfeed. Feelings of maternal guilt and shame related to use of infant formula are associated with judgmental attitudes or encounters with healthcare professionals (Jackson et al., 2021). Formula feeding also requires parental commitment to learning and responding to infant cues, which can be more difficult to discern with infants affected by NOWS. Healthcare professionals' support for families and knowledge of best practices regarding formula feeding can optimize nutrition, growth, and development.

6.9.1 Formula Choices

Parents who feed their infant either partially or completely with formula are faced with a myriad of choices about formula brands, types, and forms. Parents want to provide optimal nutrition and health benefits for their child while most must also weigh the additional factors of cost, ease, and availability when deciding which infant formula to use. Physical effects such as diarrhea, vomiting, and a general hypermetabolic state mean that infants with NOWS are at higher risk for weight loss (Kaplan et al., 2020). Given the large number of infant feeding formulas available, research has begun exploring whether specialized formulas can help decrease gastrointestinal symptoms, feeding intolerance, and fussiness associated with NOWS. Findings indicate that low lactose and lactose-free formulas did not decrease the length of hospital stay, length of treatment, or weight loss for infants with NAS (Alsaleem et al., 2021; Lembeck et al., 2021). In contrast, high-calorie infant formula (ranging from 22 to 24kcal/oz) may be beneficial to decrease weight loss, treatment failure, and length of hospital stay (Bogen et al., 2018; Kaplan et al., 2020). One of the potential benefits of high-calorie formula for infants with NOWS is the ability to deliver a smaller volume of formula which may decrease risk of vomiting and diarrhea.

Currently, there is no recommendation for a specialized formula type for infants with NOWS; instead, formula is chosen based on infant symptoms and tolerability. Standard cow's milk–based formula is most commonly used for term infants. Although each brand has its own formulation and differences in tolerability occur, all standard infant formulas are designed to support normal growth and development of the newborn. In addition, standard formulas are fortified with iron to prevent deficiency, and most have added fatty acids (DHA & ARA) to support early eye and brain development. Continuation with one brand and type of formula is commonplace for infants unless the product is unavailable or a decision is made to transition to a new product. When changing types or brands, a period of gradual transition (if possible) may minimize the potential for gastrointestinal upset such as altered stool frequency and consistency.

6.9.2 Formula Preparation

In addition to brand and type, infant formula comes in a range of forms such as ready-to-feed, liquid concentrate, and powder. The ready-to-feed form is often made available to parents in the hospital and only requires parents to add a nipple or pour the container contents into a prepared bottle with a nipple. Ready-to-feed formula is available in a range of container/bottle sizes and is convenient and easy to use for parents, particularly in the first days or weeks following birth. Cost is the most common limiting factor for prolonged use of this form, which is often more than three times the amount per ounce as powder concentrate. Powder concentrate is the cheapest form of infant formula, with liquid concentrate being in the middle of the cost continuum between ready-to-feed and powder concentrate. Both liquid and powdered concentrates require dilution with water prior to feeding. Preparation of infant formula should begin with the parents washing their hands and the workspace thoroughly with soap and water. All reusable bottles, nipples, caps, rings, and utensils should be washed and sterilized prior to each use. Water used for dilution should be from a clean, safe source and be boiled for 2 minutes and cooled before use. More rigorous preparation directions may be recommended for infants younger than 2 months or those with weakened immune systems (Centers for Disease Control and Prevention, 2023). Proportions for dilution vary between powder and liquid concentrate and should be noted on the directions for each product. Parents using formula should be encouraged to double-check all dilution directions to avoid errors such as diluting ready-to-use formula, accidentally feeding undiluted liquid concentrate, or improper dilution of the concentrate. Prepared infant formula can be safely stored in the fridge for 24 hours. After feeding the infant, any unused formula in the bottle should be discarded rather than returned to the fridge (Centers for Disease Control and Prevention, 2023).

6.10 Vitamin D Supplement

Vitamin D supplementation is recommended for infants after birth. Current recommendations indicate that all infants 12 months of age and younger should receive a supplement of 400IU daily (Porto & Abu-Alreesh, 2022). For infants who consume formula, supplementation should continue until the baby drinks at least 32 ounces of formula daily. For infants fed human milk, supplementation should continue to at least 12 months of age and until the child's diet contains a variety of vitamin D–rich foods. Older infants and toddlers aged 12 months and over require at least 600IU of vitamin D daily, and if their diet does not provide adequate sources of vitamin D–rich foods, supplementation should continue (Porto & Abu-Alreesh, 2022). Infants and children whose mothers did not have adequate levels of vitamin D, who have darker skin, whose skin may be covered with clothing or sunscreen most of the time, or who live in communities where vitamin D deficiency is prevalent are at higher risk for vitamin D deficiency (Canadian Paediatric Society, 2021). Vitamin D supplementation is an important topic for family education and support, since research has found that less than 40% of infants in the United States meet the recommended daily intake of vitamin D (Simon & Ahrens, 2020).

A prescription for vitamin D is not required but may be offered to families to emphasize the importance and may increase the rate of supplementation (Le, 2019). Vitamin D is available in liquid form for infants with concentrations varying by product; thus directions for dosing should be verified before administration.

6.11 Complementary Feeding

Complementary feeding refers to the period of transition when an infant is introduced to solid foods while gradually decreasing their intake of human milk or formula. Principles of the responsive feeding approach recommended for early infancy remain relevant for older infants as they transition from liquid nutrition. The shift from a milk-based diet to include solids with a variety of tastes and textures is an important period for the development of healthy eating skills that can last throughout childhood and adolescence. Specifically, responsive feeding for both milk-based and complementary diets is thought to promote healthy eating habits and positive weight outcomes, with the potential to decrease the risk of obesity (Redsell et al., 2021).

Introduction of complementary foods is typically recommended after the age of 4 months and not beyond 6 months (Fewtrell et al., 2017). Infant cues for readiness to add complementary foods include ability to sit up independently with steady head control, ability to pick up objects and move towards or into mouth, demonstrating interest in mealtimes and other people eating, and being hungry between feedings. Initially, the infant's nutritional needs continue to be met with a milk-based diet, while increasing the number of times each day that complementary foods are offered (Canadian Paediatric Society, 2023). Foods with a range of tastes and textures should gradually be included in the child's diet, with lumpy textures being offered no later than 9 months of age (Canadian Paediatric Society, 2023). Given the potential for infants with NOWS to demonstrate hyperreactivity to stimuli and challenges with coordination of suck, swallow, and breathe, support for safe feeding practices and a focus on textural variety may be helpful during the transition to complementary feeding. Parents can be encouraged to offer finger foods that allow for self-feeding, provide repeated exposures to different tastes and textures, and avoid pressuring or coercing an infant during feeding. Lastly, parents can also be supported to maintain a responsive feeding approach that avoids the use of food as a reward or feeding for comfort (D'Auria et al., 2020). Iron-rich foods such as meat and iron-fortified foods offered multiple times daily may decrease the risk of iron-deficiency anemia. Furthermore, introduction to cow's milk should be delayed until 12 months of age (Canadian Paediatric Society, 2023; Fewtrell et al., 2017).

6.12 Nutrition and Feeding Beyond Early Infancy

Although there is significant evidence exploring the symptoms and outcomes associated with NOWS, a clear understanding of the long-term effects of the condition has been difficult to generate. Research examining the long-term follow-up for families of an opioid-exposed infant has begun but remains complicated due to the influence of poly-substance use, institutional variations in care, biological variables, social and physical environments, parenting, and many more factors (Conradt et al., 2019; Larson et al., 2019). Evidence suggests that babies of opioid-dependent mothers may experience adverse neurodevelopmental effects until at least middle childhood (Lee et al., 2020). Additional challenges beyond the early infancy period may be hypothesized to include ongoing hypersensitivity to stimuli and motor discoordination potentially affecting speech, feeding, nutrition, and respiration.

Future research about the long-term outcomes for opioid-exposed babies is urgently needed given the significant amount of opioid use amongst child-bearing individuals (Conradt et al., 2019). In the absence of specific evidence for long-term strategies about how best to care for infants and families affected by opioid use, an overarching principle of multi-disciplinary, long-term support is reasonable. Despite the many questions that remain unanswered, it is most likely that babies exposed to opiates will have the potential to thrive when their families are well supported at every stage (Larson et al., 2019). Contributions from a variety of health professions, including (but not limited to) speech-language therapy, occupational therapy, physical therapy, social work, psychology, and dietetics, may be needed to support families with an opioid-exposed infant throughout the childhood years. Lastly, a lens of long-term care rather than episodic or acute intervention may be most appropriate as we learn more about the sequelae of opioid exposure for infants and children.

6.13 Summary

This chapter describes the complexity surrounding infant feeding among infants with NOWS. In particular, infants with NOWS are at risk for poor feeding, increased weight loss, and extended hospital length of stay. The literature is further summarized regarding the benefits of breastfeeding for infants and families, the recommendations and contraindications for breastfeeding, challenges of breastfeeding with NOWS, and strategies to support breastfeeding. Overall, we emphasize that breastfeeding has unequivocal advantages for newborns, which may be further enhanced for infants with NOWS. However, breastfeeding is not universally recommended with NOWS and there are several factors that need to be considered for women who use substances and their opioid-exposed newborns. Thus, the decision of infant feeding method should be based on maternal choice in collaboration with the care team. For families who cannot breastfeed or select to formula feed, best practices regarding formula feeding should be implemented to promote optimal nutrition and growth and development. We also stress the importance of the family and the multi-disciplinary team in the care of feeding the opioid-exposed infant. Optimally, the support provided to the family should begin during pregnancy and extend past hospital discharge.

References

Alsaleem, M., Dusin, J., & Akangire, G. (2021). Effect of low lactose formula on the short-term outcomes of Neonatal Abstinence Syndrome: A systematic review. *Global Pediatric Health, 8.* https://doi.org/10.1177/2333794X211035258

American Academy of Pediatrics. (2023, April 28). *Is your baby hungry or full? Responsive feeding explained.* HealthyChildren.Org. https://www.healthychildren.org/English/ages-stages/baby/feeding-nutrition/Pages/Is-Your-Baby-Hungry-or-Full-Responsive-Feeding-Explained.aspx

Best Start Health Nexus. (2020). *Signs that feeding is going well.* https://resources.beststart.org/wp-content/uploads/2018/11/B02-E.pdf

Bogen, D. L., Hanusa, B. H., Baker, R., Medoff-Cooper, B., & Cohlan, B. (2018). Randomized clinical trial of standard- versus high-calorie formula for methadone-exposed infants: A feasibility study. *Hospital Pediatrics, 8*(1), 7–14. https://doi.org/10.1542/hpeds.2017-0114

Bogen, D. L., & Whalen, B. L. (2019). Breastmilk feeding for mothers and infants with opioid exposure: What is best? *Seminars in Fetal and Neonatal Medicine, 24*(2), 95–104. https://doi.org/10.1016/j.siny.2019.01.001

Brockway, M., Benzies, K., & Hayden, KA. (2017). Interventions to improve breastfeeding self-efficacy and resultant breastfeeding rates: A systematic review and meta-analysis. *Journal of Human Lactation, 33*(3), 489–499. https://doi.org/10.1177/0890334417707957

Canadian Paediatric Society. (2021, July). *Vitamin D.* https://caringforkids.cps.ca/handouts/pregnancy-and-babies/vitamin_d

Canadian Paediatric Society. (2023, February 24). *Nutrition for healthy term infants, six to 24 months: An overview.* https://cps.ca/en/documents/position/nutrition-healthy-term-infants-6-to-24-months

Centers for Disease Control and Prevention. (2023, May 19). *Infant formula preparation and storage.* https://www.cdc.gov/nutrition/infantandtoddlernutrition/formula-feeding/infant-formula-preparation-and-storage.html

Cheng, F., McMillan, C., Morrison, A., Berkwitt, A., & Grossman, M. (2021). Neonatal Abstinence Syndrome: Management advances and therapeutic approaches. *Current Addiction Reports, 8*(4), 595–604. https://doi.org/10.1007/s40429-021-00387-3

Chu, L., McGrath, J. M., Qiao, J., Brownell, E., Recto, P., Cleveland, L. M., Lopez, E., Gelfond, J., Crawford, A., & McGlothen-Bell, K. (2022). A meta-analysis of breastfeeding effects for infants with Neonatal Abstinence Syndrome. *Nursing Research, 71*(1), 54–65. https://doi.org/10.1097/NNR.0000000000000555

Cleveland, L., Bonugli, R. J., & McGlothen, K. S. (2016). The mothering experiences of women with substance use disorders. *Advances in Nursing Science, 39*(2), 119–129. https://doi.org/10.1097/ANS.0000000000000118

Cleveland, L., Hill, C. M., Pulse, W. S., DiCioccio, H. C., Field, T., & White-Traut, R. (2017). Systematic review of skin-to-skin care for full-term, healthy newborns. *Journal of Obstetric, Gynecologic & Neonatal Nursing, 46*(6), 857–869. https://doi.org/10.1016/j.jogn.2017.08.005

Conradt, E., Flannery, T., Aschner, J. L., Annett, R. D., Croen, L. A., Duarte, C. S., Friedman, A. M., Guille, C., Hedderson, M. M., Hofheimer, J. A., Jones, M. R., Ladd-Acosta, C., McGrath, M., Moreland, A., Neiderhiser, J. M., Nguyen, R. H. N., Posner, J., Ross, J. L., Savitz, D. A., ... Lester, B. M. (2019). Prenatal opioid exposure: Neurodevelopmental consequences and future research priorities. *Pediatrics, 144*(3). https://doi.org/10.1542/peds.2019-0128

Crook, K., & Brandon, D. (2017). Prenatal breastfeeding education: Impact on infants with Neonatal Abstinence Syndrome. *Advances in Neonatal Care, 17*(4), 299–305. https://doi.org/10.1097/ANC.0000000000000392

D'Auria, E., Borsani, B., Pendezza, E., Bosetti, A., Paradiso, L., Zuccotti, G. V., & Verduci, E. (2020). Complementary feeding: Pitfalls for health outcomes. *International Journal of Environmental Research and Public Health, 17*(21), 7931. https://doi.org/10.3390/ijerph17217931

DiTomasso, D., Wambach, K. A., Roberts, M. B., Erickson-Owens, D. A., Quigley, A., & Newbury, J. M. (2022). Maternal worry about infant weight and its influence on artificial milk supplementation and breastfeeding cessation. *Journal of Human Lactation, 38*(1), 177–189. https://doi.org/10.1177/0890334421 1000284

Enger, L., & Hurst, N. (2023). *Patient education: Pumping breast milk (Beyond the basics).* UpToDate. https://medilib.ir/uptodate/show/1220

Favara, M. T., Smith, J., Friedman, D., Lafferty, M., Carola, D., Adeniyi-Jones, S., Greenspan, J., & Aghai, Z. H. (2022). Growth failure in infants with Neonatal Abstinence Syndrome in the Neonatal Intensive Care Unit. *Journal of Perinatology, 42*(3), 313–318. https://doi.org/10.1038/s41372-021-01183-7

Fewtrell, M., Bronsky, J., Campoy, C., Domellöf, M., Embleton, N., Fidler Mis, N., Hojsak, I., Hulst, J. M., Indrio, F., Lapillonne, A., & Molgaard, C. (2017). Complementary feeding: A position paper by the European Society for Paediatric Gastroenterology, Hepatology, and Nutrition (ESPGHAN) Committee on Nutrition. *Journal of Pediatric Gastroenterology and Nutrition, 64*(1), 119. https://doi.org/10.1097/MPG.0000000000001454

Grossman, M., & Berkwitt, A. (2019). Neonatal Abstinence Syndrome. *Seminars in Perinatology, 43*(3), 173–186. https://doi.org/10.1053/j.semp eri.2019.01.007

Harries, V., & Brown, A. (2019). The association between baby care books that promote strict care routines and infant feeding, night-time care, and maternal–infant interactions. *Maternal & Child Nutrition, 15*(4). https://doi.org/10.1111/mcn.12858

Holmes, A. P., Schmidlin, H. N., & Kurzum, E. N. (2017). Breastfeeding considerations for mothers of infants with Neonatal Abstinence Syndrome. *Pharmacotherapy, 37*(7), 861–869. https://doi.org/10.1002/phar.1944

Jackson, L., De Pascalis, L., Harrold, J., & Fallon, V. (2021). Guilt, shame, and postpartum infant feeding outcomes: A systematic review. *Maternal & Child Nutrition, 17*(3). https://doi.org/10.1111/mcn.13141

Kaplan, H. C., Kuhnell, P., Walsh, M. C., Crowley, M., McClead, R., Wexelblatt, S., Ford, S., Provost, L. P., Lannon, C., Macaluso, M., & Ohio Perinatal Quality Collaborative. (2020). Orchestrated testing of formula type to reduce length of stay in Neonatal Abstinence Syndrome. *Pediatrics, 146*(4). https://doi.org/10.1542/peds.2019-0914

Larson, J. J., Graham, D. L., Singer, L. T., Beckwith, A. M., Terplan, M., Davis, J. M., Martinez, J., & Bada, H. S. (2019). Cognitive and behavioral impact on children exposed to opioids during pregnancy. *Pediatrics, 144*(2). https://doi.org/10.1542/peds.2019-0514

Le, B. (2019). Vitamin D patient education with a provided prescription prior to newborn discharge improves adherence to Vitamin D recommendation in infants returning to clinic for follow-up. *Pediatrics, 144*, 162. https://doi.org/10.1542/peds.144.2MA2.162

Lee, S. J., Bora, S., Austin, N. C., Westerman, A., & Henderson, J. M. T. (2020). Neurodevelopmental outcomes of children born to opioid-dependent mothers: A systematic review and meta-analysis. *Academic Pediatrics, 20*(3), 308–318. https://doi.org/10.1016/j.acap.2019.11.005

Lembeck, A. L., Tuttle, D., Locke, R., Lawler, L., Jimenez, P., Mackley, A., & Paul, D. A. (2021). Breastfeeding and formula selection in Neonatal Abstinence Syndrome. *American Journal of Perinatology, 38*(14), 1488–1493. https://doi.org/10.1055/s-0040-1713754

Little, E. E., Legare, C. H., & Carver, L. J. (2018). Mother–infant physical contact predicts responsive feeding among U.S. breastfeeding mothers. *Nutrients, 10*(9), 1251. https://doi.org/10.3390/nu10091251

MacMillan, K. D. L., Rendon, C. P., Verma, K., Riblet, N., Washer, D. B., & Volpe Holmes, A. (2018). Association of rooming-in with outcomes for Neonatal Abstinence Syndrome: A systematic review and meta-analysis. *JAMA Pediatrics, 172*(4), 345. https://doi.org/10.1001/jamapediatrics.2017.5195

MacVicar, S., Humphrey, T., & Forbes-McKay, K. E. (2018). Breastfeeding and the substance-exposed mother and baby. *Birth, 45*(4), 450–458. https://doi.org/10.1111/birt.12338

Maguire, D. J., Rowe, M. A., Spring, H., & Elliott, A. F. (2015). Patterns of disruptive feeding behaviors in infants with Neonatal Abstinence Syndrome. *Advances in Neonatal Care, 15*(6), 429–439. https://doi.org/10.1097/ANC.0000000000000204

Maguire, D. J., Shaffer-Hudkins, E., Armstrong, K., & Clark, L. (2018). Feeding infants with Neonatal Abstinence Syndrome: Finding the sweet spot. *Neonatal Network, 37*(1), 11–17. https://doi.org/10.1891/0730-0832.37.1.11

McFadden, A., Gavine, A., Renfrew, M. J., Buchanan, P., Taylor, J. L., Veitch, E., Rennie, A. M., Crowther, SA., Neiman, S., & MacGillivray, S. (2017). Support for healthy breastfeeding mothers with healthy term babies. *Cochrane Database of Systematic Reviews, 2.* https://doi.org/10.1002/14651858.CD001141.pub5

McGlothen-Bell, K., Cleveland, L., Recto, P., Brownell, E., & McGrath, J. (2020). Feeding behaviors in infants with prenatal opioid exposure: An integrative review. *Advances in Neonatal Care, 20*(5), 374–383. https://doi.org/10.1097/ANC.0000000000000762

McQueen, K., Taylor, C., & Murphy-Oikonen, J. (2019). Systematic review of newborn feeding method and outcomes related to Neonatal Abstinence Syndrome. *Journal of Obstetric, Gynecologic & Neonatal Nursing, 48*(4), 398–407. https://doi.org/10.1016/j.jogn.2019.03.004

Meek, J. Y., Noble, L., & Section on Breastfeeding. (2022). Policy statement: Breastfeeding and the use of human milk. *Pediatrics, 150*(1). https://doi.org/10.1542/peds.2022-057988

Messina, S., Reisz, S., Hazen, N., & Jacobvitz, D. (2020). Not just about food: Attachments representations and maternal feeding practices in infancy. *Attachment & Human Development, 22*(5), 514–533. https://doi.org/10.1080/14616734.2019.1600153

Nagy, S., Dow, K., & Fucile, S. (2023). Oral feeding outcomes in infants born with Neonatal Abstinence Syndrome. *Journal of Perinatal & Neonatal Nursing, Publish Ahead of Print.* https://doi.org/10.1097/JPN.0000000000000741

Patrick, S. W., Barfield, W. D., Poindexter, B. B., Committee on fetus and newborn, Committee on Substance use and Prevention, Cummings, J., Hand, I., Adams-Chapman, I., Aucott, S. W., Puopolo, K. M., Goldsmith, J. P., Kaufman, D., Martin, C., Mowitz, M., Gonzalez, L., Camenga, D. R., Quigley, J., Ryan, S. A., & Walker-Harding, L. (2020). Neonatal Opioid Withdrawal Syndrome. *Pediatrics, 146*(5). https://doi.org/10.1542/peds.2020-029074

Porto, A., & Abu-Alreesh, S. (2022, August 24). *Vitamin D for Babies, Children & Adolescents.* HealthyChildren.Org. https://www.healthychildren.org/English/healthy-living/nutrition/Pages/Vitamin-D-On-the-Double.aspx?gclid=CjwKCAjwqZSlBhBwEiwAfoZUIA31cmUmKkYQuG01RNA9mV4RTU0PgnwHqcGg8-L7mPG9oRJrDG1_BoCFS8QAvD_BwE

Redsell, S. A., Slater, V., Rose, J., Olander, E. K., & Matvienko-Sikar, K. (2021). Barriers and enablers to caregivers' responsive feeding behaviour: A systematic review to inform childhood obesity prevention. *Obesity Reviews, 22*(7). https://doi.org/10.1111/obr.13228

Reece-Stremtan, S., & Marinelli, K. A. (2015). ABM clinical protocol #21: Guidelines for breastfeeding and substance use or substance use disorder. *Journal of the Academy of Breastfeeding Medicine, 10*(3), 135–141. https://doi.org/10.1089/bfm.2015.9992

Ryan, G., Dooley, J., Gerber Finn, L., & Kelly, L. (2019). Nonpharmacological management of Neonatal Abstinence Syndrome: A review of the literature. *The Journal of Maternal-Fetal & Neonatal Medicine, 32*(10), 1735–1740. https://doi.org/10.1080/14767058.2017.1414180

Shaker, C. S. (2013). Cue-based feeding in the NICU: Using the infant's communication as a guide. *Neonatal Network, 32*(6), 404–408. https://doi.org/10.1891/0730-0832.32.6.404

Short, V. L., Abatemarco, D. J., & Gannon, M. (2021). Breastfeeding intention, knowledge, and attitude of pregnant women in treatment for opioid use disorder. *American Journal of Perinatology.* https://doi.org/10.1055/s-0041-1740145

Simon, A. E., & Ahrens, K. A. (2020). Adherence to Vitamin D intake guidelines in the United States. *Pediatrics, 145*(6). https://doi.org/10.1542/peds.2019-3574

Taylor, K., & Maguire, D. (2020). A review of feeding practices in infants with Neonatal Abstinence Syndrome. *Advances in Neonatal Care, 20*(6), 430–439. https://doi.org/10.1097/ANC.0000000000000780

Victora, C. G., Bahl, R., Barros, A. J. D., França, G. V. A., Horton, S., Krasevec, J., Murch, S., Sankar, M. J., Walker, N., Rollins, N. C., & Lancet Breastfeeding Series Group. (2016). Breastfeeding in the 21st century: Epidemiology, mechanisms, and lifelong effect. *Lancet, 387*(10017), 475–490. https://doi.org/10.1016/S0140-6736(15)01024-7

World Health Organization & United Nations Children's Fund (UNICEF). (2018). *Implementation guidance: Protecting, promoting and supporting breastfeeding in facilities providing maternity and newborn services: The revised baby-friendly hospital initiative.* World Health Organization. https://apps.who.int/iris/handle/10665/272943

7 Neonatal Opioid Withdrawal Syndrome and the Role of the Speech-Language Pathologist

Communication and Associated Domains of Development

Pam Holland

7.1 Introduction

Communication and the multifaceted domains that comprise its foundation are essential to the field of speech-language pathology. Increasingly, speech-language pathologists (SLPs), allied health professionals, and educators find themselves supporting family members who are raising young children who have been substance exposed. As noted by Rutherford et al. (2022, p. 1801),

> "Research is scarce for a group of children that many speech-language pathologists (SLPs) now serve – children with a history or suspected history of opioid exposure." Neonatal opioid withdrawal syndrome (NOWS), formerly referred to as neonatal abstinence syndrome (NAS), refers to a drug withdrawal syndrome seen following birth in infants exposed to opioids and other substances in utero (Hudak et al., 2012).

Infants often demonstrate clinical symptoms within the first few days following birth and include symptoms originating in the central nervous system, gastrointestinal system, and autonomic system (Patrick et al., 2020). The myriad symptoms demonstrated post birth are more widely researched than how this prenatal exposure to opioids translates across the child's early life and even through high school.

Additionally, Rutherford et al. (2022) noted that the Appalachian region, specifically, has been hit hard by the opioid epidemic and its effects (Brown et al., 2017; Sanlorenzo et al., 2018) in infants exposed to opioids and other substances in utero (Hudak et al., 2012). SLPs nationwide are finding larger numbers of children with NOWS on their caseloads (Proctor-Williams, 2018) who are at increased risk for a variety of challenges

DOI: 10.4324/9781003397267-7

relevant to the SLP, including speech and language delays (Hall et al., 2019; Miller et al., 2020), concerns with cognitive functioning (Beckwith & Burke, 2015; Konijnenberg & Melinder, 2016; Nygaard et al., 2015), mental health symptoms associated with attention-deficit/hyperactivity disorder (ADHD) and/or autism spectrum disorder (ASD) (Ornoy et al., 2001; Sandtorv et al., 2018), behavioral and/or emotional disorders (Hall et al., 2019), hearing and vision deficits (Maguire et al., 2016; Rigg & Rigg, 2020; Walhovd et al., 2015), and memory deficits (Sundelin Wahlsten & Sarman, 2013). Studies suggest that these challenges may persist well past the neonatal and infancy stages (Conradt et al., 2019; Miller et al., 2020; Oei et al., 2017), with some studies showing the delays extending into the middle school and high school years in a segment of the population (Miller et al., 2020; Oei et al., 2017).

Even the most experienced SLPs have much to learn when providing services to children with history of opioid exposure. It is essential SLPs re-examine how their scope of practice can be realigned when collaborating with a team of providers who are delivering clinical and academic support for children prenatally exposed to opioids. Addressing the needs of the family unit is of equal importance. The research team supported by the West Virginia Department of Education coined a term that encompasses this dynamic population (Holland et al., 2023). Children with a history of opioid exposure (CHOE) does not just represent the infant prenatally exposed to opioids, but rather includes the many confounding variables that include children:

- exposed to opioids prenatally, whether they required pharmacological treatment or not;
- diagnosed with NOWS (Patrick et al., 2020) following birth;
- who have one or more members of their family who use or have used opioids;
- who have been displaced due to a parent or caregiver who uses or has used opioids;
- whose lives have been affected by the trauma associated with a familial environment that includes opioid use, misuse, or medically assisted treatment for opioid use;
- who have caregivers in recovery from opioid use.

This broader definition may provide insight into why there has been a reported increase in the caseloads of SLPs working in the schools, and suggests additional research and training is necessary for positive outcomes in language, learning, and ultimately academic and social success.

The complexities of children with a history of prenatal opioid exposure and those with a diagnosis of NOWS highlighted above is noteworthy. The basics of communication is presented by utilizing a bottom-up approach to explore variables associated with this emerging and growing population. A basic definition of communication resembles: *communication – the exchange of information/messages from a sender to a receiver.* A more in-depth description of communication includes how one may choose to send a message (orally, graphically, or gesturally) and how one receives a message (aurally, visually, or tactilely).

What this basic premise of communication fails to include is the continuity between the intent of sender and the receiver's perception of the message; for example, when a friend approaches one and says "You look tired." The intent of that message is often well-meaning and said out of concern for a friend. However, the one on the receiving end of that comment may perceive it to mean, for example, that they don't look well, they look bad, or even they should have spent more time getting ready that morning. The intent of the comment may have been benign, but it may have resulted in hurt feelings. This example relates to the later discussion surrounding stigma and the importance of including perception in the context of communication and care.

According to the Council for Clinical Certification in Audiology and Speech-Language Pathology of the American Speech-Language-Hearing Association (2018), communication includes "The Big Nine." As noted in the Standards for Certification, Standard IV-C, the nine areas all certified SLPs must demonstrate knowledge in, include: 1) speech sound production; 2) fluency and fluency disorders; 3) voice and resonance; 4) receptive and expressive language with inclusion of prelinguistic communication, paralinguistic communication, and literacy in speaking, listening, reading, and writing; 5) hearing; 6) swallowing/feeding; 7) cognitive aspects of communication, including attention, memory, sequencing, problem solving, and executive functioning; 8) social aspects of communication, including challenging behavior, ineffective social skills, and lack of communication opportunities; and 9) augmentative and alternative communication modalities.

While each of these holds value for the practicing SLP, this chapter focuses primarily on speech sound production, receptive and expressive language, cognitive aspects of communication, and social aspects of communication.

7.2 Pre- and Postnatal Development: Timing Matters, Environment Matters

There is a growing body of research associated with effects of opioids on the developing fetus, the immediate challenges infants experience post birth, and the short- and long-term outcomes of children prenatally exposed to opioids. The impact NOWS has on communication development is complex and multifaceted, and therefore the specific substance(s), as well as the timing of substance exposure prenatally, need to be considered. Not only does timing of exposure matter; the manner in which a mother receives opioids is also of importance. Mothers may be enrolled in a structured Medically Assisted Treatment (MAT) program during pregnancy or may be making independent decisions about the substances they use. Skeide and Friederici (2016) provide an overview of the ontology of the cortex from utero to 7 years of age. The authors offer data on the earliest detection of phonological and prosodic features of language at 28 weeks' gestation via the bilateral superior temporal sulcus, as well as later detection of syntactically complex sentences and prosodic processing at the sentence level via anterior superior temporal gyrus, anterior superior temporal sulcus, Brodmann area, frontal opercular cortex, posterior superior temporal gyrus, and posterior superior temporal sulcus (Skeide & Friederici, 2016). While not specific to brain development with prenatal exposure to opioids, the discussion provides depth and insight into cortical development and its relationship to the complexities of learning language. At a minimum, this provides a foundation for SLPs to understand why children with prenatal opioid exposure to the developing cortex may have challenges with language development.

SLPs may begin collaborating with families as soon as an infant is born to address feeding challenges which infants prenatally exposed to opioids may experience. Often hospitals utilize an interprofessional perspective and a nurse, SLP, occupational therapist (OT), or physical therapist (PT) provides support in this area. Regardless of the professionals involved in the early care of the infant and family/caregivers, it is best practice for infants prenatally exposed to opioids to be routinely referred to an early intervention program and other wraparound programs of care prior to discharge from the hospital (Patrick et al., 2020). It is essential that early intervention becomes as consistent as newborn hearing screenings.

It is well documented that early identification and early intervention can decrease the severity of deficits and improve behavioral outcomes (Nordhov et al., 2012). According to the American Speech-Language-Hearing Association (ASHA) (n.d.a), "early intervention is the process of providing services and supports to infants, toddlers, and their families when a child has, or is at risk for, a developmental delay, disability, or health condition that may affect typical development and learning." Children with prenatal exposure to opioids are at risk for such developmental delays, and it may be prudent that federal regulations support states in including NAS and NOWS in the current list of diagnoses which allow a child to be routinely eligible to receive early intervention services, even if only on a consultative basis.

Eligibility for services is not the only factor to be considered when collaborating with families and caregivers who have a child with NOWS. Peacock-Chambers et al. (2020) noted five central themes related to the early intervention services specific to families with opioid use disorder. These included mothers' emotions as barriers to enrollment; mothers' and caregivers' questioning the need for early intervention services; perceived stigma; building partnerships with providers; and the need for personal connections. It is clear that even after an infant/child has been determined eligible for services, providers may feel ill-equipped to address each of these variables. This research supports the need for an early intervention team to be willing to, and competent to provide emotionally, and perhaps trauma sensitive, care (Peacock-Chambers et al., 2020). Moreover, ample time for education and counselling surrounding a child's developmental concerns and for the development of collaborative relationships is warranted.

7.3 Sustainable Relationships

Relationships between the child and his/her caregiver and between the clinician and caregivers are critical to the SLP to better understand the dynamics of the situation; the variables that impact all levels of development; and how important relationships are in contributing to positive developmental outcomes for children with a history of opioid exposure.

7.3.1 Child–Caregiver Relationship

Following discharge from the hospital, infants with NOWS may remain with their biological parents, live with their grandparents, be placed in other kinship care, enter the foster care system, and/or potentially be adopted. It is not uncommon that they experience more than one of these family scenarios, which has the potential to diminish the opportunity for the establishment of a safe and consistent environment with a person or group of people. As social emotional development is the foundation for executive function skills, the child's social history needs to be investigated upon initial referral (Schmidt et al., 2019).

The placement of an infant with NOWS is based on a myriad of factors. There are many confounding variables that should be considered. Where a child resides and who become their primary caregivers can play a role in their developmental progress and long-term communication outcomes. Infants who have established an emotional connection with a caregiver have the advantage of learning in a safe and supported environment. Relationships with caregivers are the first relationships infants experience and create the foundation for Social-Emotional Learning (SEL)

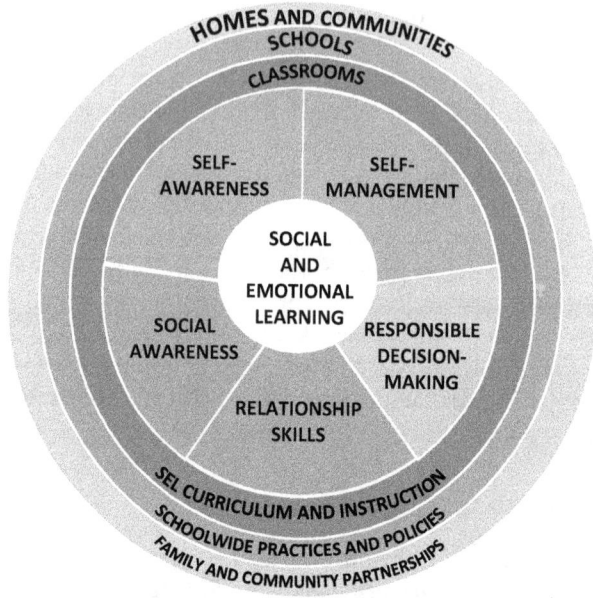

Figure 7.1 Social Emotional Learning (CASEL, 2020)

(Collaborative for Academic, Social, and Emotional Learning [CASEL], 2020). Healthy relationships between infants and children and those who are charged with their care (e.g., parents, foster parents, grandparents, childcare workers) support healthy social emotional development, lead to age-appropriate self-regulation, and executive function skills necessary for academic success. Trauma can have lasting, adverse impacts on learning, development, and even health outcomes (Harris-Burke, 2021). Furthermore, it is important to recognize that trauma also contributes to poor social emotional development. Figures 7.1 and 7.2 are examples of how healthy relationships support self-regulation, positive social emotional skills, and ultimately support academic success.

7.3.2 Clinician–Caregiver Relationship

The relationship between a child and their caregiver is not the only relationship that is critical for healthy brain development. Relationships between providers and caregivers are essential for successful early intervention outcomes. This relationship, if positively established, can assist in decreasing stigma associated with substance use disorder (SUD) and

NOWS, thereby preventing communication disorders and improving outcomes related to communication deficits. If a mutually respective relationship fails to develop between a caregiver and a provider, it can have the exact opposite effect. It is for this reason that relationships which support social emotional learning should be at the forefront of SLPs practice, as it sets the stage for executive function skills necessary for academic success, assists students develop socially, by improving decision-making skills as well as ability to set goals for themselves as they grow and develop.

The importance of collaboration, communication, and connection has been emphasized. The timing of such relationships is of equal importance. The relationship of opioids to the developing brain in utero, the relationship between infants and children and their caregivers, and finally the provider–caregiver relationship play a role in a child's overall development. An examination of the infant/child across the age span will provide additional consideration in the discussion on development in neurotypical infants and children and the differences children with NOWS may demonstrate.

7.4 Developmental Considerations

It is essential that SLPs are well versed in the developmental process of speech and language. Neurotypical children follow a fairly predictable pattern for developing language with individual difference, which often does not interfere with establishing communication skills supportive of later academic achievement. Neurodiverse children often communicate effectively and are successful in the academic arena; however, they may experience a "natural human variation" (Jaarsma & Welin, 2012). Children with NOWS may be a neurodiverse group whose developmental outcomes are yet to be fully understood. The following sections will therefore present a developmental approach to children with NOWS from birth through high school.

7.4.1 The Birth to 3 Years

Research has found that children prenatally exposed to opioids may experience challenges in the following domains: delayed cognitive, linguistic, and speech development, delayed fine and gross motor development, atypical self-regulation, and sensory seeking, strabismus, and hearing concerns (Beckwith & Burke, 2015; Fill et al., 2018; Hall et al., 2019; Hunt et al., 2008; Konijnenberg et al., 2016; Maguire et al., 2016; Miller et al., 2020; Nygaard et al., 2015; Oei et al., 2017). The importance of families establishing a relationship with a full complement of providers is of utmost importance (Schmidt et al., 2019). There is also growing evidence to support an association between NOWS and cleft lip and palate (CLP) suggesting that prenatal exposure to opioids may be an environmental risk factor in the development of CLP (Danis et al., 2021). SLPs may also see an increase in CLP on their caseload and may consider increasing their knowledge base of cleft lip and palate, specifically submucosal cleft that is often overlooked in the NAS and non-NAS populations (Danis et al., 2021; Proctor-Williams & Louw, 2022).

The neurotypical infant at 4 months demonstrates a social smile, looks at the faces of caregivers, begins to coo, cries to indicate different needs, and often will quiet or smile when a parent or caregiver talks to them (ASHA, n.d.b). Differences in infants prenatally exposed to opioids at this age can be related to time the infant spent in the neonatal intensive care unit (NICU) or how their central nervous system (CNS) adapts to the world and how much they are exposed to social interaction.

At 6 months of age, infants begin babbling and speech sounds emerge; they giggle, move their eyes in the direction of sound, and are quick to vocalize when they are happy or upset (ASHA, n.d.b). For infants with a history of prenatal exposure, visual deficits are more common, and nystagmus and strabismus are well documented (Cornish et al., 2013). SLPs should integrate this knowledge into their practice and refer infants to vision specialists as warranted.

Infants between the ages of 8 and 12 months begin using gestures to communicate, engage in pointing, look at what others point to, respond when their name is called, start to respond to simple phrases, and understand common words (ASHA, n.d.b). The primary difference between the NOWS population and neurotypical children at this age is decreased use of gestures. Gestures is one of the earliest methods an infant uses to demonstrate intentional communication, and the lack of gestures signals to providers a potential concern in development (Goldin-Meadow, 2020). As noted by Anagnostou et al. (2014), Zwaigenbaum et al. (2015), Thurm et al. (2018), and Zwaigenbaum and Penner (2018), the absence of compensatory gestures such as pointing can be a sign of autism spectrum disorder (ASD). It is of extreme importance that SLPs and the diagnostic teams they collaborate with recognize that children with NOWS should not be provided this diagnosis until a complete medical and social history and dynamic assessment is completed. Providing such hasty diagnoses to children would prove a disservice to both children with ASD and NOWS.

Neurotypical children begin to say their first words between the ages of 12 and 18 months of age. They often recognize the names of familiar people, objects, and body parts; and follow simple directions when accompanied by gestures (ASHA, n.d.b). These milestones emerge at a later date for children with history of opioid exposure. Anecdotal evidence from early intervention providers in rural Appalachia also notes a decrease in development of joint attention with prolonged use of jargon (D. Smith, personal communication, April 20, 2023). This should be further investigated for validation across all geographical regions.

By the time a child reaches 18 to 24 months of age, they should begin making animal and other environmental sounds, using at least 50 words, producing 2-word utterances, and using simple pronouns (ASHA, n.d.b). For children with prenatal exposure to opioids and other elicit substances, all of these milestones are generally delayed. Specifically, they have been noted to score on the low end of scales when participating in the *Bayley Scales of Infant and Toddler Development, Third Edition* (Bayley, 2005) at 2 years of age (Merhar et al., 2018) and demonstrate overall lower language skills (McGlone & Mactier, 2015).

As discussed earlier, relationships and environment need to be considered when assessing language development of children with a history of opioid exposure. Over the last decade, incidences of grandparents raising grandchildren have increased exponentially. According to Baime (2023), 7.1 million American grandparents are living with their grandchildren and 2.3 million are the sole caregivers. Of those who are the sole caregivers, approximately one-third of children they are raising are younger than 6 years of age. As grandparents' roles shift to that of parents and primary caregivers, they experience social stigma and isolation that contribute to negative health outcomes. This is often further complicated by raising children with adverse childhood experiences (ACEs), including trauma, which can lead to physical, psychological, or behavioral challenges. Providers must recognize the differences in parenting styles of grandparents as compared to parents. These differences may include unclear boundaries and lack of sensitivity to their grandchildren's needs (Hayslip et al., 2019). It is essential that SLPs consider this multifaceted family dynamic prior to evaluating communication skills and creating a plan of care for ongoing service provision.

As a child transitions from early intervention programs to preschool programs, informed care can be supported by ensuring there is an appropriate connection between medical and educational systems. The Adherence to Health Insurance Portability and Accountability Act (HIPAA) and the Family Educational Rights and Privacy Act (FERPA) are federally mandated. However, as stigma surrounding SUD decreases, the transition from early intervention to preschool can be supported if documentation is maintained. In addition to streamlining documentation, the World Health Organization (WHO) (2010) has associated interprofessional practice and collaborative care to improved outcomes in family health, infectious disease, humanitarian efforts, responses to epidemics, and noncommunicable diseases. Communication between providers across settings and organizations is essential to creating positive relationships and can support positive outcomes for children with a history of NOWS and the families who are responsible for their care.

7.4.2 Preschool Age – 3 to 5 Years

Hart and Risley (1995) noted disparities in parent–child interactions of families of low socioeconomic status with documented effect of these disparities on children's vocabulary and later intellectual performance. Their study described the differences in the vocabulary of children aged 3 years when provided a language rich environment. Specifically, if children hear 3,000 words per hour, by the age of 3, they have heard 33 million words. If they only hear 500 words per hour, by the age of 3, they have heard only 9 million words (Hart & Risley, 1995). Providing families with this easy-to-understand concept is a first step in improving language development. This is essential in helping children develop age-appropriate skills such as using pronouns, plurals and other morphological endings, spatial concepts, descriptive words, categories, and answering questions (Paul, 2020; Stanford Children's Health, n.d.). Hunt et al. (2008) indicated that children with a history of opioid exposure assessed using the *Reynell Developmental Language Scales III* exhibited reduced expressive language and verbal comprehension at 3 years of age.

The connection between social emotional development and language has already been noted, but should be at the forefront of any discussion as children enter preschool. It is at this time they begin consistent peer

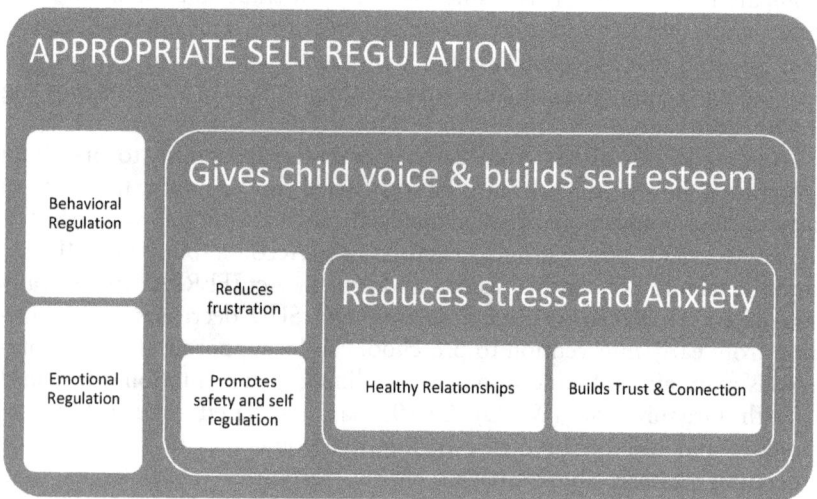

Figure 7.2 Relationships and regulations (Foley & Hochman, 2006)

interaction while simultaneously having to manage emotional arousal and demonstrate one of their first milestones with academic success. The challenges preschoolers face within a classroom environment include the need to initiate prosocial behaviors (e.g., sharing, helping others, cooperating, taking turns, understanding rules) and build friendships while simultaneously staying connected with adults, and this can be overwhelming. The 3–5-year-old child must demonstrate an awareness of basic emotional expressions, develop management of their own emotions, and make early attempts to solve interpersonal problems with peers (Foley & Hochman, 2006) (see Figure 7.2).

7.4.3 Elementary School Age

Rutherford et al. (2022) conducted focus groups with SLPs working in the schools in rural Appalachia as participants. SLPs indicated an increase in the number of children on their caseloads overall. The question arises whether this increase is in part due to the growth of children with a history of NOWS or suspected history of prenatal exposure to opioids within this region. The perceptions of the SLPs who participated in the focus groups indicated that the children on their caseloads with a known or suspected history of prenatal opioid exposure exhibit deficits with speech, language, and cognitive/executive function skills, and demonstrate overall developmental delays. Regarding "hallmark characteristics" of the child with NOWS, there was a report of children with a greater severity of needs, inconsistent performance, and atypical manifestations once they reached elementary school (Rutherford et al., 2022). Regarding social emotional well-being, additional external factors reported included safety and well-being with their home environment and the transient nature of families resulting in changing school environments (Rutherford et al., 2022).

SLPs working in the school setting are well known for addressing speech sound disorders. Rutherford et al. (2022) indicated that articulation errors in children with a history of opioid disorder were reported to be idiosyncratic with unusual error patterns and inconsistent across settings. The SLP participants questioned if this was secondary to challenges with impulsivity, self-regulation, and attention, which they often believed to be a contributing factor to progress.

Classroom teachers report attention concerns, hyperactivity, and impulsivity leading to higher rates of referral for special services and the need for academic accommodations (Fill et al., 2018; Sundelin Wahlsten & Sarman, 2013). When teachers were asked to complete ADHD scales, serious challenges in these same areas were noted along with motor and memory skills with children aged 5 and 6 (Sundelin Wahlsten & Sarman, 2013).

7.4.4 Secondary School Age

Nygaard et al. (2018) reported that magnetic resonant imaging (MRI) scans of teenagers who were exposed to opioids in utero demonstrated a 10% reduction in total brain volume and 10% reduction in cerebral cortex and cerebral white matter. Deficits for this age group were noted specifically in the pre-frontal cortex, which is essential for executive functioning skills, the occipital lobe, which is required for visual processing, and segments of the temporal lobe, which is essential for language (Weismer et al., 2005).

The gaps identified in elementary school persisted and widened in middle and high school years, and the academic gap widens as the years progress (Oei et al., 2017). These students demonstrate a higher rate of executive function and cognitive concerns, motor issues, difficulties with behavioral regulation, emotional concerns, speech and language delays, and hearing deficits as well as ophthalmic issues (Beckwith & Burke, 2015; Fill et al., 2018; Hall et al., 2019; Hunt et al., 2008, Konijnenberg et al., 2016; Maguire et al., 2016; Miller et al., 2020; Nygaard et al., 2015; Oei et al., 2017). This may translate to the middle and high school students who remain on the caseloads of SLPs and contribute to the reported higher caseloads as noted from the focus groups (Rutherford et al., 2022).

SLPs working within this setting and with this age group must be vigilant and continue the collaborative process with other educators due to the evidence of this academic gap. A potential solution is to examine the history of middle and high school students who are struggling academically. A request for language assessment and/or psychological evaluation may identify underlying language deficits as contributors to difficulties in behavioral regulation and necessitate and support an Individual Education Plan (IEP) through high school.

Describing the characteristics of a child with NOWS from infant to high school is a challenge, as the child moves through many developmental stages. The SLP must be cognizant of the domains of language and how they evolve within various social settings and ages. As noted previously, the child with NOWS may have a neurodiverse CNS and they may also have family dynamics that one must consider prior to making a differential diagnosis and creating a collaborative, individualized plan of care. These external factors may also contribute to the challenges for ensuring the plan of care is sustainable.

7.5 Translational Research

According to ASHA (n.d.c), evidence-based practice (EBP) is the process of applying current, best evidence, client/patient/caregiver perspectives, and clinical expertise to make decisions about assessment and treatment.

The researcher–clinician gap has led to a delay in applying new research knowledge to clinical practice, which is challenging to EBP. Translational research is the translation of new knowledge and techniques generated by advances in basic science research to inform and develop new approaches for assessment and intervention. Collaboration between scientists and clinicians from various disciplines can advance translational research and address the researcher–clinician gap (Rubio et al., 2010; National Institutes of Health, 2009).

Research evidence, clinical expertise, and caregiver perspectives are the building blocks of developing an evidence base of characteristics of children with a history of prenatal opioid exposure. In order to inform assessment and intervention approaches for SLPs serving this new population, an example of translational research will be described in two parts. First, for therapeutic application, clinician expertise will be presented through the lens of the perspectives of speech-language pathologists working in the schools in rural Appalachia (Maxwell et al., 2022), with a triangular conclusion including caregiver perspectives with a particular focus on stigma associated with this relatively new but growing population surrounding SUD. Second, reflections regarding the implications for developing SLP curricula and specialized training to address the needs of mothers with SUD and children with NOWS will be discussed.

7.5.1 Therapeutic Application

In Table 7.1 seven family units are presented. They are used to emphasize the validity of research findings about developmental challenges children with a history of opioid exposure may demonstrate. These cases highlight timing of referral and the referral source, clinical characteristics across the Big 9, and confounding variables which spotlight, once again, the need for an interprofessional team approach and establishing trusting relationships. In Table 7.1 Ramey's length of relationship with the provider and the associated stigma is important to note. This is where the team of providers must begin to ensure positive outcomes for a child with a history of opioid exposure.

The focus group with 20 SLPs from West Virginia was an attempt to begin a dialogue between what is being seen in the schools and what the growing body of literature indicates (Rutherford et al., 2022). The results of this small, qualitative study were consistent with the current literature and highlights perceived clinical characteristics, perceived significant differentiators; both internal to the child and perceived confounding factors external to the child (e.g., safety and well-being, home environment, effects on school environment). These confounding variables perceived by the SLPs in this study relate to the factors outside of the school system,

Table 7.1 Case studies; upon examination of the evidence, clinician's expertise, family's experiences, and perspectives presented in the case studies, it is clear that there is growing evidence regarding communication challenges with this population

	Mandi & Gibson	Markey & Ramey	Bonnie & Sarah	Alys & Kevin	Katie & Liam	Heidi & Deon	Aaron & Timothy
Referral/Age	IP clinic 1 m	BTT 7 m Virtual Relationship	BTT 12 m	BTT 13 m	IP clinic 15 m	BTT 15 m	OP clinic 22 m
Perceived Clinical Characteristics	F/M	F/M	S/L/C/F/M SI	F/S/L/C/SE/M	S/L	F/S/L/C/ M/SI Concerns for ASD	S/L/C/M/SI/ F/SE/V
Perceived Significant Differentiators		Inconsistent performance	Greater severity of needs	Greater severity of needs	Greater severity of needs	Greater severity of needs	Greater severity of needs
Perceived Confounding Factors	First-time mom Enrolled in Recovery program Family history of SUD Trauma and active recovery	Stigma Did not want providers in house	Grandparents fostering to adopt	Foster care with visitation with biological father	Trauma Family history of SUD Active recovery	Stigma Challenging family dynamics	Adopted Collaborating with multiple agencies
Length of Relationship	15 m	2 m	18 m	12 m	15 m	7 m	24 m

F = Feeding S = Speech L = Language C = Cognition
SE = Social Emotional M = Motor SI = Sensory Integration V = Vision

Table 7.2 Parent perspectives

Parent Statement	Family History	Suggestions for the SLP
"School sent home oral care instructions with a toothbrush and toothpaste. I think they still see me as someone who is using."	Karen is a 24-year-old mother who was raised by a family with generations of SUD. She has experienced significant trauma associated with this and became involved with a man who was physically abusive. When her oldest son was 2, he witnessed his father being shot and killed and also has significant trauma. Her younger son's father is incarcerated. At the time of this statement, her oldest son was 4 and her youngest son 18 months; she had graduated from an inpatient rehabilitation program, was living independently, and was working full-time. Both boys were in daycare. While her youngest son has a full set of age-appropriate teeth, her eldest had all deciduous teeth pulled due to prolonged poor oral hygiene when she was still with his father when she admitted to using multiple substances. Despite the fact that all children received the same oral care instructions and had a toothbrush and toothpaste sent home as part of a school-wide curriculum, she associated this with a time she was not at her best. She felt singled out and judged by those working at the daycare.	Listen to your families. Recognize how trauma plays a role in parent and child relationships. Consider how you can make families feel special but not different or stigmatized.

(Continued)

Table 7.2 (Continued)

Parent Statement	Family History	Suggestions for the SLP
"Every time I go to the doctor, I feel judged because I have to disclose my son was prenatally exposed to opioids. I know they see that in his chart. Then I feel like I have to say, he was adopted so they know it wasn't me."	Diana is a foster mom who began fostering at birth and then adopted. Her anxiety with going to the doctor is high due to the continued feeling of feeling judged. What bothers her the most is she is an early intervention provider and is working every day with moms in recovery. She is on a journey to improve her biases surrounding pregnant mothers who are exposing their babies to substances. She has seen first-hand the challenges her son experienced, which include all of the disruptions of the CNS following birth, including tremors, gastrointestinal difficulty, poor feeding, and excessive, high-pitch crying. This was followed by developmental delays requiring occupational therapy, physical therapy, developmental therapy, and speech therapy. Her son just finished kindergarten and does have an IEP for reading support and speech therapy for articulation errors. He continues to be "high energy" but was academically successful and is moving forward to first grade.	Reconnect with the idea that families are diverse. Create foster family, grandparent, or other kinship care support group with multiple providers to offer guidance.

"I want to bring him to therapy because I know he needs it, but I don't have heat in my car. He doesn't want to put clothes on and then he has a meltdown and cries non-stop when we get home."

Mom knows her son needs therapy. It is winter and her car does not have heat. Her son has AUD-Level 3, is non-verbal, and has severe sensory aversions with visual perceptual challenges that prevent him from walking without holding someone's hand. He has been at home secondary to COVID-19 for over a year. He does not like to wear clothes and the only thing he "eats" is milk from a certain bottle. He will only eat when he is alone in his room and wearing only a diaper. So yes! He needs therapy but what is the priority for this family right now? The team chose to help her find funding to fix the heat in her car and not remove her from the outpatient schedule due to poor attendance. Spring came, school started. He is attending school regularly, attending all outpatient therapy sessions regularly, and mom has developed strong relationships with all of his teachers and therapists. He is exploring more tastes and smiling, not crying!

Consider how socioeconomic status and social determinants of health force families to make decisions.

Refer to outside resources (e.g., social work, department of health and human services).

At a minimum, reconsider attendance policies for outpatient clinics.

Investigate resources for telehealth options.

Send strategies that can be easily implemented at home when families don't have transportation; use text, email, or social media platforms to distribute information.

but have also been noted in the literature to be contributors to challenges children prenatally exposed to opioids face when entering school (Coggins et al., 2007).

In order to decrease and ultimately eliminate any long-term effects of prenatal exposure to opioids, mothers must feel supported by their health care providers so they can safely seek health and educational services for their children without feeling judged. Statements made by mothers to a SLP working in early intervention in West Virginia demonstrate mothers' perspectives.

How can SLPs improve family experiences? As stories and parent perspectives are shared, providers are reminded of how essential relationships are in improving developmental outcomes for children with a history of opioid exposure.

SLPs, along with the health and education teams they work with, must advocate for what they need to ensure this population of infants, children, and their families is best served. This may include requesting specific trauma-informed professional development, embracing the complexity of what evaluation and treatment looks like outside of standardized assessments, and prioritizing the foundations for language and learning by placing social emotional development and executive functioning at the forefront of all treatment plans (e.g., Individualized Family Service Plans [IFSP], IEPs, and 504 Plans). All professionals must regularly participate in a self-evaluation of stigma and biases to ensure relationships between provider and caregivers are mutually positive.

7.5.2 Communication Sciences and Disorders Programs – Curriculum and Clinical Reflections

According to the Council for Clinical Certification in Audiology and Speech-Language Pathology of the American Speech-Language-Hearing Association (2018), academic programs in communication sciences and disorders (CSD) prioritize educational outcomes surrounding prevention, assessment, and intervention for individuals with communication disorders. The emerging data surrounding children with NOWS indicate a need for a curriculum and specialized training which encompasses trauma-informed care, and educational practices that reconceptualize the SLP scope of practice. Providers must understand the complexity of children with NOWS and should include the whole child, and the family dynamic. Understanding the perspective and experiences of mothers with a history of SUD when seeking care for their child must be at the foundation of future professional development activities in order to ensure interprofessional, compassionate, and interactional health and educational services.

CSD programs and other educational and health professions must ensure their students graduate as informed providers. Suggested activities include: 1) starting a faculty–student book club and possibly making it a component of the university's IPE program; inviting alumni and other professionals in the community to learn alongside one another; 2) offering a Special Topics course with a Community-Based Learning (CBL) theme; 3) inviting guest speakers (e.g., providers from various recovery programs, peer recovery coaches, nurses from the Neonatal Therapeutic Unit [NTU], early intervention providers); 4) applying for university-supported research or other state and federal grants to add to the body of research. While these suggestions are focused on academia, all apply to SLPs working in any health and educational settings and are applicable to other disciplines.

7.6 Summary

Improving understanding of how trauma effects the brain and how that translates to learning and other health outcomes is essential for SLPs and allied health professionals and is long overdue. Timing, environment, relationships, and perspectives are the central themes SLPs should integrate into their dynamic assessment and intervention practices with children with NOWS. These concepts are directly related to the healthy development of a child's social emotional skills and are indeed the foundation for learning. Children and families need engagement that includes two-way communication and considers the perspectives of mothers in recovery from substance use or families who have experienced traumatic situations.

It is essential to start at the beginning. This means gathering as much information about a child's prenatal and social history as possible and doing so in a trauma-sensitive and destigmatizing manner. This will allow professionals to continue to build the body of evidence for understanding communication skills for this unique and growing population. There is a need for guidelines and specialized programing. However, there are simple suggestions may consider integrating into their practice now.

SLPs are challenged to use routines more consistently to allow children predictable environments for learning and ensure that children have developed age appropriate social emotional skills, and if there are deficits, start with this aspect of cognition and executive functioning, for without them improvements in other domains such as speech sound production and language skills may prove futile. Acknowledge emotions and feelings of children so that children can not only feel heard but provided with language concepts that teach them to express their thoughts, feelings, and ideas other than through overt behaviors. A functional, wholistic, and relationship-based approach is well documented in the literature surrounding ASD (Astington, 1994; Greenspan & Wieder, 2009; Perkins, 2005; Rollins, 2016; Rydell, 2012) and may prove to be appropriate strategies for children with a history of opioid exposure while SLPs continue to participate in research specific to this group of children.

Additionally, SLPs are encouraged to participate in annual stigma training, refer to psychologists who can provide services such a parent child interaction therapy (PCIT), and maintain open dialogue with all caregivers and family members involved in the care of children. The child with a history of opioid exposure must have wraparound care that follows them wherever they go to ensure long-term outcomes that are positive for communication.

Acknowledgments

The information presented in this chapter would not have been possible without the following friends, colleagues, and students: Lee Ann Brammer, Dr. Lisa Fry, Dr. Jamie Maxwell, Dr. Kelly Rutherford, Audrey Lankford, Teagan Beitzel, Lauren Downing, and Haley Black. A final and most sincere appreciation to the students who enrolled in our first independent study with Dr. Mary Weidner.

References

American Speech-Language-Hearing Association. (n.d.a). *Early Intervention.* (Practice Portal). Retrieved September 9, 2023, from www.asha.org/Practice-Portal/Professional-Issues/Early-Intervention/

American Speech-Language-Hearing Association. (n.d.b). *Birth to one year.* ASHA. Retrieved September 9, 2023, from https://www.asha.org/public/developmental-milestones/communication-milestones-birth-to-1-year/

American Speech-Language-Hearing Association. (n.d.c). *Evidence-Based Practice (EBP).* ASHA. Retrieved September 9, 2023. https://www.asha.org/research/ebp/

Anagnostou, E., Zwaigenbaum, L., Szatmari, P., Fombonne, E., Fernandez, B. A., Woodbury-Smith, M., Brian, J., Bryson, S., Smith, I. M., Drmic, I., Buchanan, J. A., Roberts, W., & Scherer, S. W. (2014). Autism spectrum disorder: Advances in evidence-based practice. *Canadian Medical Association Journal, 186*(7), 509–519. https://doi.org/10.1503/cmaj.121756

Astington, J. W. (1994). Children's developing notions of others' minds. In J. Duchan, L. E. Hewitt, & R. M. Sonnenmeier (Eds.), *Pragmatics: From theory to practice.* Prentice Hall.

Baime, A. J. (2023, March 2). *When Grandparents are called to parent – Again.* AARP https://www.aarp.org/home-family/friends-family/info-2023/grandparents-become-parents-again.html

Bayley, N. (2005). *Bayley Scales of Infant and Toddler Development, Third Edition (Bayley – III®)* [Database record]. APA PsycTests. https://doi.org/10.1037/t14978-000

Beckwith, A. M., & Burke, S. A. (2015). Identification of early developmental deficits in infants with prenatal heroin, methadone, and other opioid exposure. *Clinical Pediatrics*, *54*(4), 328–335. https://doi.org/10.1177/000992281 4549545

Brown, J. D., Goodin, A. J., & Talbert, J. C. (2017). Rural and Appalachian disparities in neonatal abstinence syndrome incidence and access to opioid abuse treatment. *Journal of Rural Health*, *34*(1), 6–13. https://doi.org/10.1111/jrh.12251

Coggins, T. E., Timler, G. R., & Olswang, L. B. (2007). A state of double jeopardy: Impact of prenatal alcohol exposure and adverse environments on the social communicative abilities of school-age children with fetal alcohol spectrum disorder. *Language, Speech, and Hearing Services in Schools*, *38*(2), 117–127. https://doi.org/10.1044/0161-1461(2007/012)

Collaborative for Academic, Social, and Emotional Learning. (2020). *What is social emotional learning?* https://schoolguide.casel.org/what-is-sel/what-is-sel/

Conradt, E., Flannery, T., Aschner, J. L., Annett, R. D., Croen, L. A., Duarte, C. S., Friedman, A. M., Guille, C., Hedderson, M. M., Hofheimer, J. A., Jones, M. R., Ladd-Acosta, C., McGrath, M., Moreland, A., Neiderhiser, J. M., Nguyen, R. H. N., Posner, J., Ross, J. L., Savitz, D. A., … Lester, B. M. (2019). Prenatal opioid exposure: Neurodevelopmental consequences and future research priorities. *Pediatrics*, *144*(3). https://doi.org/10.1542/peds.2019-0128

Cornish, K. S., Hrabovsky, M., Scott, N. W., Myerscough, E., & Reddy, A. R. (2013). The short-and long-term effects on the visual system of children following exposure to maternal substance misuse in pregnancy. *American Journal of Ophthalmology*, *156*(1), 190–194.

Council for Clinical Certification in Audiology and Speech-Language Pathology of the American Speech-Language-Hearing Association. (2018). *2020 Standards for the Certificate of Clinical Competence in Speech-Language Pathology.* ASHA. www.asha.org/certification/2020-SLP-Certification-Standards.

Danis, D. O., 3rd, Bachrach, K., Piraquive, J., Marston, A. P., & Levi, J. R. (2021). Cleft lip and palate in newborns diagnosed with neonatal abstinence syndrome. *Otolaryngology – Head and Neck Surgery*, *164*(1), 199–205. https://doi.org/10.1177/0194599820944899

Fill, M.-A., Miller, A. M., Wilkinson, R. H., Warren, M. D., Dunn, J. R., Schaffner, W., & Jones, T. F. (2018). Educational disabilities among children born with neonatal abstinence syndrome. *Pediatrics*, *142*(3). https://doi.org/10.1542/peds.2018-0562

Foley, G., & Hochman, J. (2006). *Mental health in early intervention: Achieving unity in principles and practice.* Paul H. Brookes Publishing Co.

Goldin-Meadow, S. (2020). Using gesture to identify and address early concerns about language and pragmatics. *Pediatrics*, *146*(3), 278–283. https://doi.org/10.1542/peds.2020-0242G

Green, R. (2014). *Lost at school: Why our kids with behavioral challenge are falling through cracks and how we can help them.* Scribner Publishing.

Greenspan, S. I., & Wieder, S. (2009). *Engaging autism: Using the floortime approach to help children relate, communicate, and think.* De Capo Lifelong Books.

Hall, E. S., McAllister, J. M., & Wexelblatt, S. L. (2019). Developmental disorders and medical complications among infants with subclinical intrauterine opioid exposures. *Population Health Management, 22*(1), 19–24. https://doi.org/10.1089/pop.2018.0016

Harris-Burke, N. (2021). *The deepest well: Healing the long-term effects of childhood trauma and adversity.* Mariner Books.

Hart, B., & Risley, T. (1995). *Meaningful differences in the everyday experience of young American children.* Paul H. Brookes Publishing Co.

Hayslip, B., Fruhauf, C. A., & Dolbin-MacNab, M. L. (2019). Grandparents raising grandchildren: What have we learned over the past decade? *The Gerontologist, 59*(3), 152–163. https://doi.org/10.1093/geront/gnx106

Holland, P., Fry, L., Maxwell, J., Rutherford, K. (2023, February 15–17). *NAS, NOWS, CHOE: Acronyms SLPs need to know and why!* [Oral Presentation]. 2023 KSHA Convention: IGNITE: Be the Spark for Positive Impact.

Hudak, M. L., Tan, R. C., The Committee on Drugs, The Committee on Fetus and Newborn, Frattarelli, D. A. C., Galinkin, J. L., Green, T. P., Neville, K. A., Paul, I. M., Van Den Anker, J. N., Papile, L.-A., Baley, J. E., Bhutani, V. K., Carlo, W. A., Cummings, J., Kumar, P., Polin, R. A., Wang, K. S., & Watterberg, K. L. (2012). Neonatal drug withdrawal. *Pediatrics, 129*(2), 540–560. https://doi.org/10.1542/peds.2011-3212

Hunt, R. W., Tzioumi, D., Collins, E., & Jeffery, H. E. (2008). Adverse neurodevelopmental outcome of infants exposed to opiate in-utero. *Early Human Development, 84*(1), 29–35. https://doi.org/10.1016/j.earlhumdev.2007.01.013

Jaarsma, P., & Welin, S. (2012). Autism as a natural human variation: Reflections on the claims of the neurodiversity movement. *Health Care Analysis, 20*(1), 20–30. https://doi.org/10.1007/s10728-011-0169-9

Konijnenberg, C., Sarfi, M., & Melinder, A. (2016). Mother–child interaction and cognitive development in children prenatally exposed to methadone or buprenorphine. *Early Human Development, 101,* 91–97. https://doi.org/10.1016/j.earlhumdev.2016.08.013

Maguire, D. J., Taylor, S., Armstrong, K., Shaffer-Hudkins, E., Germain, A. M., Brooks, S. S., Cline, G. J., & Clark, L. (2016). Long-term outcomes of infants with neonatal abstinence syndrome. *Neonatal Network, 35*(5), 277–286. https://doi.org/10.1891/0730-0832.35.5.27

Maxwell, J., Rutherford, K., Holland, P., Fry, L., Rigon, A., & Lankford, A. (2022). Perceptions of speech-language pathologists' service provision in the opioid epidemic: A focus group. *American Journal of Speech-Language Pathology.* https://doi.org/10.1044/2022_AJSLP-21-00337

McGlone, L., & Mactier, H. (2015). Infants of opioid-dependent mothers: Neurodevelopment at six months. *Early Human Development, 91*(1), 19–21. https://doi.org/10.1016/j.earlhumdev.2014.10.006

Merhar, S. L., McAllister, J. M., Wedig-Stevie, K. E., Klein, A. C., Meinzen-Derr, J., & Poindexter, B. B. (2018). Retrospective review of neurodevelopmental outcomes in infants treated for neonatal abstinence syndrome. *Journal of Perinatology, 38*(5), 587–592. https://doi.org/10.1038/s41372-018-0088-9

Miller, J. S., Anderson, J. G., Erwin, P. C., Davis, S. K., & Lindley, L. C. (2020). The effects of neonatal abstinence syndrome on language delay from birth to 10 years. *Journal of Pediatric Nursing*, 51, 67–74. https://doi.org/10.1016/j.pedn.2019.12.011

National Institutes of Health. (2009). Translational research. Retrieved from http://nihroadmap.nih.gov/clinicalresearch/ overview-translational.asp. https://doi.org/10.1177/1609406917733847

Nordhov, S. M., Rønning, J. A., Ulvund, S. E., Dahl, L. B., & Kaaresen, P. I. (2012). Early intervention improves behavioral outcomes for preterm infants: Randomized controlled trial. *Pediatrics*, 129(1), 9–16. https://doi.org/10.1542/peds.2011-0248

Nygaard, E., Moe, V., Slinning, K., & Walhovd, K. B. (2015). Longitudinal cognitive development of children born to mothers with opioid and polysubstance use. *Pediatric Research*, 78(3), 330–335. https://doi.org/10.1038/pr.2015.95

Nygaard, E., Slinning, K., Moe, V., Due-Tønnessen, P., Fjell, A., & Walhovd, K. B. (2018). Neuroanatomical characteristics of youths with prenatal opioid and poly-drug exposure. *Neurotoxicology and Teratology*, 68, 13–26. https://doi.org/10.1016/j.ntt.2018.04.004

Oei, J. L., Melhuish, E., Uebel, H., Azzam, N., Breen, C., Burns, L., Hilder, L., Bajuk, B., Abdel-Latif, M. E., Ward, M., Feller, J. M., Falconer, J., Clews, S., Eastwood, J., Li, A., & Wright, I. M. (2017). Neonatal abstinence syndrome and high school performance. *Pediatrics*, 139(2). https://doi.org/10.1542/peds.2016-2651

Ornoy, A., Segal, J., Bar-Hamburger, R., & Greenbaum, C. (2001). Developmental outcome of school-age children born to mothers with heroin dependency: Importance of environmental factors. *Developmental Medicine and Child Neurology*, 43(10), 668–675. https://doi.org/10.1017/s0012162201001219

Patrick, S. W., Barfield, W. D., Poindexter, B. B., AAP Committee on Fetus and Newborn, Committee on Substance Use and Prevention, Cummings, J., Hand, I., Adams-Chapman, I., Aucott, S. W., Puopolo, K. M., Goldsmith, J. P., Kaufman, D., Martin, C., Mowitz, M., Gonzalez, L., Camenga, D. R., Quigley, J., Ryan, S. A., & Walker-Harding, L. (2020). Neonatal opioid withdrawal syndrome. *Pediatrics*, 146(5). https://doi.org/10.1542/peds.2020-029074

Paul, R. (2020, January 28). *Understanding language development milestones*. Yale School of Medicine. https://medicine.yale.edu/news-article/understanding-language-development-milestones/

Peacock-Chambers, E., Feinberg, E., Senn-McNally, M., Clark, M., Jurkowski, B., Suchman, N., Byatt, N., & Friedmann, P. (2020). Engagement in early intervention services among mothers in recovery from opioid use disorders. *Pediatrics*, 145(2), 1–8. https://doi.org/10.1542/peds.2019-1957

Perkins, M. R. (2005). Pragmatic ability and disability as emergent phenomena. *Clinical Linguistics & Phonetics*, 19(5), 367–377. https://doi.org/10.1080/02699200400027155

Proctor-Williams, K. (2018). The opioid crisis on our caseloads. *The ASHA Leader*, 23(11), 42–49. https://doi.org/10.1044/leader.FTR1.23112018.42

Proctor-Williams, K., & Louw B. (2022). Cleft lip and/or palate in infants prenatally exposed to opioids. *The Cleft Palate Craniofacial Journal*, 59(4), 513–521. doi:10.1177/10556656211013687

Rigg, K. K., & Rigg, M. S. (2020). Opioid-induced hearing loss and neonatal abstinence syndrome: Clinical considerations for audiologists and recommendations for future research. *American Journal of Audiology, 29*(4), 701–709. https://doi.org/10.1044/2020_AJA-20-00054

Rollins, P. R. (2016). Words are not enough. *Topics in Language Disorders, 36*(3), 198–216. https://doi.org/10.1097/TLD.0000000000000095

Rubio, D. M., Schoenbaum, E. E., Lee, L. S., Schteingart, D. E., Marantz, P. R., Anderson, K. E., Platt, L. D., Baez, A., & Esposito, K. (2010). Defining translational research: Implications for training. *Academic Medicine, 85*(3), 470–475. https://doi.org/10.1097/ACM.0b013e3181ccd618

Rutherford, K., Maxwell, J., Fry, L., Holland, P., Rigon, A., & Lankford, A. (2022). Perceived clinical characteristics of children with history of opioid exposure: A speech-language pathology perspective. *American Journal of Speech-Language Pathology, 31*(4), 1801–1816. https://doi.org/10.1044/2022_AJSLP-21-00336

Rydell, P. J. (2012). *Learning style profile for children with autism spectrum disorders* [Audiobook]. Northern Speech Services.

Sandtorv L. B., Fevang S. K. E., Nilsen S. A., et al. (2018). Symptoms associated with attention deficit/hyperactivity disorder and autism spectrum disorders in school-aged children prenatally exposed to substances. *Substance Abuse: Research and Treatment, 12*, 117822181876577. https://doi:10.1177/1178221818765773

Sanlorenzo, L. A., Stark, A. R., & Patrick, S. W. (2018). Neonatal abstinence syndrome: An update. *Current Opinion in Pediatrics, 30*(2), 182–186. https://doi.org/10.1097/MOP.0000000000000589

Schmidt, R., Wolfson, L., Stinson, J., Poole, N., & Greaves, L. (2019). *Mothering and opioids: Addressing stigma and acting collaboratively.* Centre of Excellence for Women's Health. www.bccewh.bc.ca

Skeide, M. A., & Friederici, A. D. (2016). The ontogeny of the cortical language network. *Nature Reviews Neuroscience, 17*(5), 323–332. https://doi.org/10.1038/nrn.2016.23

Stanford Children's Health (n.d.) *Age-appropriate speech and language milestones.* Lucile Packard Children's Hospital Stanford. https://www.stanfordchildrens.org/en/topic/default?id=age-appropriate-speech-and-language-milestones-90-P02170

Sundelin Wahlsten, V., & Sarman, I. (2013). Neurobehavioural development of preschool-age children born to addicted mothers given opiate maintenance treatment with buprenorphine during pregnancy. *Acta Paediatrica, 102*(5), 544–549. https://doi.org/10.1111/apa.12210

Thurm, A., Powell, E. M., Neul, J. L., Wagner, A., & Zwaigenbaum, L. (2018). Loss of skills and onset patterns in neurodevelopmental disorders: Understanding the neurobiological mechanisms. *Autism Research, 11*(2), 212–222. https://doi.org/10.1002/aur.1903

Walhovd, K. B., Bjørnebekk, A., Haabrekke, K., Siqveland, T., Slinning, K., Nygaard, E., Fjell, A. M., Due-Tønnessen, P., Bjørnerud, A., & Moe, V. (2015). Child neuroanatomical, neurocognitive, and visual acuity outcomes with maternal opioid and polysubstance detoxification. *Pediatric Neurology, 52*(3), 326–332. https://doi.org/10.1016/j.pediatrneurol.2014.11.008

Weismer, S. E., Plante, E., Jones, M., & Tomblin, J. B. (2005). A functional magnetic resonance imaging investigation of verbal working memory in adolescents with specific language impairment. *Journal of Speech, Language, and Hearing Research, 48*(2), 405–425. https://doi.org/10.1044/1092-4388(2005/028)

World Health Organization. (2010). *Framework for Action on Interprofessional Education and Collaborative Practice.* https://apps.who.int/iris/handle/10665/70185

Zwaigenbaum, L., Bauman, M. L., Stone, W. L., Yirmiya, N., Estes, A., Hansen, R. L., McPartland, J. C., Natowicz, M. R., Choueiri, R., Fein, D., Kasari, C., Pierce, K., Buie, T., Carter, A., Davis, P. A., Granpeesheh, D., Mailloux, Z., Newschaffer, C., Robins, D., ... Wetherby, A. (2015). Early identification of autism spectrum disorder: Recommendations for practice and research. *Pediatrics, 136*(1), 10–40. https://doi.org/10.1542/peds.2014-3667C

Zwaigenbaum, L., & Penner, M. (2018). Autism spectrum disorder: Advances in diagnosis and evaluation. *BMJ, 361.* https://doi.org/10.1136/bmj.k1674

8 The Role of Occupational Therapy and the Interprofessional Approach to Mitigating Developmental Sequelae Associated With Neonatal Opioid Withdrawal Syndrome

Jenene W. Craig and Christy Gliniak

8.1 Introduction

Occupational therapy (OT) provides important contributions in the management of neonatal opioid withdrawal syndrome (NOWS) and the mitigation of developmental sequelae, from the earliest developmental opportunity in the Neonatal Intensive Care Unit (NICU) extending through the formative years of early childhood. NOWS is a medical condition that occurs when a newborn baby is exposed to opioids during the prenatal period, imposing significant risk of gestational complications for both mother and developing infant(s) (Centers for Disease Control and Prevention [CDC], 2023; Patrick et al., 2020). An increasing number of infants experiencing in-utero opioid exposure and withdrawal between 2000 to 2016 prompted a terminology shift from neonatal abstinence syndrome (NAS) to NOWS for more accurate diagnosis, incidence, and treatment (Grossman & Berkwitt, 2019; Jilani et al., 2022; Klaman et al., 2017). NOWS, a subset of NAS, has become a more widespread term for infant withdrawal from opioids or prescribed medications that a mother received to address opioid substance use disorder while pregnant (Grossman & Berkwitt, 2019; Jilani et al., 2022; Schiff & Grossman, 2019). The traditional term NAS has been used to describe intra-uterine drug exposure to include both opioids and non-opioids such as antidepressants, methamphetamine, barbiturates, and other psychotropic substances (Grossman & Berkwitt, 2019; Patrick et al., 2020). This is important because specific screening and treatment protocols can be used to promote the best outcomes for NOWS infants, whereas infants not exposed to opioids may require different assessment and management (Grossman & Berkwitt, 2019; Patrick et al., 2020). In this chapter, discussion will be specific to NOWS unless otherwise stated.

DOI: 10.4324/9781003397267-8

NOWS is characterized by a range of symptoms including tremors, seizures, irritability, and feeding difficulties, among others. The condition is associated with long-term developmental sequelae that can have significant impact on both the child's and parent's well-being. NOWS is a heterogeneous condition that consists of central nervous system hyperactivity, autonomic nervous system dysfunction, and gastrointestinal problems, with symptoms typically beginning 24–72 hours after birth (Weller et al., 2021). Through a sensory-based and family-centered trauma-informed care approach, OT practitioners can promote better long-term outcomes for both the infant and parent/caregiver. This chapter will address an overview of NOWS, integrated collaborative care, and the role occupational therapy.

8.2 Overview of NOWS

Maternal substance use continues to be a global health problem of significant proportions, with the incidence of NOWS increasing more than seven-fold in the last decade, growing from 1.2 to 8.8 per 1,000 hospital births (Grossman & Berkwitt, 2019; Patrick et al., 2020; Rose-Jacobs et al., 2019). This requires an urgent response, not only to ameliorate the significant effects on child development but also to address the tremendous social and economic costs to society (Fraser et al., 2007; Weller et al., 2021). Intrauterine drug exposure alters the chemistry and structural formation of the brain, leading to subsequent cognitive and behavioral challenges (Behnke & Smith, 2013; Benninger et al., 2020) as evidenced in later infant and child assessments. Researchers are looking to identify the detrimental influences of NOWS on the brain with the hope of informing early intervention strategies and optimizing developmental outcomes (Benninger et al., 2020; Kocherlakota, 2014; Rosenblum et al., 2018).

Nearly all drugs are known to cross the placenta and can have significant teratogenic effects, especially early in the embryonic stage (Behnke & Smith, 2013; Merhar et al., 2021). Illicit substances alter brain structure and circuitry in varying degrees based on the type, timing, and frequency of the substance(s) used (Behnke & Smith, 2013; Oei, 2019). Research indicates an altered maturation of neuronal connective tracts and smaller neuroanatomic volumes in infants born to opioid-addicted mothers (Kocherlakota, 2014; Merhar et al., 2021). Opioid exposure can cause neuronal apoptosis and inhibit the uptake of neurotransmitters such as dopamine and norepinephrine, resulting in deleterious effects on the structural formation and function of the brain (Kocherlakota, 2014; Oei, 2019). Additionally, insults to the nervous system during these critical periods of neurogenesis are more devastating in comparison to exposure to the mature brain with fully operational regulatory systems (Behnke & Smith, 2013; Merhar et al., 2021).

Infants exposed to opioids during pregnancy endure a high allostatic load of toxic stress when considering the biological, psychological, and environmental stressors of intrauterine drug exposure, including violence, parental mood disturbances, and poverty (Glantz & Chambers, 2006; Oei, 2019; Shonkoff et al., 2012). Additionally, infants who have been exposed to illicit substances in utero have a higher instance of prematurity, lower birth weights, reduced head circumference, and impaired fetal brain growth (Glantz & Chambers, 2006; Merhar et al., 2021; Patrick et al., 2020). Relatedly, infants with acute opioid withdrawal experience a cascade of symptoms and often have impairments in neuropsychological function and poor attachment in their early relationships (Benninger et al., 2022; Glantz & Chambers, 2006). As these infants grow, resulting pathological consequences on the developing brain presents greater propensity towards long-term developmental impairments, particularly in behavioral and cognitive domains (Behnke & Smith, 2013; Benninger et al., 2022; Oei, 2019). In a recent study, using *Bayley Scales of Infant and Toddler Development, Third Edition* (Bayley, 2005) at 3–4 months, 9–12 months, and 15–18 months, neurodevelopmental scores of infants with NOWS were not significantly different from published norms in the first year of life; however, they were lower than published norms in the second year of life in areas of language and cognition (Benninger et al., 2020). Jilani et al. (2022) describe alterations in neurodevelopment as "dysregulation in 4 dimensional and interactional neurobehavioral domains: autonomic control, attention/state control, motor/tone control, and sensory processing/modulation" (p. 33), all of which fall within the domain of occupational therapy. Furthermore, "children with intrauterine opioid exposure demonstrated behavioral challenges at school age, particularly with deficits in attention and hyperactivity, executive function, and inhibitory control" (Benninger et al., 2020, p. 2).

Infants with NOWS experience withdrawal signs that may interfere with their occupational performance in activities of daily living (ADLs). In turn, occupational therapy intervention, as early as the NICU, offers potential to improve future occupational performance and engagement with caregivers. Partnering with parents, family members, and other supportive caregivers is critical, as early neurostructural changes can significantly impact the necessary co-occupations of infancy vital to building healthy infant–parent relationships. Parental opioid use disorder (OUD) can also disrupt sensitive parenting strategies required for regulation, healthy attachment, and buffering stress, further interfering with social–emotional development and learning (Martin et al., 2022; Valadez et al., 2020). Considering these combined physiologic and environmental barriers, resources are needed to address developmental needs, reduce toxic stress, and promote nurturing early relationships for these high-risk parent/caregiver–infant dyads (Shan et al., 2020). Occupational therapists are well positioned for service of this special population in the context of infant–parent co-occupation and optimizing development (Price & Miner, 2009; Richter et al., 2023).

8.3 Integrated Collaborative Care

The interprofessional approach to healthcare involves collaboration among healthcare professionals from multiple disciplines, each contributing from varying scopes of practice in order to provide comprehensive care to patients. The interprofessional team may include neonatologists, pediatricians, other physicians, nurses, therapists, dieticians, pharmacists, psychologists, social workers, lactation specialists, and other consultants who play a crucial role in the care of infants with NOWS. The word "collaborative" implies communication among two or more healthcare professionals who are working toward a common goal to deliver care (Elkington, 2023). Integrated collaborative care (ICC) is a term that describes how healthcare professionals manage, organize, and integrate patient care coordination with an aim to ensure patient wellness (Elkington, 2023; Heath et al., 2013; Nancarrow et al., 2013; Schot et al., 2020). The authors would like to acknowledge the importance of family involvement in the care of their child and as part of the collaborative team as evinced in research around Family Integrative Collaborative Care (Franck & O'Brien, 2019). The focus of this chapter will be on integrative collaborative care specific to Occupational therapists (OTs), physical therapists (PTs), and speech-language pathologists (SLPs), who often coordinate care across disciplines, various lifespan populations, and settings.

Starting as early as the NICU, OT, PT, and SLP practitioners who have advanced clinical knowledge in gestational and infant development can work as neonatal therapists (NT) offering important holistic direct patient care and consultative services to premature and medically complex infants and their parents/caregivers (National Association of Neonatal Therapists [NANT], 2023). Each NT, regardless of discipline of training, must possess shared foundational knowledge and skills in order to work in the NICU. However, beyond the fundamental knowledge and skills required, each discipline (OT, PT, and SLP) brings a unique professional perspective and their own discipline-specific knowledge and training. Inferred roles for NTs would include those that would fall within the practice guidelines outlined by each neonatal therapy professional discipline of OT, PT, and SLP (American Speech-Language-Hearing Association, 2004; Craig et al., 2018; NANT, 2023; Sweeney et al., 2009).

8.4 Occupational Therapy Overview

The scope of practice for occupational therapists is based on the American Occupational Therapy Association (AOTA) Practice Framework and the Philosophical Base of Occupational Therapy (AOTA, 2017), which states that "the use of occupation to promote individual, family, community, and population health is the core of OT practice, education, research, and advocacy" (p. 1). Occupations are the everyday activities that people do as individuals, in families, and with communities to occupy time and bring meaning and purpose to life and are categorized as "activities of daily living (ADLs), instrumental activities of daily living (IADLs), health management, rest and sleep, education, work, play, leisure, and social participation" (AOTA, 2020). As such, "occupations include things people need to, want to and are expected to do" (World Federation of Occupational Therapists [WFOT], 2012, p. 2).

Occupational science is important to the practice of occupational therapy and "provides a way of thinking that enables an understanding of occupation, the occupational nature of humans, the relationship between occupation, health and well-being, and the influences that shape occupation" (WFOT, 2012, p. 2). Unique to OT and its holistic approach is a strong educational foundation in mental health, enabling occupational therapists to assess clients' psychosocial needs and strengths for individualized interventions.

Occupational therapy services are provided across the lifespan for habilitation, rehabilitation, and promotion of health and wellness for clients with disability and non-disability-related needs. These services include acquisition and preservation of occupational identity for clients who have or are at risk for developing an illness, injury, disease, disorder, condition, impairment, disability, activity limitation, or participation restriction (AOTA, 2020). The work of OT is described through two primary areas: the *domain*, the profession's purview and areas in which therapists have knowledge and expertise; and the *process*, which describes actions therapists take when providing services that are client-centered and focused on engagement in occupations (see Figure 8.1).

Occupations and co-occupations include bathing, diapering/toileting, dressing, eating and swallowing, feeding, functional mobility, child rearing, religious and spiritual expression, health management, social and emotional health promotion and maintenance, communication with the healthcare system, rest and sleep, education, and play exploration and participation (AOTA, 2020). Within OT practice areas of the NICU and pediatrics, the *client* is viewed as the infant/child–parent/caregiver and is further described through the perspective of co-occupation.

Achieving health, well-being, and participation in life through engagement in occupation

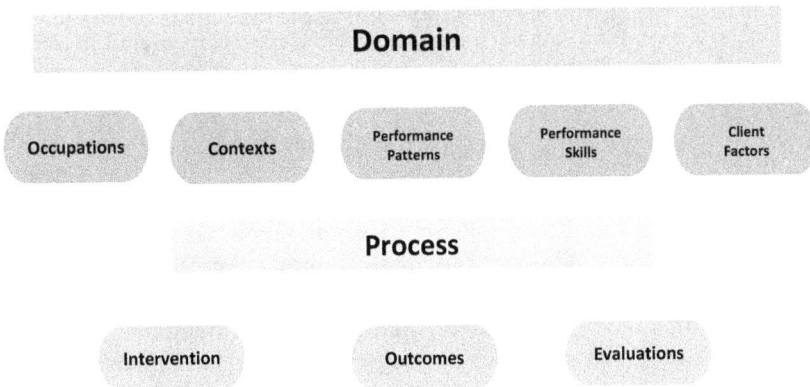

Figure 8.1 Occupational therapy domain and process

8.4.1 Infant–Parent Co-Occupation

Co-occupation is a term used in occupational therapy referring to the shared participation of two or more individuals in a specific activity, involving not only the parent/caregiver's participation, but also the infant's (Esdaile & Olson, 2004; Pierce, 2009). This includes any task/activity valued by the family culture in which the parent/caregiver and infant are expected to engage in together. Theoretically, it is thought that participation in co-occupation contributes to quality of life, with deprivation in co-occupational opportunities seen as disruptive to health and well-being (Pickens & Pizur-Barnekow, 2009). This is particularly relevant to the stressful environment of the NICU where the earliest opportunity for parent–infant co-occupation such as dressing, bathing or feeding is often met with medical and psychosocial constrictions. For OTs, these occupations exist on a continuum beginning with requirements for infant survival, to more complex activities involving shared plans and coordinated actions as evinced in toddlers, children, and adolescents (Craig & Smith, 2020; Pickens & Pizur-Barnekow, 2009; Richter et al., 2023). Overall, co-occupation is an important part of OT, as it recognizes the infant's active role in their own care and promotes the development of meaningful relationships between the infant and caregivers (Richter et al., 2023).

The work of co-occupation, supported by occupational therapists, serves to couple infant mental health and milestone progression, to foster parent/family–infant attachment, sensitive parenting, regulation, and sensory-motor skill development. This OT therapeutic approach continues throughout early intervention services, into preschool play-based services, later school occupational performance, and preparation for adult ADLs and IADLs across the lifespan.

8.5 Role of the OT in the Neonatal Intensive Care Unit (NICU)

When working with infants in the NICU, it is imperative to use a family-centered, age-appropriate, neuroprotective, developmental care approach to guide treatment planning and interventions (Piccotti et al., 2019). These principles are outlined within the Guidelines for the Institutional Implementation of Developmental Neuroprotective Care in the NICU and influential models of care such as the Universe of Developmental Care Model and the Neonatal Integrative Developmental Care Model (Altimier & Phillips, 2013; Coughlin, 2021; Gibbins et al., 2008; Milette et al., 2019; Piccotti et al., 2019). OT interventions align with these developmental care models as they coincide directly with areas of infant occupation and age-appropriate ADLs.

Occupational therapy services in the acute treatment and management of NOWS include, but are not limited to, nonpharmacological interventions such as: therapeutic handling, developmental positioning, infant massage, feeding and swallowing, sensory modulation, and engagement of parents in co-occupations and ADL interventions such as swaddle bathing, dressing, skin care, baby wearing, protection/promotion of sleep, and discharge readiness planning. The advanced-level knowledge required for practice in the NICU includes familiarity with relevant medical conditions, procedures, and equipment; an understanding of the individualized developmental abilities and vulnerabilities of preterm and full-term infants; an understanding of relevant theories; working knowledge of family systems, early social–emotional development, infant mental health, neuroprotection, pain and stress, and the NICU environment; and an understanding of multidisciplinary team collaboration (Altimier & Phillips, 2013; Coughlin et al., 2009; Craig et al., 2018; Craig et al., 2015; NANT, 2023).

8.5.1 OT and Infant Mental Health

Occupational therapy's multifaceted and holistic approach to patients experiencing NOWS includes comprehensive management of the infant/

child and parent/family including mental health (AOTA, 2020; Oostlander et al., 2019). Underlying principles of infant mental health include:

> the ability to develop effective physical, social and emotion regulation as well as to establish and depend on reciprocal relationships with primary care providers, and for those providers to be able to reflect on the baby's experience, in order to provide safe, individualized, nurturing and regulating opportunities for growth.
>
> (Browne, 2021, p. 1)

Substance use disorders can interfere with a mother's interpersonal skills, parenting competencies, and attachment style, creating severe repercussions for the child's future psychosocial development (Brancato & Cannizzaro, 2018; Parolin & Simonelli, 2016). As such, the OT's role around infant–caregiver psychosocial development is essential to support confidence and competence in early parenting skills (Craig et al., 2015; Lee et al., 2012).

8.5.2 Nonpharmacological Interventions

The American Academy of Pediatrics (AAP) recommends a nonpharmacological approach to care as the preferred treatment method for NOWS during hospitalization (Patrick et al., 2020). More commonly, NICUs use a systematic Eat, Sleep, Console approach, capitalizing on the co-regulatory qualities of the parent together with nonpharmacological strategies to decrease the length of hospitalization and need for medication (Grisham et al., 2019; McRae et al., 2021; Rhoads & Waskosky, 2022). There are circumstances, however, where withdrawal becomes more severe and the combination of pharmacological and nonpharmacological interventions are required (Patrick et al., 2020; Piccotti et al., 2019).

When caring for these high-risk dyads, occupational therapists bring strong skills in the area of nonpharmacological interventions and a unique developmental perspective. The OT recognizes impactful elements to long-term development and keeps this central to their clinical reasoning using formal and informal assessments related to neurobehavioral skills and functional performance. OTs are trained to evaluate an infant's movement quality and muscle tone, and to detect any variances within their primitive reflexes. This is relevant considering the symptomatology of NOWS and propensity for tremors, clonus, hypertonicity, and hyperreflexia. Although it is beyond the scope of this chapter to describe all advanced practice OT interventions, the following section highlights a few as examples.

8.5.2.1 Therapeutic Handling

Therapeutic handling is commonly used by occupational therapists to support an infant's neurobehavioral organization and to optimize behavioral state control. The style of handling selected can either "up-regulate" to increase arousal or "down-regulate" from a hyper-alert or crying state to obtain a quiet alert state, which is best for social exchanges and functional activities such as feeding. Therapeutic handling, as a modality, capitalizes on positive human touch as opposed to procedural touch. It is best to initiate therapeutic handling first by using a static touch, accompanied by a soft voice. This "hand-hug" can prepare the infant for movement and is often an effective calming strategy with a dysregulated infant. Therapists use their whole hands, with mild pressure and deliberately slow movement. When working with infants in withdrawal, an OT will avoid light stroking and often facilitate non-nutritive sucking during a handling session. During handling, graded movement may be introduced as a form of vestibular input – rhythmic, vertical rocking is preferred and holding in a prone vs. supine position can also be beneficial.

Due to prolonged postures of flexion and hypertonia, the OT will evaluate and provide range of motion (ROM) exercises while engaged in therapeutic handling. These therapeutic interventions additionally afford an opportunity to evaluate skin integrity, particularly in the creases of the axilla, elbow, and palms. These are areas at risk for skin breakdown when infants have high muscle tone. An OT will help monitor skin for excoriations that can occur on the elbows and knees as a result of restlessness and excessive movements in the crib. Therapeutic handling is used to support ADLs such as diapering or pre/post feeding, but also for intervention to address sensory-motor system stress or activated sympathetic nervous system responses, to balance muscle tone relaxation/activation and restore postural alignment. When a parent is present, an OT will prioritize coaching support of the parent's therapeutic handling, to include transfers to skin-to-skin holding or a smooth state transition to sleep.

8.5.2.2 Sleep Protection

Sleep is an important occupation impacting both physical and mental health. Chronic opioid withdrawal impacts opioid receptors, located in the same nuclei used in sleep regulation, resulting in significant insomnia, frequent arousals, and decreased REM sleep (Wang & Teichtahl, 2007). Infants experiencing acute NOWS often have a difficult time falling asleep and maintaining sleep, prompting mothers with OUD to adjust their sleep practices to minimize withdrawal symptoms (Morrison et al., 2023). These persistent sleep disturbances can cause safe sleep protocols to be difficult to adhere to. OTs are often utilized for state and sleep recommendations/ interventions including approaches around handling and positioning.

Trained cuddle team volunteers and staff nurses are often utilized when family members cannot be available.

8.5.2.3 Positioning

Swaddling is considered an effective non-pharmacological intervention in the management of NOWS to decrease arousal, improve motor organization, and promote sleep (Mangat et al., 2019). OTs provide therapeutic positioning recommendations regarding swaddling and devices used for areas of postural support, proprioceptive input, sleep management, and pain relief. When actively in withdrawal, an infant with NOWS can also have difficulty with thermoregulation. OTs can assist with containment strategies that reduce overheating and offer developmentally appropriate movement patterns for the term baby as opposed to those utilized for the premature infant.

8.5.2.4 Feeding

Occupational therapists with advanced training conduct comprehensive feeding evaluations to provide recommendations and educational support for families, often influencing decisions regarding pharmacological interventions and/or readiness for discharge home. During bottle feeding between opioid exposed mother–infant dyads, higher maternal stress and decreased maternal sensitivity led to the decreased ability by the mother to read and respond to infant cues, which resulted in poor co-regulation during feeding (Rinaldi et al., 2023). For infants with NOWS or NAS, neurobehavioral dysregulation of autonomic, sleep/attentional state, motor/muscle tone, and sensory processing/modulation influences feeding performance, resulting in frantic, uncoordinated feeding and leading to inadequate nutrition (Isbell, 2022; McGlothen-Bell et al., 2020; Velez et al., 2021). Feeding behaviors can range from flailing limbs, turning away, pushing or spitting out the nipple, crying, hyperphagia, and hyper/hypo-tonicity (Isbell, 2022; Rinaldi et al., 2023). Currently, there is a paucity of literature related to the complex feeding challenges experienced by infants with NOWS as compared to NAS (McQueen et al., 2019; Nagy et al., 2023). However, breastfeeding is the most studied nonpharmacological intervention for lactating mothers who take methadone or buprenorphine used to reduce withdrawal symptoms and foster bonding and attachment (McQueen et al., 2019; Patrick et al., 2020). McQueen et al. (2019) explored correlations between feeding methods and outcomes for infants exposed to opioids. Findings highlighted breastfeeding outcomes related to decreased incidence and duration of pharmacological intervention, shorter hospitalization, and reduced severity of NAS/NOWS symptoms. A NT can be a powerful advocate for breastfeeding when working with opioid-exposed dyads.

8.5.2.5 Additional Interventions

There are multiple systems addressed by occupational therapy related to NOWS to include the environment, family/psychosocial, sensory, neurobehavioral, neuromotor, and musculoskeletal systems. Environmental modifications are frequently necessary to reduce overstimulation and prevent behavioral disturbances from visual, auditory, tactile, olfactory, gustatory vestibular, proprioceptive, and interoceptive sensations. In general, quiet environments with low lighting and minimal activity are most supportive especially in early weeks, during feeding or transition to sleep. Interventions are provided when sensory input exceeds an infant's threshold, resulting in dysregulation, poor consolability, and problems with sensory modulation (Jilani et al., 2022). Once leaving the NICU, outpatient OT may be necessary for continued support for infants with persistent dysregulation and limited ability to engage in age-appropriate social experiences and ADLs.

8.5.3 Trauma-Informed Care With Infants Experiencing NOWS

Neonatal opioid withdrawal is a form of childhood adversity and can constitute an adverse childhood experience (ACE) due to prolonged toxic stress, sleep fragmentation, noxious stimuli/pain, and parent separation (Bartlett & Sacks, 2019; Coughlin, 2021; D'Agata et al., 2016). Research in genetics, neuroscience, and epidemiology all provide evidence that "these experiences have effects at the molecular, cellular, and organ level, with consequences on physical, emotional, developmental, and behavioral health across the lifespan" (Forkey et al., 2021, p. 1). Toxic stress responses during early brain development negatively influence the function of the hypothalamic–pituitary–adrenal axis, sympathetic nervous system, and gene expression, leading to long-term dysregulation (D'Agata et al., 2018; Forkey et al., 2021; Montirosso et al., 2015). For these reasons, it is essential for interprofessional team members working with individuals with OUD and NOWS to use a trauma-informed approach.

The National Child Traumatic Stress Network defines trauma-informed care (TIC) as "medical care in which all parties involved assess, recognize, and respond to the effects of traumatic stress on children, caregivers, and health care providers" (Forkey et al., 2021, p.1). This includes efforts to prevent re-traumatization and recognize secondary traumatic stress which results from witnessing first-hand trauma experiences of others (Forkey et al., 2021; Substance Abuse and Mental Health Services Administration [SAMHSA], 2014). This philosophical view requires a caregiver to move away from the traditional, medical model approach of "What is wrong with you?" to "What happened to you?" (Forkey et al., 2021). The underpinning of a TIC approach is to utilize the buffering effect of parental presence, co-regulation, and early infant–parent attachment to optimize long-term neurodevelopmental outcomes (Coughlin, 2021; Sanders & Hall, 2018).

The developmental risks of children with intrauterine drug exposure include the potential for intergenerational trauma transmission. Many mothers with OUD have experienced early adversity, anxiety, depression, and other psychiatric disorders (SAMHSA, 2018). Research has found that "the majority of women entering treatment for OUD have a history of sexual assault, trauma, or domestic violence and/or come from homes where their caregivers used drugs (SAMHSA, 2018, p. 42). Up to 85% of pregnancies of opioid-using women are unintended (Auerbach et al., 2021), adding to the risk for adverse maternal and infant outcomes like postpartum depression, preterm birth, low birthweight, and interpersonal violence (Nelson et al., 2022). A retrospective study of children born to mothers with greater than four ACEs found that they were 40% less likely to avoid an adverse childhood experience and 4.76 times more likely to have four or more ACEs themselves (Schickedanz et al., 2021).

Occupational therapists who provide infant mental health interventions recognize the importance of critical early relationships and empowering parents. Punitive, stigmatizing, and judgmental behaviors towards mothers with OUD dismantle feelings of safety and prevent self/co-regulation, openness to important healthcare education, and parental presence. A TIC approach creates a safe, positive, and supportive environment to facilitate parent empowerment and resilience in the infant–parent relationship (Cleveland et al., 2016; Forkey et al., 2021; Gliniak, 2022). TIC upon discharge also incorporates cross-agency collaboration, coordinated care, and protective wrap-around services to help families in recovery and to disrupt the intergenerational trauma cycle (Duffee et al., 2021). Health systems are often slow to adopt policies related to TIC and subsequently teams lack the knowledge, time, and resources required for successful implementation (Forkey et al., 2021; Gliniak, 2022). Gliniak (2022) highlights the individual and systemic barriers and facilitators toward TIC integration in the NICU (see Figure 8.2).

Discussions related to the complexities of TIC implementation are beyond the scope of this chapter. However, prioritizing trauma-informed practices when working with NOWS holds tremendous potential to

Neonatal Trauma-Informed Care Implementation Determinants

Systemic Facilitators:
Supportive Management & Programs

Individual Facilitators:
Qualities of a Trauma-Informed Professional

Systemic Barriers

Individual Barriers

Individual Facilitators

Systemic Facilitators

Trauma-Informed Care Integration

Trauma-Informed Care Not Understood or Prioritized

Systemic Barriers:
Poor Psychological Support
Lack of Clinical Guidelines
Comunication Gaps
Staffing Shortages

Individual Barriers:
Task-Oriented Caregiving
Caregiver Burnout
Depersonalization
Education Gaps

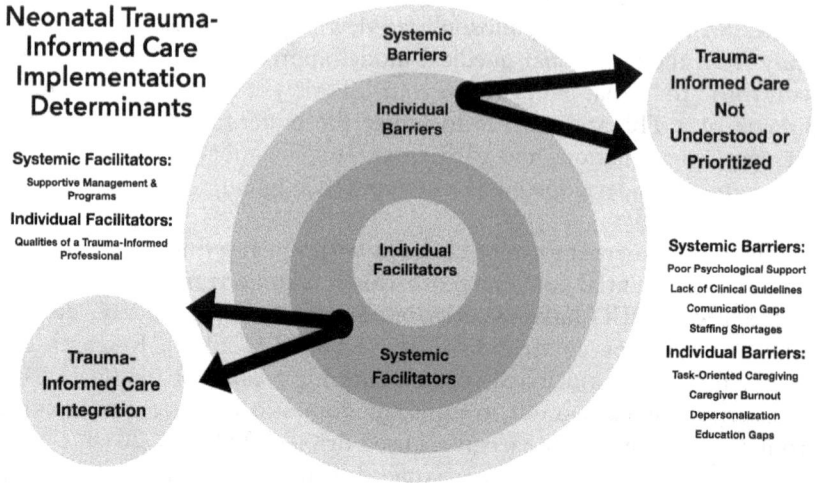

Figure 8.2 Neonatal Trauma Informed-Care Implementation Determinants

improve patient experiences, reduce staff burnout, and optimize infant neurodevelopmental outcomes across the continuum of care.

8.6 Occupational Therapy Post NICU

Risks for developmental sequelae persist well beyond the NICU for infants with intrauterine opioid exposure. As a result, interventions should include "home visiting, screening, parent education, and connecting families to additional community support to reduce harm, mitigate childhood trauma, and support the entire family" (Voss et al., 2023, p. 1288). Occupational therapy is required for targeted interventions to address developmental, academic, or functional performance concerns.

8.6.1 Early Intervention

Early childhood (birth–5 years) is a critical period in which foundational life occupations are nurtured (e.g., eating, dressing, play, learning, social participation, rest and sleep, and chores). The development of cognitive, motor, social–emotional, and self-care skills are important to support these occupations through the delivery of early OT services (Kingsley & Clark, 2020). As such, hospital-based healthcare teams who care for infants with NOWS are particularly well positioned to initiate early intervention (EI) referrals, given the elevated developmental risk factors inherent to NOWS. Unfortunately, only approximately 25% of all eligible children across the United States receive EI services. In addition, public systems, such as child welfare and early intervention, are increasingly stretched by increasing numbers of children affected by the opioid crisis (Patrick et al., 2020).

8.6.2 School-Aged Children

Maternal drug use during pregnancy has the potential for long-term negative implications on neurodevelopment, physical health, and social and psychological well-being (Shan et al., 2020). Limited longitudinal studies exist related to infants with opioid and polysubstance exposure due to poor reporting, variability in substances, and limitations in tracking research participants (Benninger et al., 2020; Nygaard et al., 2015). Despite this, some researchers have successfully isolated clusters of observable behaviors that correspond to associated maternal drugs of choice. Behnke and Smith (2013) report long-term consequences of opioid exposure including difficulties in arousal, attention, and memory with a specific vulnerability identified in parts of the brain that support regulation and executive functions. Hayatbakhsh et al. (2012) identify additional outcomes related to lower performance in attention, memory, and impulse control in older children. Developmental surveillance of infants with NOWS is recommended, including the use of validated screening and assessment tools during the first year, followed by standardized neurodevelopmental and multi-domain assessments at later time points (i.e., 18–24 and 33–36 months) when higher-order functions, such as cognition, language, and behavior, emerge and can be more accurately tested (Benninger et al., 2020; Nygaard et al., 2016; Wong & Leland, 2016).

Children with NOWS may develop special needs due to neurobiological factors, which can influence their ability to participate and enjoy early emotional interactions with parents or complex social exchanges with school-aged peers. Early engagement in shared interactions are positive interventions that support learning to communicate and regulate emotions for future complex thinking and social interaction. Powerful interventions for young children, derived from developmental theory, focus on the relationship between a caregiver's level of responsiveness and the child's development of social communication (Hyman et al., 2020). One such approach is known as the Developmental, Individual Differences, and Relationship-Based model (DIR®). Through DIR®, OTs, PTs, and SLPs provide coaching to help increase responsiveness to the parent or caregiver through imitating, expanding on, or joining in to child-initiated play activities. This approach supports developmental capacities of the child such as joint attention, imitation, and affective social engagement (Hyman et al.,

2020). DIR® as an intervention can help parents partner with their child to promote foundational skill development, including regulation, joint attention, communication and language, motor skills, cognition, ideation and execution, and social problem-solving.

8.7 Summary

The integrated collaborative care approach is crucial to mitigating the developmental sequelae associated with NOWS and promoting the best possible outcomes for high-risk infants and families (McCarty & Braswell, 2022; McDaniel et al., 2021). OT plays an important role by contributing a rich developmental perspective and advanced practice skills that foster age-appropriate neuromotor, cognitive, sensory, and psychosocial development. These nonpharmacological relationship-based interventions often begin in the NICU during early infant–parent co-occupations and extend through critical stages of early development and beyond. Related to NOWS, occupational therapists provide evidence-based therapeutic interventions in a wide range of clinical settings (e.g., mental health, substance use, and perinatal care) and prioritize habilitative approaches of infant mental health services to promote healthy early relationship with their developing baby prenatally and after birth (AOTA, 2020; Branjerdporn et al., 2020). A family-centered approach is used whenever possible to boost parental autonomy and confidence using hands-on learning opportunities and non-judgmental dialogue. Occupational therapy practitioners emphasize a holistic approach and incorporate both individual and cultural contexts to maximize developmental capacities and promote principles of autonomy throughout the lifespan.

References

Altimier, L., & Phillips, R. M. (2013). The neonatal integrative developmental care model: Seven neuroprotective core measures for family-centered developmental care. *Newborn and Infant Nursing Reviews, 13*(1), 9–22. https://doi.org/10.1053/j.nainr.2016.09.030

American Occupational Therapy Association. (2017). Philosophical base of occupational therapy. *American Journal of Occupational Therapy, 71*(2). https://doi.org/10.5014/ajot.2017.716S06

American Occupational Therapy Association. (2020). Occupational therapy practice framework: Domain and process. *The American Journal of Occupational Therapy, 74*(2), 1–87. https://doi.org/10.5014/ajot.2020.74S2001

American Speech-Language-Hearing Association. (2004). Knowledge and skills needed by speech-language pathologists providing services to infants and families in the NICU environment. https://www.asha.org/policy/KS2004-00080/

Auerbach, S. L., Agbemenu, K., Ely, G. E., & Lorenz, R. (2021). A review of unintended pregnancy in opioid-using women: Implications for nursing. *Journal of Addictions Nursing, 32*(2), 107–114.

Bartlett, J. D., & Sacks, V. (2019). Adverse childhood experiences are different than child trauma, and it's critical to understand why. *Child Trends.*

Bayley, N. (2005). *Bayley Scales of Infant and Toddler Development, Third Edition* (Bayley – III®) [Database record]. APA PsycTests. https://psycnet.apa.org/doi/10.1037/t14978-000

Behnke, M., & Smith, V. C. (2013). Prenatal substance abuse: Short- and long-term effects on the exposed fetus. *Pediatrics, 131*(3), 1009–1024. https://doi.org/10.1542/peds.2012-3931

Benninger, K. L., Borghese, T., Kovalcik, J. B., Moore-Clingenpeel, M., Isler, C., Bonachea, E. M., Stark, A. R., Patrick, S. W., & Maitre, N. L. (2020). Prenatal exposures are associated with worse neurodevelopmental outcomes in infants with neonatal opioid withdrawal syndrome. *Frontiers in Pediatrics, 8,* 462. https://doi.org/10.3389/fped.2020.00462

Benninger, K. L., Richard, C., Conroy, S., Newton, J., Taylor, H. G., Sayed, A., Pietruszewski, L., Nelin, M. A., Batterson, N., & Maitre, N. L. (2022). *One-year neurodevelopmental outcomes after neonatal opioid withdrawal syndrome (Benninger et al., 2022)* (p. 889932 Bytes) [Data set]. ASHA journals. https://doi.org/10.23641/ASHA.20044403.V1

Brancato, A., & Cannizzaro, C. (2018). Mothering under the influence: How perinatal drugs of abuse alter the mother-infant interaction. *Rev Neurosci, 29*(3), 283–294. https://doi.org/10.1515/revneuro-2017-0052

Branjerdporn, G., Meredith, P., Wilson, T., & Strong, J. (2020). Prenatal predictors of maternal–infant attachment. *Canadian Journal of Occupational Therapy, 87*(4), 265–277. https://doi.org/10.1177/0008417420941781

Browne, J. V. (2021). Infant mental health in intensive care: Laying a foundation for social, emotional and mental health outcomes through regulation, relationships and reflection. *Journal of Neonatal Nursing, 27*(1), 33–39. https://doi.org/10.1016/j.jnn.2020.11.011

Centers for Disease Control and Prevention. (2023, November 4). *Alcohol use in pregnancy.* https://www.cdc.gov/ncbddd/fasd/alcohol-use.html

Cleveland, L. M., Bonugli, R. J., & McGlothen, K. S. (2016). The mothering experiences of women with substance use disorders. *Advances in Nursing Science, 39*(2), 119–129. https://doi.org/10.1097/ANS.0000000000000118

Coughlin, M. E. (2021). *Transformative nursing in the NICU: Trauma-informed, age-appropriate care.* Springer Publishing Company.

Coughlin, M., Gibbins, S., & Hoath, S. (2009). Core measures for developmentally supportive care in Neonatal Intensive Care Units: Theory, precedence and practice. *Journal of Advanced Nursing, 65*(10), 2239–2248. https://doi.org/10.1111/j.1365-2648.2009.05052.x

Craig, J. W., Carroll, S., Ludwig, S., & Sturdivant, C. (2018). Occupational therapy's role in the Neonatal Intensive Care Unit. *American Journal of Occupational Therapy, 72*(2), 1–9.

Craig, J. W., Glick, C., Phillips, R., Hall, S. L., Smith, J., & Browne, J. (2015). Recommendations for involving the family in developmental care of the NICU baby. *Journal of Perinatology, 35*(1), 5–8. https://doi.org/10.1038/jp.2015.142

Craig, J. W., & Smith, C. R. (2020). Risk-adjusted/neuroprotective care services in the NICU: The elemental role of the neonatal therapist (OT, PT, SLP). *Journal of Perinatology, 40*(4), 549–559. https://doi.org/10.1038/s41372-020-0597-1

D'Agata, A. L., Coughlin, M., & Sanders, M. R. (2018). Clinician perceptions of the NICU infant experience: Is the NICU hospitalization traumatic? *American Journal of Perinatology, 35*(12), 1159–1167. https://doi.org/10.1055/s-0038-1641747

D'Agata, A. L., Young, E. E., Cong, X., Grasso, D. J., McGrath, J. M., & Forsythe, P. L. (2016). Infant Medical Trauma in the Neonatal Intensive Care Unit (IMTN). *Advances in Neonatal Care, 16*(4), 289–297. https://doi.org/10.1097/ANC.0000000000000309

Duffee, J., Szilagyi, M., Forkey, H., Kelly, E. T., & Council on Community Pediatrics, Council on Foster Care, Adoption, and Kinship Care, Council on Child Abuse and Neglect, Committee on Psychosocial Aspects of Child and Family Health (2021). Trauma-informed care in child health systems. *Pediatrics, 148*(2). https://doi.org/10.1542/peds.2021-052579

Elkington, S. (2023). *Neonatal therapists' perceptions of using integrated collaborative care in the Neonatal Intensive Care Unit.* [Doctoral dissertation, The University of Texas at El Paso]. Scholarworks.

Esdaile, S. A., & Olson, J. A. (2004). *Mothering occupations: Challenge, agency, and participation.* F. A. Davis.

Forkey, H., Szilagyi, M., Kelly, E. T., Duffee, J., & Council on Foster Care, Adoption, and Kinship Care, Council on Community Pediatrics, Council on Child Abuse and Neglect, Committee on Psychosocial Aspects of Child and Family Health. (2021). Trauma-informed care. *Pediatrics, 148*(2). https://doi.org/10.1542/peds.2021-052580

Franck, L. S., & O'Brien, K. (2019). The evolution of family-centered care: From supporting parent-delivered interventions to a model of family integrated care. *Birth Defects Research, 111*(15), 1044–1059. https://doi.org/10.1002/bdr2.1521

Fraser, J. A., Barnes, M., Biggs, H. C., & Kain, V. J. (2007). Caring, chaos and the vulnerable family: Experiences in caring for newborns of drug-dependent parents. *International Journal of Nursing Studies, 44*(8), 1363–1370. https://doi.org/10.1016/j.ijnurstu.2006.06.004

Gibbins, S., Hoath, S. B., Coughlin, M., Gibbins, A., & Franck, L. (2008). The universe of developmental care: A new conceptual model for application in the Neonatal Intensive Care Unit. *Advances in Neonatal Care, 8*(3), 141–147. https://doi.org/10.1097/01.ANC.0000324337.01970.76

Glantz, M. D., & Chambers, J. C. (2006). Prenatal drug exposure effects on subsequent vulnerability to drug abuse. *Development and Psychopathology, 18*(3), 893–922. https://doi.org/10.1017/S0954579406060445

Gliniak, C. (2022). *Cultivating trauma-informed care in the Neonatal Intensive Care Unit (NICU): A qualitative look at perceived determinants to implementation* (Order No. 29162995). [Doctoral dissertation, Fielding Graduate University, Santa Barbara, CA,]. ProQuest Dissertations & Theses Global. (2656860290).

Grisham, L. M., Stephen, M. M., Coykendall, M. R., Kane, M. F., Maurer, J. A., & Bader, M. Y. (2019). Eat, Sleep, Console approach: A family-centered model for the treatment of neonatal abstinence syndrome. *Advances in Neonatal Care, 19*(2), 138–144. https://doi.org/10.1097/ANC.0000000000000581

Grossman, M., & Berkwitt, A. (2019). Neonatal abstinence syndrome. *Seminars in Perinatology, 43*(3), 173–186. https://doi.org/10.1053/j.semperi.2019.01.007

Hayatbakhsh, M. R., Flenady, V. J., Gibbons, K. S., Kingsbury, A. M., Hurrion, E., Mamun, A. A., & Najman, J. M. (2012). Birth outcomes associated with cannabis use before and during pregnancy. *Pediatric Research, 71*(2), 215–219. https://doi.org/10.1038/pr.2011.25

Heath, B., Wise Romero, P., & Reynolds, K. (2013, March). *A standard framework for levels of integrated healthcare.* SAMHSA-HRSA Center for Integrated Health Solutions. https://thepcc.org/sites/default/files/resources/SAMHSA-HRSA%202013%20Framework%20for%20Levels%20of%20Integrated%20Healthcare.pdf

Hyman, S. L., Levy, S. E., Myers, S. M., Kuo, D., Apkon, S., Brei, T., Davidson, L. F., Davis, B. E., Ellerbeck, K. A., & Noritz, G. H. (2020). Executive summary: Identification, evaluation, and management of children with autism spectrum disorder. *Pediatrics, 145*(1). https://doi.org/10.1542/peds.2019-3447

Hynan, M. T., & Hall, S. L. (2015). Psychosocial program standards for NICU parents. *Journal of Perinatology, 35*(1), 1–4. https://doi.org/10.1038/jp.2015.141

Isbell, C. (2022) Feeding in infants born substance exposed: A sensory-based, family-centered approach. *SIS Quarterly Practice Connections, 7*(4).

Jilani, S. M., Jones, H. E., Grossman, M., Jansson, L. M., Terplan, M., Faherty, L. J., Khodyakov, D., Patrick, S. W., & Davis, J. M. (2022). Standardizing the clinical definition of opioid withdrawal in the neonate. *The Journal of Pediatrics, 243*, 33–39. https://doi.org/10.1016/j.jpeds.2021.12.021

Kingsley, K. L., & Clark, G. F. (2020). Occupational therapy interventions for children ages birth–5 years. *The American Journal of Occupational Therapy, 74*(5). https://doi.org/10.5014/ajot.2020.745001

Klaman, S. L., Isaacs, K., Leopold, A., Perpich, J., Hayashi, S., Vender, J., Campopiano, M., & Jones, H. E. (2017). Treating women who are pregnant and parenting for opioid use disorder and the concurrent care of their infants and children: Literature review to support national guidance. *J Addict Med, 11*(3), 178–190. https://doi.org/10.1097/adm.0000000000000308

Kocherlakota, P. (2014). Neonatal abstinence syndrome. *Pediatrics, 134*(2), 547–561. https://doi.org/10.1542/peds.2013-3524

Lee, Y., Garfield, C., & Kim, H. (2012). Self-efficacy theory as a framework for interventions that support parents of NICU infants. *Proceedings of the 6th International Conference on Pervasive Computing Technologies for Healthcare.* 6th International Conference on Pervasive Computing Technologies for Healthcare, San Diego, United States. https://doi.org/10.4108/icst.pervasivehealth.2012.248710

Mangat, A. K., Schmölzer, G. M., & Kraft, W. K. (2019). Pharmacological and non-pharmacological treatments for the Neonatal Abstinence Syndrome (NAS). *Semin Fetal Neonatal Med, 24*(2), 133–141. https://doi.org/10.1016/j.siny.2019.01.009

Martin, C., Chen, H.-W. B., & Dozier, M. (2022). Intervening with opioid-exposed newborns: Modifying an evidence-based parenting intervention.

Delaware Journal of Public Health, 8(2), 94–98. https://doi.org/10.32481/djph.2022.05.014

McCarty, T., & Braswell, E. (2022). Implementation of interprofessional rounds decreases neonatal abstinence syndrome length of stay. *The Journal of Pediatric Pharmacology and Therapeutics*, 27(2), 157–163. https://doi.org/10.5863/1551-6776-27.2.157

McDaniel, C. E., Jacob-Files, E., Deodhar, P., McGrath, C. L., & Desai, A. D. (2021). Strategies to improve the quality of team-based care for neonatal abstinence syndrome. *Hospital Pediatrics*, 11(9), 968–981. https://doi.org/10.1542/hpeds.2020-003830

McGlothen-Bell, K., Cleveland, L., Recto, P., Brownell, E., & McGrath, J. (2020). Feeding behaviors in infants with prenatal opioid exposure: An integrative review. *Adv Neonatal Care*, 20(5), 374–383. https://doi.org/10.1097/anc.0000000000000762

McQueen, K., Taylor, C., & Murphy-Oikonen, J. (2019). Systematic review of newborn feeding method and outcomes related to neonatal abstinence syndrome. *Journal of Obstetric, Gynecologic & Neonatal Nursing*, 48(4), 398–407. https://doi.org/10.1016/j.jogn.2019.03.004

McRae, K., Sebastian, T., Grossman, M., & Loyal, J. (2021). Parent perspectives on the Eat, Sleep, Console approach for the care of opioid-exposed infants. *Hospital Pediatrics*, 11(4), 358–365. https://doi.org/10.1542/hpeds.2020-002139

Merhar, S. L., Kline, J. E., Braimah, A., Kline-Fath, B. M., Tkach, J. A., Altaye, M., He, L., & Parikh, N. A. (2021). Prenatal opioid exposure is associated with smaller brain volumes in multiple regions. *Pediatric Research*, 90(2), 397. https://doi.org/10.1038/s41390-020-01265-w

Milette, I., Martel, M.-J., da Silva, M. R., & Coughlin, M. (2019). Guidelines for the institutional implementation of developmental neuroprotective care in the NICU: A joint position statement from CANN, CAPWHN, NANN and COINN. *Advances in Neonatal Care*, 19(1), 9–10. https://doi.org/10.1177/0844562117708126

Montirosso, R., Provenzi, L., Tavian, D., Morandi, F., Bonanomi, A., Missaglia, S., Tronick, E., & Borgatti, R. (2015). Social stress regulation in 4-month-old infants: Contribution of maternal social engagement and infants' 5-HTTLPR genotype. *Early Human Development*, 91(3), 173–179. https://doi.org/10.1016/j.earlhumdev.2015.01.010

Morrison, T. M., Standish, K. R., Wanar, A., Crowell, L., Safon, C. B., Colvin, B. N., Friedman, H., Schiff, D. M., Wachman, E. M., Colson, E. R., Drainoni, M. L., & Parker, M. G. (2023). Drivers of decision-making regarding infant sleep practices among mothers with opioid use disorder. *J Perinatol*, 43(7), 923–929. https://doi.org/10.1038/s41372-023-01701-9

Nagy, S., Dow, K., & Fucile, S. (2023). Oral feeding outcomes in infants born with neonatal abstinence syndrome. *Journal of Perinatal & Neonatal Nursing*, *Publish Ahead of Print*. https://doi.org/10.1097/JPN.0000000000000741

Nancarrow, S. A., Booth, A., Ariss, S., Smith, T., Enderby, P., & Roots, A. (2013). Ten principles of good interdisciplinary team work. *Human resources for Health*, 11(1), 1–11. https://doi.org/10.1186/1478-4491-11-19

National Association of Neonatal Therapists. (2023) *2023 Neonatal Therapy Core Scope of Practice*. NANT Professional Collaborative. Retrieved July 14, 2023, from https://neonataltherapists.com/resources/

Nelson J. L., Winston, K., Bloch, E., & Craig J. W. (2022). What is the lived experience of mothers in a Level-IV Neonatal Intensive Care Unit? *British Journal of Occupational Therapy, 85*(11), 910–917. https://doi.org/10.1177/0308022622 1097302

Nygaard, E., Moe, V., Slinning, K., & Walhovd, K. B. (2015). Longitudinal cognitive development of children born to mothers with opioid and polysubstance use. *Pediatric Research, 78*(3), 330–335. https://doi.org/10.1038/pr. 2015.95

Nygaard, E., Slinning, K., Moe, V., & Walhovd, K. B. (2016). Behavior and attention problems in eight-year-old children with prenatal opiate and polysubstance exposure: A longitudinal study. *PLoS One, 11*(6), https://doi.org/ 10.1371/journal.pone.0158054

Oei, J. L. (2019). Introduction. *Seminars in Fetal and Neonatal Medicine, 24*(2), 85. https://doi.org/10.1016/j.siny.2019.01.005

Oostlander, S. A., Falla, J. A., Dow, K., & Fucile, S. (2019). Occupational therapy management strategies for infants with neonatal abstinence syndrome: Scoping review. *Occupational Therapy in Health Care, 33*(2), 197–226. https://doi.org/ 10.1080/07380577.2019.1594485

Parolin, M., & Simonelli, A. (2016). Attachment theory and maternal drug addiction: The contribution to parenting interventions. *Frontiers in Psychiatry, 7*. https://doi.org/10.3389/fpsyt.2016.00152

Patrick, S. W., Barfield, W. D., & Poindexter, B. B. (2020). Neonatal opioid withdrawal syndrome. *Pediatrics, 146*(5). https://doi.org/10.1542/peds.2020-029074

Piccotti, L., Voigtman, B., Vongsa, R., Nellhaus, E. M., Rodriguez, K. J., Davies, T. H., & Quirk, S. (2019). Neonatal opioid withdrawal syndrome: A developmental care approach. *Neonatal Network, 38*(3). https://doi.org/10.1891/ 0730-0832.38.3.160

Pickens, N. D., & Pizur-Barnekow, K. (2009). Co-occupation: Extending the dialogue. *Journal of Occupational Science, 16*(3), 151–156. https://doi.org/ 10.1080/14427591.2009.9686656

Pierce, D. (2009). Co-occupation: The challenges of defining concepts original to occupational science. *Journal of Occupational Science, 16*(3), 203–207. https:// doi.org/10.1080/14427591.2009.9686663

Price, P., & Miner, S. (2009). Extraordinarily ordinary moments of co-occupation in a Neonatal Intensive Care Unit. *Occupation, Participation and Health, 29*(2), 72–78. https://doi.org/10.3928/15394492-20090301-04

Rhoads, S. C., & Waskosky, A. (2022). Eat, Sleep, Console method and the management of neonatal opioid withdrawal syndrome: A literature review. *Journal of Neonatal Nursing, 28*(4), 236–239. https://doi.org/https://doi.org/10.1016/ j.jnn.2021.10.006

Richter, M, Angell, A., Kellner, P., Smith, J., Pineda, R. (2023). Infant and parent outcomes related to NICU-based co-occupational engagement. *Occupational Therapy Journal of Research.* https://doi.org/10.1177/15394492231160690

Rinaldi, K., Brown, L. F., & Maguire, D. (2023). Evaluating maternal–infant feeding interactions in dyads with opioid exposure. *Journal of Neonatal Nursing*, *29*(5), 767–772. https://doi.org/10.1016/j.jnn.2023.02.009

Rose-Jacobs, R., Trevino-Talbot, M., Lloyd-Travaglini, C., Cabral, H. J., Vibbert, M., Saia, K., & Wachman, E. M. (2019). Could prenatal food insecurity influence neonatal abstinence syndrome severity? *Addiction*, *114*(2), 337–343. https://doi.org/10.1111/add.14458

Rosenblum, K., Lawler, J., Alfafara, E., Miller, N., Schuster, M., & Muzik, M. (2018). Improving maternal representations in high-risk mothers: A randomized, controlled trial of the mom power parenting intervention. *Child Psychiatry Human Development*, *49*(3), 372–384. https://doi.org/10.1007/s10578-017-0757-5

Sanders, M. R., & Hall, S. L. (2018). Trauma-informed care in the newborn intensive care unit: Promoting safety, security and connectedness. *Journal of Perinatology*, *38*(1), 3–10. https://doi.org/10.1038/jp.2017.124

Schickedanz, A., Escarce, J. J., Halfon, N., Sastry, N., Chung, P. J. (2021). Intergenerational associations between parents' and children's adverse childhood experience scores. *Children*, *8*(9), 747. https://doi.org/10.3390/children8090747

Schiff, D. M., & Grossman, M. R. (2019). Beyond the Finnegan scoring system: Novel assessment and diagnostic techniques for the opioid-exposed infant. *Seminars in Fetal and Neonatal Medicine*, *24*(2), 115–120. https://doi.org/10.1016/j.siny.2019.01.003

Schot, E., Tummers, L., & Noordegraaf, M. (2020). Working on working together. A systematic review on how healthcare professionals contribute to interprofessional collaboration. *Journal of Interprofessional Care*, *34*(3), 332–342. https://doi.org/10.1080/13561820.2019.1636007

Shan, F., MacVicar, S., Allegaert, K., Offringa, M., Jansson, L. M., Simpson, S., Moulsdale, W., & Kelly, L. E. (2020). Outcome reporting in neonates experiencing withdrawal following opioid exposure in pregnancy: A systematic review. *Trials*, *21*(1), 1–14. https://doi.org/10.1186/s13063-020-4183-9

Shonkoff, J. P., Garner, A. S., Siegel, B. S., Dobbins, M. I., Earls, M. F., Garner, A. S., McGuinn, L., Pascoe, J., & Wood, D. L. (2012). The lifelong effects of early childhood adversity and toxic stress. *Pediatrics*, *129*(1), 232–246. https://doi.org/10.1542/peds.2011-2663

Substance Abuse and Mental Health Services Administration. (2014). *SAMHSA's Concept of trauma and guidance for a trauma-informed approach*. https://ncsacw.samhsa.gov/userfiles/files/SAMHSA_Trauma.pdf

Substance Abuse and Mental Health Services Administration. (2018). *NSDUH Annual National Report*. https://www.samhsa.gov/data/report/2018-nsduh-annual-national-report

Sweeney, J. K., Heriza, C. B., & Blanchard, Y. (2009). Neonatal physical therapy. Part I: Clinical competencies and Neonatal Intensive Care Unit clinical training models. *Pediatric Physical Therapy*, *21*(4), 296–307. https://doi.org/10.1097/pep.0b013e3181bf75ee

Valadez, E. A., Tottenham, N., Tabachnick, A. R., & Dozier, M. (2020). Early parenting intervention effects on brain responses to maternal cues among high-risk children. *Am J Psychiatry, 177*(9), 818–826. https://doi.org/10.1176/appi. ajp.2020.20010011

Velez, M. L., Jordan, C., & Jansson, L. M. (2021). Reconceptualizing non-pharmacologic approaches to neonatal abstinence syndrome (NAS) and neonatal opioid withdrawal syndrome (NOWS): A theoretical and evidence-based approach. Part II: The clinical application of nonpharmacologic care for NAS/NOWS. *Neurotoxicology and Teratology, 88.* https://doi.org/10.1016/j.ntt.2021.107020

Voss, M. W., Barrett, T. S., Campbell, A. J., & Van Komen, A. (2023). Parenting and the opioid epidemic: A systematic scoping review. *Journal of Child and Family Studies, 32*(5), 1280–1293. https://doi.org/10.1007/s10826-023-02576-2

Wang, D., & Teichtahl, H. (2007). Opioids, sleep architecture and sleep-disordered breathing. *Sleep Medicine Reviews, 11*(1), 35–46. https://doi.org/10.1016/j.smrv.2006.03.006

Weller, A. E., Crist, R. C., Reiner, B. C., Doyle, G. A., & Berrettini, W. H. (2021). Neonatal opioid withdrawal syndrome (NOWS): A transgenerational echo of the opioid crisis. *Cold Spring Harbor Perspectives in Medicine, 11*(3), https://doi.org/10.1101/cshperspect.a039669

Wong, C., & Leland, N. E. (2016). Non-pharmacological approaches to reducing negative behavioral symptoms: A scoping review. *Occupation, Participation and Health, 36*(1), 34–41. https://doi.org/10.1177/1539449215627278

World Federation of Occupational Therapists. (2012). *Occupational Science.* [Position statement]. https://www.wfot.org/resources/occupational-science

9 Neonatal Opioid Withdrawal Syndrome (NOWS)

The Impact on the Movement System and the Role of the Physical Therapist

Dana McCarty and Kara Boynewicz

9.1 Introduction

Neonatal opioid withdrawal syndrome (NOWS) is a group of neonatal clinical symptoms from prolonged in-utero exposure to illicit or prescribed drugs (Malcolm, 2015). The term NOWS is often used interchangeably neonatal abstinence syndrome (NAS), but the use of NOWS more recently refers to infants born with opioid exposure, and NAS has been used to refer to infants with polysubstance exposure (Weller et al., 2021).

An interprofessional approach to caring for the infant with NOWS optimizes outcomes (Spence et al., 2020). Early physical therapy (PT) referral affords prompt identification of individual infant neurobehavioral and motor needs and caregiver education before clinical symptoms of NOWS worsen and become difficult to manage. Regardless of whether an infant requires pharmacological intervention, the PT can assist with development of an individualized plan for supportive care. The purpose of this chapter is to outline infant clinical manifestations of NOWS that may indicate PT referral, the role of PT in the management of NOWS, including appropriate evaluation and treatment, parent education and interaction, and developmental outcomes.

9.2 Clinical Manifestations of NOWS Impacting the Movement System

The infant may manifest signs of clinical withdrawal in a variety of ways based on the amount of exposure and to what drug. Below, in Table 9.1, signs and symptoms of withdrawal impacting the PT evaluation will be discussed based on the categories of autonomic instability, motor system, and neurobehavior. (Haddad et al., 2005; Malcolm, 2015).

DOI: 10.4324/9781003397267-9

Table 9.1 Clinical manifestations of neonatal withdrawal

Opioids

Autonomic Instability	Motor System	Neurobehavior
Temperature instability Increased sweating Nasal stuffiness Frequently yawning Sneezing Mottling Exaggerated Moro reflex	Tremors Hypertonia Hyperactive deep tendon reflexes Seizures	Irritability Increased wakefulness High-pitched cry

Cocaine

Autonomic Instability	Motor System	Neurobehavior
Temperature instability Nasal stuffiness Bradycardia Respiratory distress	Tremors Hypertonia Seizures	Irritability Difficult arousing Hyperalertness High-pitched cry

Selective Serotonin Reuptake Inhibitors

Autonomic Instability	Motor System	Neurobehavior
Temperature instability Tachypnea Respiratory distress	Jitteriness and/or restlessness Tremors Hypertonia or rigidity Seizures	Continuous crying Irritability Sleep disturbance

9.2.1 Autonomic Instability

During the PT examination, autonomic system manifestations of withdrawal, such as skin mottling, tremors, startles, and frequent yawning and sneezing, can be present (Malcolm, 2015). Addressing autonomic instability through motor system support is the foundation for PT examination and treatment (Sweeney et al., 2010). The PT must employ a variety of techniques to assess and treat autonomic instability during the evaluation for the infant safety and accurate assessment (McCarty et al., 2019).

9.2.2 Motor System

Abnormal movement patterns can be appreciated, especially during early withdrawal in the first 6 weeks of life, but may vary based on degree of withdrawal and infant's state regulation skills (Heller et al., 2017; Jones et al., 2010; Velez et al., 2009). Movement quality is impacted by neurological excitability during active withdrawal and can appear rigid, tremulous, or ballistic (Velez et al., 2009). Increased muscle tone, or hypertonia, is often present during active withdrawal (Johnson et al., 2001) and may limit active range of motion, leading to muscle contractures and delayed acquisition of gross motor milestones (Hoare & Imms, 2004).

Typical movement characteristics of infants with NOWS include increased neurological excitability, hypertonicity, and hyperactivity, but evidence shows that some infants present with low muscle tone and abnormal movements (Belcher et al., 1999). Withdrawing infants are also at greater risk for developing torticollis and plagiocephaly due to a combination of factors including frequent containment and swaddling, length of hospital stay, and increased muscle tone in the upper extremities and neck (McAllister et al., 2018).

9.2.3 Neurobehavior

Stress signs are infant behaviors used to communicate needs and may include facial grimacing, color changes of the skin, and fluctuations in heart rate and breathing (Velez et al., 2021b). More stress behaviors indicate greater difficulty regulating response to environmental stimuli (Pineda et al., 2020), which further limits the infant's ability to move their body with control.

Behavioral state regulation has a significant impact on the motor system because infants struggle to transition between states of awareness (Velez et al., 2018). Infants in withdrawal may have difficulty maintaining a calm alert state and shift abruptly from crying to sleep (Hart et al., 2019), which impacts vital aspects of growth and development such as eating. The PT's assessment of infant response to developmental strategies to facilitate a calm alert state supports the infant's overall plan of care. The infant's state of arousal is an important consideration during the PT evaluation. Withdrawing infants usually demonstrate hypertonicity when awake (Velez et al., 2018; McAllister et al., 2018), so muscle tone should be continually assessed throughout the examination to account for these fluctuations.

9.3 Differences Between Full-Term and Preterm Infant Withdrawal

Clinical manifestations of NOWS as described above are most common in full-term infants. Preterm infants, however, do not develop classic signs of NOWS due to developmental immaturity of the central nervous system, lower total drug exposure duration compared with full-term infants, and less adipose tissue for lipophilic drug storage (Allocco et al., 2016; Amiri &

Nair, 2022). Preterm infants, both with and without NOWS, demonstrate distinct movements and behaviors related to developmental immaturity such as tremulous uncoordinated movements, hyperactive startle reflexes, irritability, and poor feeding; therefore, signs of clinical withdrawal may be easily missed (Amiri & Nair, 2022).

Because NOWS assessment tools were designed for use in full-term infants, extrapolation to preterm infants can be difficult (Allocco et al., 2016). Full-term infants score significantly higher than preterm infants for sleep disturbances (Allocco et al., 2016; Amiri & Nair, 2022), tremors, muscle tone, sweating, nasal stuffiness, and loose stools than preterm infants, and preterm infants were scored more regularly for hyperactive Moro reflex, tachypnea, and poor feeding using the Neonatal Abstinence Scoring System (NASS) (Allocco et al., 2016). These results indicate that clinical presentations in full-term and preterm infants are different and support the need to develop new tools to better measure NOWS symptoms in preterm infants.

9.4 Role of the Physical Therapist in NOWS Management

The PT has an important role on the NOWS care team and offers important evaluation and treatment approaches for movement dysfunction related to opioid exposure (McCarty et al., 2019).

9.4.1 Physical Therapy Examination of the Movement System

9.4.1.1 Time of Examination

Scheduling a PT examination requires flexibility of all involved caregivers. The timing of the initial examination and ongoing treatments depends on the infant's state regulation, response to pharmacological management, and clinical symptoms. Ideally, the infant should be in a calm alert state for accurate musculoskeletal assessment. However, these windows of time can be short and unpredictable, and therefore good communication with the nurse and other team members, as well as scheduling flexibility, are fundamental. If the infant feeds on demand, being paged to the bedside affords observation of natural sleep–wake transitions and the infant's neurobehavioral skills. Necessary observations for the evaluation such as the infant's required positioning aids and environmental supports, muscle tone (McAllister et al., 2018; Velez & Jansson, 2008), postures (Maguire et al., 2015), preferred movement patterns (Velez et al., 2009), motor asymmetries (McAllister et al., 2018), and quality of movement (Velez et al., 2009) may be completed concurrently with nursing care to reduce physical stimulation of the infant.

Timing the examination immediately following medication may improve tolerance to therapeutic handling but can mask the infant's ability to self-regulate during active withdrawal. It is therefore important to consult the nurse who may provide additional context to the infant's presentation.

Timing of the PT examination is also important to reduce gastrointestinal disturbances. Handling the infant prior to feeding can reduce risk of reflux and discomfort (Maguire et al., 2015), but many infants will be too irritable to tolerate handling while hungry and will require an examination after feeding. During the examination, the PT should note how infant neurobehavior (e.g., reactivity to sensory stimulation, abrupt sleep–wake cycles) and motor skills (e.g., hypertonia) impact feeding success (Maguire et al., 2015).

9.4.1.2 Impact of Drug Class on Clinical Presentation

Knowledge of the infant's drug exposure history is helpful, as particular drug classes may have different effects on infant movement. Clinical signs and symptoms of withdrawal can present similarly between opioids, selective serotonin reuptake inhibitors (Haddad et al., 2005), and cocaine (Conradt et al., 2013), but subtle differences can occur at specific time points over a two-week period of withdrawal (Jones et al., 2010). Velez et al. (2009) found that infants exposed to selective serotonin reuptake inhibitors did not have statistically different NICU Network Neurobehavioral Scale or NASS scores compared to controls, but also found that maternal buprenorphine dose at delivery was negatively correlated with quality of movement, and self-regulation, and positively correlated with the CNS parameters of the stress/abstinence scale.

The need for pharmacologic intervention may also have an impact on clinical presentation. For example, infants experiencing NOWS who require pharmacological intervention present with higher arousal, excitability, and hypertonicity compared to newborns with drug exposure who did not need pharmacological intervention (Velez et al., 2018), whereas infants treated with buprenorphine typically have poorer movement quality, higher excitability, and more lethargy than infants who do not need medication (Jones et al., 2010).

9.4.1.3 Standardized Assessments Used by the Physical Therapist

Standardized assessments provide objective measures of change over time, justify therapeutic intervention, and evaluate outcomes (Jones et al., 2010). They may also be useful in identifying early developmental differences so that specific interventions and parental education can be administered (Goldstein & Campbell, 2008). Although there is no "gold standard" for motor assessment in the NOWS population, many tests can provide useful information to the developmental team. The PT must use clinical judgment to determine the infant's ability to tolerate handling and additional stressors of infant testing, as well as whether the infant's performance is truly representative of overall motor function. See Table 9.2 (Als et al., 2005; Bier et al., 2015; Harris et al., 2010; Hunt et al., 2008; Jones et al., 2010; Maitre et al., 2016; Noble & Boyd, 2012; Nugent, 2013; Oyemade et al., 1994; Palchik et al., 2013; Tavasoli et al., 2014; Velez et al., 2009).

The NICU Network Neurobehavioral Scale is a comprehensive assessment of motor and sensory responses, neurological integrity, and behavioral function (i.e., neurobehavior) (Lester et al., 2014). It has been validated on healthy infants, preterm infants, and infants at high risk who are prenatally exposed to substances (Conradt et al., 2013). The NICU Network Neurobehavioral Scale is interpreted using 13 summary scores: orientation, habituation, hypertonicity, hypotonicity, excitability, arousal, lethargy, non-optimal reflexes, asymmetric reflexes, stress, self-regulation, quality of movement, and handling (Lester & Tronick, 2004), which have internal consistency (α = 0.87–0.90) (Fink et al., 2012) and good reliability (α = 0.30–0.44) (Eeles et al., 2017). Studies demonstrate that the NICU Network Neurobehavioral Scale is sensitive enough in the NOWS population to detect differences in infant neurobehavior based on the infant's need for pharmacological management (Jones et al., 2010; Velez et al., 2009).

The Test of Infant Motor Performance (TIMP) measures functional motor behavior of infants and provides norm-references for motor development from 34 weeks postmenstrual age to 4 months corrected age (Campbell et al., 2006). The TIMP can discriminate among infants with varying risk for poor motor performance in early infancy and successfully detects change in motor performance over time (Campbell & Hedeker, 2001). The TIMP has been used to measure motor performance in infants with prenatal cocaine (Gasparin et al., 2012) and polysubstance (Benninger et al., 2020), and buprenorphine exposure (Boynewicz et al., 2023), and identifies infants with substance exposure that may benefit from PT (e.g., infants scoring in the low average range compared to age-matched peers). See Table 9.2 (Boynewicz et al., 2023; Censullo, 1994; Gewolb et al., 2004; Grossman et al., 2017; Harris et al., 2010; Nugent, 2013; Maguire et al., 2015; McAllister et al., 2018; Mouradian & Als, 1994; Velez & Jansson, 2008).

Table 9.2 Neonatal standardized assessments for potential use in infants with NAS

Motor Assessment	Age	Brief Description	Infant/Toddler Characteristics Tested
TIMP	32 weeks PMA– 4 months	Evaluates motor control and organization of posture and movement for functional activities	Orientation head in space, response to auditory and visual stimuli, body alignment, spontaneous limb movements
GMA	Preterm– 4 months	Documents spontaneous movements to identify early CNS dysfunction	Movement patterns
NBO	Birth– 3 months	Relationship-based tool, designed to sensitize parents to their baby's behavior and foster positive parent–infant interactions	Autonomic and physiologic stability, motor regulation, organization of state, responsiveness
APIB	28 weeks PMA– 1 month post-term	A comprehensive systematic assessment of the preterm and full-term newborn based on NBAS, but greater focus on self-regulation and disorganization	Autonomic, motor, state, attention, and self-regulation assessed via maneuvers that increase in vestibular and tactile demands on the infant
Dubowitz	30 weeks PMA– 4 months	Provides a detailed profile of neurological status and identifies infants with neurological abnormalities	Posture and tone, reflexes, movements, neurobehavioral responses
NBAS	36 weeks PMA–6 weeks post-term	Identifies full range of individual neurobehavioral functioning and identifies areas of difficulty	Autonomic, motor and reflexes, state, social/ attentional
NNNS	30 weeks PMA– 4 months	Assesses at-risk infants (particularly substance exposed), documenting neurological integrity and broad range of behavioral functioning	Neurological (tone, reflexes), behavioral, stress/abstinence items

Table 9.2 (Continued)

Parent Component	Formal Training Required?	Administration Time (minutes)	Studies Describing Use of Assessment in Drug-Exposed Infants
No	No – instructional DVD and infant handling experience recommended	20–40	TIMP identifies infants with substance exposure that may benefit from PT (e.g., infants scoring in the low average range compared to age-matched peers)
No	Yes – 4–5-day training with GMs Trust	10–30	Associations between abnormal GMs and long-term developmental outcomes in infants exposed to opioids and HIV
Yes	2-day training followed by telementoring	Variable – infant led	No studies specifically using NBO in NOWS population. May be a particularly helpful tool to assess parent–infant interaction in the setting of NAS
No, but parent presence during testing encouraged	Yes – ~2 years, including preparatory competencies, on-site and independent practice, and established reliability with trainer prior to use	Up to 60	
No	No	10–15	
No	Yes – training sessions, complete 20 exams, must achieve agreement of 90% with scoring	20–30	Maternal self-reported chronic illicit drug use positively correlated with poor habituation (response to stimuli) scores in full-term infants using the NBAS
No	Yes – training programs available, practice until ready for certification	30	Established reliability and validity in NAS population. Motor development deficits in 1-month-old infants exposed to cocaine in utero and improvements in motor scores in the BSID (2nd edition) at 12 months and the PDMS (1st edition) at 18 months, reflecting an early neurotoxic effect

Table 9.2 (Continued)

Motor Assessment	Age	Brief Description	Infant/Toddler Characteristics Tested
HINT	2.5–12.5 months	Screening tool to identify neuromotor differences in infants	Pregnancy, delivery, and infant health history; parental perceptions of how their infant moves and plays; 21 motor, cognitive, and behavioral items
HINE	2–24 months	Used to identify early signs of cerebral palsy and other neuromotor disorders	Items include cranial nerve function, posture, quality and quantity of movements, tone, and reflexes
AIMS	Birth–18 months	Performance-based observational tool for infant gross motor development	4 positions observed: prone, supine, sitting, standing
PDMS-2	0–71 months	Scored based on norm-referenced motor activities to detect infants and children with motor delays	Gross motor (reflexes, stationary, locomotion, object manipulation) and fine motor (grasping, visual motor integration)
BSID-III	1–42 months	Scored based on norm-referenced activities to detect infants and toddlers at risk for delay	5 subscales: cognitive, receptive and expressive language, fine and gross motor, 2 parent questionnaires: social-emotional and adaptive behavior
Dyadic Mutuality Code (DMC)	0–6 months	Synchrony of mother–child interaction. Score-based categories are "low responsivity" (6–8 points), "moderate responsivity" (9 points), and "high responsivity" (10–12 points)	Responsiveness of infant and mother in the early parent–infant relationship 6 items that measure mutual attention, positive affect, maternal pauses, turn-taking, infant clarity of cues, and maternal sensitive responsiveness

Table 9.2 (Continued)

Parent Component	Formal Training Required?	Administration Time (minutes)	Studies Describing Use of Assessment in Drug-Exposed Infants
Yes: questionnaire	No – instructional DVD and infant handling experience recommended	30	Comparative predictive validity to the AIMS and predictive correlations to the BSID-III in at-risk infant population (not exclusively, but including drug-exposed) at multiple follow-up ages
No	No	15	Decreased trunk and limb muscle tone in 41–42-week full-term infants exposed to antiepileptic drugs in utero as compared to controls
No	No	20–30	AIMS scores at 4 months were significantly different between infants exposed to high doses vs. low doses of methadone
No	Recommended for clinicians with training in tests and measures	45–60	Significantly lower gross and fine motor scores on PDMS (1st edition) at 24 months in infants with history of cocaine exposure in utero as compared to controls considering confounding variables
Yes: questionnaire	No	50–90	Significantly lower scores in all subscales of the BSID-III in toddlers at 18 months, 2 years, and 3 years with history of NAS
Yes	No	5-minute observation	

9.4.2 Physical Therapy Intervention

As part of the NOWS interprofessional team approach, early PT that addresses both the motor and sensory needs of infants may include handling tolerance, midline orientation, therapeutic exercises, and behavioral organization (Franco et al., 2005).

9.4.2.1 Environmental Supports

The environment can greatly aid in recovery, reduce length of hospital stay, and prolong sleep periods in infants with NOWS (Maguire, 2014; Ryan et al., 2019). Infants with NOWS rely heavily on external supports to self-regulate. Self-regulation, which has been described as a cornerstone in healthy development, is necessary for the infant's autonomic stability, physical growth, and participation in appropriate feeding and sleep/wake cycles (Velez et al., 2021a). Reducing lighting and sound (Maguire, 2014), keeping sounds levels below 45 dB, and positioning cribs away from high-volume areas of the unit can all help reduce overstimulation (White-Traut et al., 2002).

9.4.2.2 Sensory-Motor Interventions

Providing sensory inputs in a graded manner such as approaching the bedside using a gentle voice prior to touching the infant is recommended to prevent infant hyper-responsiveness to external stimulation (Velez & Jansson, 2008). Infants with NOWS also have difficulty regulating vestibular input (Velez et al., 2009); therefore, caregivers should avoid quick, jerking movements to prevent infant startling. Slow, rhythmic, vertical movements decrease irritability and improve behavioral state (Ryan et al., 2019; Velez & Jansson, 2008).

9.4.2.3 Positioning

Positioning aids like blanket rolls or a tight swaddle provide boundaries and promote sleep in healthy full-term infants (Franco et al., 2005) as well as infants with NOWS. Calming strategies that enhance midline flexion such as pacifier use, hand-to-mouth positioning, or skin-to-skin contact can be incorporated into the infant's resting position (Ryan et al., 2019). Although prone and side-lying positions can improve containment and decrease infant irritability, supine positioning should be encouraged in preparation for home per the American Academy of Pediatrics sleep recommendations (Gelfer et al., 2013). Use of supportive boundaries while the infant is awake can facilitate active movement of the trunk and extremities toward midline, which encourages motor organization and optimal state regulation (McCarty et al., 2019). The PT can model these positioning strategies for parents as well as other members of the care team for optimal carryover and infant benefit (Spence et al., 2020).

9.4.2.4 Therapist-Delivered Motor Intervention

Evidence supports use of auditory, tactile, visual, and vestibular interventions to improve behavioral state regulation in drug-exposed infants (White-Traut et al., 2002). The PT should use sensory-motor strategies outlined above to help the infant transition to a calm alert state prior to handling to promote a positive motor learning experience. The infant should be moved slowly through space and held closely to prevent startling during transfers (Velez & Jansson, 2008). Unswaddled, free-play opportunities may help maintain appropriate muscle length in the trunk and extremities.

9.4.2.5 Infant Massage

Massage in both preterm and healthy full-term infant populations has well-established positive effects on a variety of infant outcomes, including reduced infant stress and improved weight gain (Diego et al., 2007) and improved long-term neurodevelopmental outcomes (Onozawa et al., 2001; Procianoy et al., 2010). Infant massage also enhances parent–infant bonding (Onozawa et al., 2001) and improves maternal mood and anxiety levels (Feijó et al., 2006). In the NOWS population, parent-facilitated infant massage has been shown to reduce maternal stress and depressive symptoms (Porter et al., 2015) and improve mothers' perceptions of infant calmness and comfort (Hahn et al., 2016).

In a study by Rana et al. (2022), a small cohort of full-term opioid-exposed infants tolerated 30 minutes of full body massage daily during hospitalization and demonstrated significant improvements in measures of physiological stability (Rana et al., 2022). Porter and Porter (2004) describe infant massage as moderately firm effleurage strokes on the extremities for periods of 10–30 minutes followed by gentle passive muscle elongation (Porter & Porter, 2004). Although neurobehavioral and motor effects of massage have not been studied in infants with opioid withdrawal (Rana et al., 2022), our own clinical observations demonstrated that the use of this approach to infant massage results in improved state organization, tolerance of muscle stretch, and increased variety of active movement. During infant massage, use of upper or lower body swaddle, pacifier, and room darkening may be necessary to reduce environmental stimuli and achieve positive infant responses.

9.4.2.6 Swaddled Bathing and Hydrotherapy

Swaddled bathing and hydrotherapy have numerous benefits for infants with NOWS. Healthy newborn infants bathed while swaddled demonstrate better temperature regulation, lower heart rate, and reduced pain scores compared with infants bathed with traditional methods (Çaka & Gözen, 2018). Neonatal hydrotherapy has been used in high-risk infant populations to reduce pain and stress signs (Edraki et al., 2014) and to impact tone and movement (Vignochi et al., 2010). The buoyancy and warmth of water reduce muscle tone, improve state organization and movement patterns, and improve tolerance of muscle elongation and therapeutic handling (McManus & Kotelchuck, 2007). Most importantly, swaddled bathing and hydrotherapy provide another opportunity for a positive sensory-motor experience between parent and infant. During the hydrotherapy session, the infant should be swaddled and lowered slowly into a deep basin with water temperature between 98.5°F and 100.5°F (37°C–38°C) (Sweeney et al., 2013). Gentle elongation and guided movement in varied positions is provided for a total of 10 to 20 minutes, monitoring infant tolerance and water temperature closely. Slow, paced handling during hydrotherapy should be emphasized and practiced with the parent throughout the hospital stay.

9.5 Principles of Parent and Caregiver Interaction and Education

Within the population of mothers with substance use disorders, evidence supports the effectiveness of parent education and training programs to improve parent and infant developmental outcomes (Moreland & McRae-Clark, 2018). Educating parents and caregivers of infants with NOWS is complicated but uniquely rewarding (McCarty et al., 2019). The PT should avoid making assumptions about the parents' or caregivers' abilities, beliefs, or background experiences. In order to cultivate a meaningful relationship with the family, the PT should affirm and encourage parent and caregiver presence at the bedside as an essential part of the infant's healing process (Howard et al., 2017).

There is a large body of evidence to support the effectiveness of family-centered care approaches to parent education (Kutahyalioglu & Scafide, 2022). Family-centered care aims to involve parents in all aspects of care and provide open communication between parents and the infant's medical team to improve parent–infant bonding (Kutahyalioglu & Scafide, 2022). Individual one-on-one education at the bedside is ideal, allowing for meaningful dialogue, relationship building, and affirmation of positive parent–infant interactions (McCarty et al., 2019). In all parent interactions, it is important to not only model appropriate support of the infant's development, but also to explain behaviors and/or activities that parents are being taught (Dunst et al., 2007). For example, if a clinician enters the room while parent and infant are present and lowers the television volume and closes the shades, but does not explain the importance of these environmental modifications, the caregiver may interpret this negatively or fail to adopt these helpful strategies.

9.5.1 Psychosocial Aspects of Parent Education Content and Delivery

Parental retention of information is impacted by many factors including parental guilt, the parent's addiction treatment, and socioeconomic factors like transportation, educational level, and involvement of social services (Velez & Jansson, 2008). Other challenges some families face can include unstable housing, limited financial resources, and lack of social support (Velez & Jansson, 2008), job instability, and dealing with the stigma of addiction – all of which can result in greater mental health issues (Conradt et al., 2013).

As a result, this parent population needs consistency in both content and methods of delivery. Parents of infants with NOWS might also benefit from simple written instruction with photos to augment verbal education; however, the practice of hands-on activity with guidance is superior for reinforcement and carryover (Byrne et al., 2019).

9.5.2 Swaddling and Infant Handling

Many parents need encouragement to hold their infants. Caregiving or holding can be stressful, especially if their infant is fussy, and this may be a trigger for relapse to substance misuse (Rutherford et al., 2013). Educating parents to hold the infant skin-to-skin or swaddled can decrease infant restlessness, respiratory distress, and pain (Ryan et al., 2019). Basic gross motor skill progression and facilitation should also be discussed and practiced with parents (Byrne et al., 2019; Dusing et al., 2008). Infants with hypertonia may have a more challenging time learning to move and interact with their caregivers (Jansson & Patrick, 2019). Parents often mistake their infant's hypertonia for muscle strength. It is therefore important to distinguish the difference for caregivers in simple, nonjudgmental terms. Using opportunities to point out hypertonic movement characteristics during diapering or holding is important in the education, guidance of, and collaboration with families, nurses, and other clinicians (e.g., speech-language therapists).

9.5.3 Safety and Sleep Recommendations

PTs should be aware of potential safety concerns that might exist in the home environment, especially related to the appropriate use of seating devices (Beaudin et al., 2013) and sleep practices (Gelfer et al., 2013). Parents should be educated to provide opportunities for "free floor play" to encourage movement exploration while avoiding play on beds or other elevated surfaces. Also, because infants with a history of NOWS have a higher rate of Sudden Infant Death Syndrome (SIDS) than infants who are typically developing (Kahila et al., 2007), safe sleep education and practices should be introduced early and consistently (Gelfer et al., 2013).

9.5.4 Parent–Infant Interaction

The quality of the early interaction between infants and their caregivers is a key factor influencing child development (Rocha et al., 2020; Soares et al., 2018). As a result of sensory and motor regulation impairments, however, infants with NOWS are challenged to respond appropriately to caregiver attempts to interact (Maguire et al., 2016), and caregivers may have a difficult time interpreting infant cues. Therefore, the PT should model and explain and model appropriate social reciprocity for the parent (Velez & Jansson, 2008).

The PT may use a variety of techniques to facilitate positive parent–infant interactions during a therapy session. Censullo (1994) recommends six key strategies to support parent–infant interactions: (a) teaching the mother to identify the infant's behavioral cues and to tailor responses to match the infant's preferences, (b) guiding the mother to position the infant in her line of vision, (c) demonstrating ways to modulate the use of pauses, imitation, sequences, and combinations of her facial expression, voice, and touch, (d) encouraging practice of suggestions and trial-and-error learning, (e) reinforcing sensitive responsiveness whenever it occurred, and (f) praising success.

Family-centered care and parent training require developing an understanding of the strengths and needs of the infant's entire family. Use of parent–infant interaction assessment tools can help interventionists determine why parent training or coaching appears effective for some families but not for others (Dusing et al., 2019).

9.6 The Role of the Physical Therapist on the Interprofessional Team

As previously discussed, the role of the PT on the interprofessional NOWS care team is an essential one (McCarty et al., 2019). PTs use their knowledge of infant and child development and evidence-based parent and caregiver educational strategies to implement important contributions to infants and families affected by NOWS.

9.6.1 Hospital Setting

The medical team is encouraged to set up an automatic PT referral process for all infants admitted NOWS (Jansson & Patrick, 2019). PTs are an integral part of the interdisciplinary team, providing expert assessment of the motor system, neurobehavior, muscle tone changes, and parent education (McCarty et al., 2019). Early motor and neurobehavioral assessments can identify early differences in development so that specific therapeutic interventions and parental education can be administered (Goldstein & Campbell, 2008). PT intervention supports important infant activities such as feeding, self-regulation development, positioning, caregiver presence, swaddling, and skin-to-skin (Ryan et al., 2019). PTs can provide essential information about the infant's response to pharmacological and nonpharmacological interventions to the medical team as they seek to attenuate withdrawal symptoms. For this reason, PTs' communication with medical providers is essential to optimizing infant outcomes during hospitalization.

9.6.2 Outpatient Setting

Interdisciplinary follow-up clinics ensure that families are supported and infants are screened and referred for intervention services as needed. Infants with NOWS have higher readmission during the first year of life (Shrestha et al., 2021) and PTs following these families can play an important role with ongoing assessment and education in the first year of life.

Standardized assessments administered in the follow-up clinic that detect motor delays can assist with referral and qualification for Early Intervention services, which further support families in monitoring infant developmental needs. See Table 9.3 (Howard et al., 2017; Maguire, 2014; Ryan et al., 2019; Velez & Jansson, 2008).

9.7 Developmental Outcomes

Currently, there is more evidence to suggest long-term effects of opioid exposure on behavioral and cognitive outcomes than on motor outcomes in childhood and adolescence. However, motor development plays an important role in the emergence of cognition and behavior and is often first domain of development to demonstrate delays (Lobo et al., 2013).

Within the first 3 months of life, PT is indicated for more than 60% of infants with NOWS based on identification of abnormal movements,

Table 9.3 Outpatient follow-up considerations for the infant with history of NOWS

Examination	Intervention	Plan of Care/Coordination, Communication and Documentation
History and Review of Systems: • Are all caregivers educated on the signs of NAS and educational content presented at hospital discharge? • Does a typical day for the infant include active free play and/or appropriate use of positioning devices? • Is the caregiver utilizing appropriate calming strategies including massage, hydrotherapy, swaddled bathing, vertical sway/bounce, rhythmic patting, and non-nutritive suck? • What are caregiver concerns or goals? Tests and Measures: • Balance and Posture: assessed in a variety of positions including supine, side-lying, supported sitting, supported standing • Environmental Factors: physical, social, and attitudinal environment in which the caregiver and infant live and conduct their lives. • Motor Function: movement quality, achievement of motor milestones • Muscle Performance and Range of Motion: including infant's tolerance of gentle passive muscle elongation, changes in muscle tone with activity or rest, presence of contractures and/or asymmetries • Pain: screening for signs and symptoms of active withdrawal • Neuromotor Development and Sensory Processing: infant's ability to sustain calm alert state, visual engagement, and appropriate interactional skills and level of support required • Self-Care and Domestic Life: caregiver's ability to care for both infant and his/her health and carrying out everyday actions/tasks associated with home life	Patient Instruction: • Consider caregiver's communication ability, affect, cognition, language, and learning style/preferences • Include demonstration and return-demonstration for identified activities • Provide written handouts with images when possible • Offer for parents to use video to supplement • Include therapist contact information Motor Function Training and Therapeutic Exercise: • Gentle passive range of motion of trunk and extremities with infant in calm state to promote active and symmetric movement • Side-lying play to help assist/improve active range of motion in gravity-eliminated position and ease of midline flexion attainment to build strength/endurance • Progression of prone activities from caregiver's chest to a solid surface using supported forearm weight bearing and caudal weight shift at hips • Upright activities to progress head control, active flexion, and visual engagement	• Summarize information gathered in examination and evaluation process to create plan of care including frequency of future follow-up appointments • Referrals: including Early Intervention services, discipline-specific services (PT, OT, SLP, nutrition), social work, specialty physician (e.g., neurology) • Communication and coordination with follow-up care team regarding infant and family progress and needs • Communication of recommendations with treating therapist (PT, OT, SLP) as indicated • Documentation to capture infant's current level of function, prognosis, intervention/education provided at visit, plan of care, and recommendations

tremors, and hypotonia; however, nearly 90% of infants requiring PT during this time demonstrate typical development by 12 months of age (Tuhkanen et al., 2019). The most common motor characteristics in this population are trunk hypotonia and lower extremity hypertonia (Belcher et al., 1999). In a home monitoring program for infants who were substance-exposed, 32 infants were assessed at discharge and sequentially up to 18 months of age with the Dubowitz Infant Neurological Scale. Most infants were found to have persistent mild neurological symptoms such as trunk hypotonia and intermittent irritability. A small percentage were noted to have moderate neurological signs such as increased extensor tone, oral motor abnormalities, and persistent tremors (Belcher et al., 2005).

A recent systematic review and meta-analysis examined motor scores from infancy to 6 years of age found that lower motor scores were appreciated overall (p<0.001) in children with substance exposure (Yeoh et al., 2019). This same review also found significantly lower cognitive scores across 13 studies in children aged 3–6 years (Yeoh et al., 2019), supporting the interconnected nature of developmental domain competence and the likelihood that NOWS influences the neurodevelopmental trajectory throughout childhood (Libertus & Hauf, 2017).

9.8 Summary

In summary, PTs play an important role in the nonpharmacological management of infants with NOWS and their families and caregivers. These infants display a wide variety of motor and sensory impairments, and the pediatric PT is uniquely situated to provide interventions that optimize the infant's ability to self-regulate as well as meet developmental milestones. Most importantly, PTs can provide essential parent and caregiver education that optimize outcomes for both parents and infants.

References

Allocco, E., Melker, M., Rojas-Miguez, F., Bradley, C., Hahn, K. A., & Wachman, E. M. (2016). Comparison of neonatal abstinence syndrome manifestations in preterm versus term opioid-exposed infants. *Advances in Neonatal Care, 16*(5), 329–336. https://doi.org/10.1097/ANC.0000000000000320

Als, H., Butler, S., Kosta, S., & McAnulty, G. (2005). The Assessment of Preterm Infants' Behavior (APIB): Furthering the understanding and measurement of neurodevelopmental competence in preterm and full-term infants. *Mental Retardation and Developmental Disabilities Research Reviews, 11*(1), 94–102. https://doi.org/10.1002/mrdd.20053

Amiri, S., & Nair, J. (2022). Gestational age alters assessment of neonatal abstinence syndrome. *Pediatric Reports, 14*(1), 50–57. https://doi.org/10.3390/pediatric14010009

Beaudin, M., Maugans, T., St-Vil, D., & Falcone, R. A. (2013). Inappropriate use of infant seating devices increases risks of injury. *Journal of Pediatric Surgery*, 48(5), 1071–1076. https://doi.org/10.1016/j.jpedsurg.2013.02.022

Belcher, H. M. E., Butz, A. M., Hoon, A. H., Reeves, S. A., & Pulsifer, M. B. (2005). Spectrum of early intervention services for children with intrauterine drug exposure. *Infants and Young Children*, 18(1), 2–15.

Belcher, H. M., Shapiro, B. K., Leppert, M., Butz, A. M., Sellers, S., Arch, E., Kolodner, K., Pulsifer, M., Lears, M. K., & Kaufmann, W. E. (1999). Sequential neuromotor examination in children with intrauterine cocaine/polydrug exposure. *Developmental Medicine and Child Neurology*, 41(4), 240–246. https://doi.org/10.1017/s0012162299000511

Benninger, K. L., Borghese, T., Kovalcik, J. B., Moore-Clingenpeel, M., Isler, C., Bonachea, E. M., Stark, A. R., Patrick, S. W., & Maitre, N. L. (2020). Prenatal exposures are associated with worse neurodevelopmental outcomes in infants with neonatal opioid withdrawal syndrome, *Frontiers in Pediatrics*, 8, 462. https://doi.org/10.3389/fped.2020.00462

Bier, J. B., Finger, A. S., Bier, B. A., Johnson, T. A., & Coyle, M. G. (2015). Growth and developmental outcome of infants with in-utero exposure to methadone vs buprenorphine. *Journal of Perinatology*, 35(8), 656–659. https://doi.org/10.1038/jp.2015.22

Boynewicz, K., Campbell, S. K., & Chroust, A. (2023). Early identification of atypical motor performance of infants with prenatal opioid exposure. *Pediatric Physical Therapy*. https://doi.org/10.1097/PEP.0000000000001021

Byrne, E. M., Sweeney, J. K., Schwartz, N., Umphred, D., & Constantinou, J. (2019). Effects of instruction on parent competency during infant handling in a neonatal intensive care unit. *Pediatric Physical Therapy*, 31(1), 43–49. https://doi.org/10.1097/PEP.0000000000000557

Çaka, S. Y., & Gözen, D. (2018). Effects of swaddled and traditional tub bathing methods on crying and physiological responses of newborns. *Journal for Specialists in Pediatric Nursing*, 23(1). https://doi.org/10.1111/jspn.12202

Campbell, S. K., & Hedeker, D. (2001). Validity of the Test of Infant Motor Performance for discriminating among infants with varying risk for poor motor outcome. *The Journal of Pediatrics*, 139(4), 546–551. https://doi.org/10.1067/mpd.2001.117581

Campbell, S. K., Levy, P., Zawacki, L., & Liao, P.-J. (2006). Population-based age standards for interpreting results on the test of motor infant performance. *Pediatric Physical Therapy*, 18(2), 119–125. https://doi.org/10.1097/01.pep.000 0223108.03305.5d

Censullo, M. (1994). Strategy for promoting greater responsiveness in adolescent parent/infant relationships: Report of a pilot study. *Journal of Pediatric Nursing*, 9(5), 326–332.

Conradt, E., Sheinkopf, S. J., Lester, B. M., Tronick, E., LaGasse, L. L., Shankaran, S., Bada, H., Bauer, C. R., Whitaker, T. M., Hammond, J. A., & Maternal Lifestyle Study. (2013). Prenatal substance exposure: Neurobiologic organization at 1 month. *The Journal of Pediatrics*, 163(4), 989–994.e1. https://doi.org/10.1016/j.jpeds.2013.04.033

Diego, M. A., Field, T., Hernandez-Reif, M., Deeds, O., Ascencio, A., & Begert, G. (2007). Preterm infant massage elicits consistent increases in vagal activity and gastric motility that are associated with greater weight gain. *Acta Paediatrica*, 96(11), 1588–1591. https://doi.org/10.1111/j.1651-2227.2007.00476.x

Dunst, C. J., Trivette, C. M., & Hamby, D. W. (2007). Meta-analysis of family-centered helpgiving practices research. *Mental Retardation and Developmental Disabilities Research Reviews*, 13(4), 370–378. https://doi.org/10.1002/mrdd.20176

Dusing, S. C., Marcinowski, E. C., Rocha, N. A. C. F., Tripathi, T., & Brown, S. E. (2019). Assessment of parent–child interaction is important with infants in rehabilitation and can use high-tech or low-tech methods. *Physical Therapy*, 99(6), 658–665. https://doi.org/10.1093/ptj/pzz021

Dusing, S. C., Murray, T., & Stern, M. (2008). Parent preferences for motor development education in the neonatal intensive care unit. *Pediatric Physical Therapy*, 20(4), 363–368. https://doi.org/10.1097/PEP.0b013e31818add5d

Edraki, M., Paran, M., Montaseri, S., Razavi Nejad, M., & Montaseri, Z. (2014). Comparing the effects of swaddled and conventional bathing methods on body temperature and crying duration in premature infants: A randomized clinical trial. *Journal of Caring Sciences*, 3(2), 83–91. https://doi.org/10.5681/jcs.2014.009

Eeles, A. L., Olsen, J. E., Walsh, J. M., McInnes, E. K., Molesworth, C. M. L., Cheong, J. L. Y., Doyle, L. W., & Spittle, A. J. (2017). Reliability of neurobehavioral assessments from birth to term equivalent age in preterm and term born infants. *Physical & Occupational Therapy in Pediatrics*, 37(1), 108–119. https://doi.org/10.3109/01942638.2015.1135845

Feijó, L., Hernandez-Reif, M., Field, T., Burns, W., Valley-Gray, S., & Simco, E. (2006). Mothers' depressed mood and anxiety levels are reduced after massaging their preterm infants. *Infant Behavior & Development*, 29(3), 476–480. https://doi.org/10.1016/j.infbeh.2006.02.003

Fink, N. S., Tronick, E., Olson, K., & Lester, B. (2012). Healthy newborns' neurobehavior: Norms and relations to medical and demographic factors. *The Journal of Pediatrics*, 161(6), 1073–1079. https://doi.org/10.1016/j.jpeds.2012.05.036

Franco, P., Seret, N., Van Hees, J.-N., Scaillet, S., Groswasser, J., & Kahn, A. (2005). Influence of swaddling on sleep and arousal characteristics of healthy infants. *Pediatrics*, 115(5), 1307–1311. https://doi.org/10.1542/peds.2004-1460

Gasparin, M., Silveira, J. L., Garcez, L. W., & Levy, B. S. (2012). Oral and general motor behavior of newborns from crack and/or cocaine using mothers. *Revista Da Sociedade Brasileira de Fonoaudiologia*, 17(4), 459–463.

Gelfer, P., Cameron, R., Masters, K., & Kennedy, K. A. (2013). Integrating "Back to Sleep" recommendations into neonatal ICU practice. *Pediatrics*, 131(4), 1264–1270. https://doi.org/10.1542/peds.2012-1857

Gewolb, I. H., Fishman, D., Qureshi, M. A., & Vice, F. L. (2004). Coordination of suck–swallow–respiration in infants born to mothers with drug-abuse problems. *Developmental Medicine and Child Neurology*, 46(10), 700–705. https://doi.org/10.1111/j.1469-8749.2004.tb00984.x

Goldstein, L. A., & Campbell, S. K. (2008). Effectiveness of the Test of Infant Motor Performance as an educational tool for mothers. *Pediatric Physical Therapy, 20*(2), 152–159. https://doi.org/10.1097/PEP.0b013e3181729de8

Grossman, M. R., Berkwitt, A. K., Osborn, R. R., Xu, Y., Esserman, D. A., Shapiro, E. D., & Bizzarro, M. J. (2017). An initiative to improve the quality of care of infants with neonatal abstinence syndrome. *Pediatrics, 139*(6). https://doi.org/10.1542/peds.2016-3360

Haddad, P. M., Pal, B. R., Clarke, P., Wieck, A., & Sridhiran, S. (2005). Neonatal symptoms following maternal paroxetine treatment: serotonin toxicity or paroxetine discontinuation syndrome? *Journal of Psychopharmacology, 19*(5), 554–557. https://doi.org/10.1177/0269881105056554

Hahn, J., Lengerich, A., Byrd, R., Stoltz, R., Hench, J., Byrd, S., & Ford, C. (2016). Neonatal abstinence syndrome: The experience of infant massage. *Creative Nursing, 22*(1), 45–50. https://doi.org/10.1891/1078-4535.22.1.45

Harris, S. R., Backman, C. L., & Mayson, T. A. (2010). Comparative predictive validity of the Harris Infant Neuromotor Test and the Alberta Infant Motor Scale. *Developmental Medicine and Child Neurology, 52*(5), 462–467. https://doi.org/10.1111/j.1469-8749.2009.03518.x

Hart, B. J., Viswanathan, S., & Jadcherla, S. R. (2019). Persistent feeding difficulties among infants with fetal opioid exposure: Mechanisms and clinical reasoning. *The Journal of Maternal-Fetal & Neonatal Medicine, 32*(21), 3633–3639. https://doi.org/10.1080/14767058.2018.1469614

Heller, N. A., Logan, B. A., Morrison, D. G., Paul, J. A., Brown, M. S., & Hayes, M. J. (2017). Neonatal abstinence syndrome: Neurobehavior at 6 weeks of age in infants with or without pharmacological treatment for withdrawal. *Developmental Psychobiology, 59*(5), 574–582. https://doi.org/10.1002/dev.21532

Hoare, B. J., & Imms, C. (2004). Upper-limb injections of botulinum toxin-A in children with cerebral palsy: A critical review of the literature and clinical implications for occupational therapists. *The American Journal of Occupational Therapy, 58*(4), 389–397. https://doi.org/10.5014/ajot.58.4.389

Howard, M. B., Schiff, D. M., Penwill, N., Si, W., Rai, A., Wolfgang, T., Moses, J. M., & Wachman, E. M. (2017). Impact of parental presence at infants' bedside on neonatal abstinence syndrome. *Hospital Pediatrics, 7*(2), 63–69. https://doi.org/10.1542/hpeds.2016-0147

Hunt, R. W., Tzioumi, D., Collins, E., & Jeffery, H. E. (2008). Adverse neurodevelopmental outcome of infants exposed to opiate in-utero. *Early Human Development, 84*(1), 29–35. https://doi.org/10.1016/j.earlhumdev.2007.01.013

Jansson, L. M., & Patrick, S. W. (2019). Neonatal abstinence syndrome. *Pediatric Clinics of North America, 66*(2), 353–367. https://doi.org/10.1016/j.pcl.2018.12.006

Johnson, R. E., Jones, H. E., Jasinski, D. R., Svikis, D. S., Haug, N. A., Jansson, L. M., Kissin, W. B., Alpan, G., Lantz, M. E., Cone, E. J., Wilkins, D. G., Golden, A. S., Huggins, G. R., & Lester, B. M. (2001). Buprenorphine treatment of pregnant opioid-dependent women: Maternal and neonatal outcomes. *Drug and Alcohol Dependence, 63*(1), 97–103. https://doi.org/10.1016/s0376-8716(00)00194-0

Jones, H. E., O'Grady, K. E., Johnson, R. E., Velez, M., & Jansson, L. M. (2010). Infant neurobehavior following prenatal exposure to methadone or buprenorphine: Results from the neonatal intensive care unit network neurobehavioral scale. *Substance Use & Misuse*, *45*(13), 2244–2257. https://doi.org/10.3109/10826084.2010.484474

Kahila, H., Saisto, T., Kivitie-Kallio, S., Haukkamaa, M., & Halmesmäki, E. (2007). A prospective study on buprenorphine use during pregnancy: Effects on maternal and neonatal outcome. *Acta Obstetricia et Gynecologica Scandinavica*, *86*(2), 185–190. https://doi.org/10.1080/00016340601110770

Kutahyalioglu, N. S., & Scafide, K. N. (2022). Effects of family-centered care on bonding: A systematic review. *Journal of Child Health Care*. https://doi.org/10.1177/13674935221085799

Lester, B. M., Andreozzi-Fontaine, L., Tronick, E., & Bigsby, R. (2014). Assessment and evaluation of the high risk neonate: The NICU Network Neurobehavioral Scale. *Journal of Visualized Experiments*, *90*. https://doi.org/10.3791/3368

Lester, B. M., & Tronick, E. Z. (2004). History and description of the Neonatal Intensive Care Unit Network Neurobehavioral Scale. *Pediatrics*, *113*(3 Pt 2), 634–640.

Libertus, K., & Hauf, P. (2017). Editorial: Motor skills and their foundational role for perceptual, social, and cognitive development. *Frontiers in Psychology*, *8*, 301. https://doi.org/10.3389/fpsyg.2017.00301

Lobo, M. A., Harbourne, R. T., Dusing, S. C., & McCoy, S. W. (2013). Grounding early intervention: Physical therapy cannot just be about motor skills anymore. *Physical Therapy*, *93*(1), 94–103. https://doi.org/10.2522/ptj.20120158

Maguire, D. (2014). Care of the infant with neonatal abstinence syndrome: Strength of the evidence. *The Journal of Perinatal & Neonatal Nursing*, *28*(3), 204–211. https://doi.org/10.1097/JPN.0000000000000042

Maguire, D. J., Rowe, M. A., Spring, H., & Elliott, A. F. (2015). Patterns of disruptive feeding behaviors in infants with neonatal abstinence syndrome. *Advances in Neonatal Care*, *15*(6), 429–439. https://doi.org/10.1097/ANC.0000000000000204

Maguire, D. J., Taylor, S., Armstrong, K., Shaffer-Hudkins, E., Germain, A. M., Brooks, S. S., Cline, G. J., & Clark, L. (2016). Long-term outcomes of infants with neonatal abstinence syndrome. *Neonatal Network*, *35*(5), 277–286. https://doi.org/10.1891/0730-0832.35.5.277

Maitre, N. L., Chorna, O., Romeo, D. M., & Guzzetta, A. (2016). Implementation of the hammersmith infant neurological examination in a high-risk infant follow-up program. *Pediatric Neurology*, *65*, 31–38. https://doi.org/10.1016/j.pediatrneurol.2016.09.010

Malcolm, W. (Ed.). (2015). Neonatal abstinence syndrome. In *Beyond the NICU: Comprehensive Care of the High-Risk Infant*. McGraw-Hill Education.

McAllister, J. M., Hall, E. S., Hertenstein, G. E. R., Merhar, S. L., Uebel, P. L., & Wexelblatt, S. L. (2018). Torticollis in infants with a history of neonatal abstinence syndrome. *The Journal of Pediatrics*, *196*, 305–308. https://doi.org/10.1016/j.jpeds.2017.12.009

McCarty, D. B., Peat, J. R., O'Donnell, S., Graham, E., & Malcolm, W. F. (2019). "Choose physical therapy" for neonatal abstinence syndrome: Clinical management for infants affected by the opioid crisis. *Physical Therapy, 99*(6), 771–785. https://doi.org/10.1093/ptj/pzz039

McManus, B. M., & Kotelchuck, M. (2007). The effect of aquatic therapy on functional mobility of infants and toddlers in early intervention. *Pediatric Physical Therapy, 19*(4), 275–282. https://doi.org/10.1097/PEP.0b013e3181575190

Moreland, A. D., & McRae-Clark, A. (2018). Parenting outcomes of parenting interventions in integrated substance-use treatment programs: A systematic review. *Journal of Substance Abuse Treatment, 89*, 52–59. https://doi.org/10.1016/j.jsat.2018.03.005

Mouradian, L. E., & Als, H. (1994). The influence of neonatal intensive care unit caregiving practices on motor functioning of preterm infants. *The American Journal of Occupational Therapy, 48*(6), 527–533. https://doi.org/10.5014/ajot.48.6.527

Noble, Y., & Boyd, R. (2012). Neonatal assessments for the preterm infant up to 4 months corrected age: A systematic review. *Developmental Medicine and Child Neurology, 54*(2), 129–139. https://doi.org/10.1111/j.1469-8749.2010.03903.x

Nugent, J. K. (2013). The competent newborn and the neonatal behavioral assessment scale: T. Berry Brazelton's legacy. *Journal of Child and Adolescent Psychiatric Nursing, 26*(3), 173–179. https://doi.org/10.1111/jcap.12043

Onozawa, K., Glover, V., Adams, D., Modi, N., & Kumar, R. C. (2001). Infant massage improves mother–infant interaction for mothers with postnatal depression. *Journal of Affective Disorders, 63*(1–3), 201–207. https://doi.org/10.1016/s0165-0327(00)00198-1

Oyemade, U. J., Cole, O. J., Johnson, A. A., Knight, E. M., Westney, O. E., Laryea, H., Hill, G., Cannon, E., Fomufod, A., & Westney, L. S. (1994). Prenatal predictors of performance on the Brazelton Neonatal Behavioral Assessment Scale. *The Journal of Nutrition, 124*(6 Suppl), 1000S–1005S. https://doi.org/10.1093/jn/124.suppl_6.1000S

Palchik, A. B., Einspieler, C., Evstafeyeva, I. V., Talisa, V. B., & Marschik, P. B. (2013). Intra-uterine exposure to maternal opiate abuse and HIV: The impact on the developing nervous system. *Early Human Development, 89*(4), 229–235. https://doi.org/10.1016/j.earlhumdev.2013.02.004

Pineda, R., Wallendorf, M., & Smith, J. (2020). A pilot study demonstrating the impact of the supporting and enhancing NICU sensory experiences (SENSE) program on the mother and infant. *Early Human Development, 144*, https://doi.org/10.1016/j.earlhumdev.2020.105000

Porter, L. S., & Porter, B. O. (2004). A blended infant massage–parenting enhancement program for recovering substance-abusing mothers. *Pediatric Nursing, 30*(5), 363–372, 401.

Porter, L. S., Porter, B. O., McCoy, V., Bango-Sanchez, V., Kissel, B., Williams, M., & Nunnewar, S. (2015). Blended infant massage-parenting enhancement program on recovering substance-abusing mothers' parenting stress, self-esteem, depression, maternal attachment, and mother-infant interaction. *Asian Nursing Research, 9*(4), 318–327. https://doi.org/10.1016/j.anr.2015.09.002

Procianoy, R. S., Mendes, E. W., & Silveira, R. C. (2010). Massage therapy improves neurodevelopment outcome at two years corrected age for very low birth weight infants. *Early Human Development*, 86(1), 7–11. https://doi.org/10.1016/j.earlhumdev.2009.12.001

Rana, D., Garde, K., Elabiad, M. T., & Pourcyrous, M. (2022). Whole body massage for newborns: A report on non-invasive methodology for neonatal opioid withdrawal syndrome. *Journal of Neonatal-Perinatal Medicine*, 15(3), 559–565. https://doi.org/10.3233/NPM-220989

Rocha, N. A. C. F., Dos Santos Silva, F. P., Dos Santos, M. M., & Dusing, S. C. (2020). Impact of mother–infant interaction on development during the first year of life: A systematic review. *Journal of Child Health Care*, 24(3), 365–385. https://doi.org/10.1177/1367493519864742

Rutherford, H. J. V., Potenza, M. N., & Mayes, L. C. (2013). The neurobiology of addiction and attachment. In N. E. Suchman, M. Pajulo, & L. C. Mayes (Eds.), *Parenting and substance abuse: Developmental approaches to intervention* (pp. 3–23). Oxford University Press. https://doi.org/10.1093/med:psych/9780199743100.003.0001

Ryan, G., Dooley, J., Gerber Finn, L., & Kelly, L. (2019). Nonpharmacological management of neonatal abstinence syndrome: A review of the literature. *The Journal of Maternal-Fetal & Neonatal Medicine*, 32(10), 1735–1740. https://doi.org/10.1080/14767058.2017.1414180

Shrestha, S., Roberts, M. H., Maxwell, J. R., Leeman, L. M., & Bakhireva, L. N. (2021). Post-discharge healthcare utilization in infants with neonatal opioid withdrawal syndrome. *Neurotoxicology and Teratology*, 86. https://doi.org/10.1016/j.ntt.2021.106975

Soares, H., Barbieri-Figueiredo, M., Pereira, S., Silva, M., & Fuertes, M. (2018). Parents attending to nurse visits and birth age contribute to infant development: A study about the determinants of infant development. *Early Human Development*, 122, 15–21. https://doi.org/10.1016/j.earlhumdev.2018.05.006

Spence, K., Boedeker, R., Harhausen, M., Kaushal, G., Buchanan, P., & Josephsen, J. (2020). Avoiding NICU transfers for newborns with neonatal opioid withdrawal syndrome (NOWS): A quality improvement initiative to manage NOWS on the mother–baby unit. *Journal of Addiction Medicine*, 14(5), 401–408. https://doi.org/10.1097/ADM.0000000000000607

Sweeney, J. K., Gutierrez, T., & Brachy, J. C. (2013). Neonates and parents: Neurodevelopmental perspectives in the neonatal intensive care unit and follow-up. In D. A. Umphred, R. T. Lazaro, M. L. Roller, & G. U. Burton (Eds.), *Neurological rehabilitation* (6th ed., pp. 300–301). Elsevier.

Sweeney, J. K., Heriza, C. B., Blanchard, Y., & Dusing, S. C. (2010). Neonatal physical therapy. Part II: Practice frameworks and evidence-based practice guidelines. *Pediatric Physical Therapy*, 22(1), 2–16. https://doi.org/10.1097/PEP.0b013e3181cdba43

Tavasoli, A., Azimi, P., & Montazari, A. (2014). Reliability and validity of the Peabody Developmental Motor Scales – second edition for assessing motor development of low birth weight preterm infants. *Pediatric Neurology*, 51(4), 522–526. https://doi.org/10.1016/j.pediatrneurol.2014.06.010

Tuhkanen, H., Pajulo, M., Jussila, H., & Ekholm, E. (2019). Infants born to women with substance use: Exploring early neurobehavior with the Dubowitz neurological examination. *Early Human Development, 130*, 51–56. https://doi.org/10.1016/j.earlhumdev.2018.12.019

Velez, M., & Jansson, L. M. (2008). The opioid dependent mother and newborn dyad: Non-pharmacologic care. *Journal of Addiction Medicine, 2*(3), 113–120. https://doi.org/10.1097/ADM.0b013e31817e6105

Velez, M. L., Jansson, L. M., Schroeder, J., & Williams, E. (2009). Prenatal methadone exposure and neonatal neurobehavioral functioning. *Pediatric Research, 66*(6), 704–709. https://doi.org/10.1203/PDR.0b013e3181bc035d

Velez, M. L., Jordan, C., & Jansson, L. M. (2021a). Reconceptualizing nonpharmacologic approaches to neonatal abstinence syndrome (NAS) and neonatal opioid withdrawal syndrome (NOWS): A theoretical and evidence-based approach. Part II: The clinical application of nonpharmacologic care for NAS/NOWS. *Neurotoxicology and Teratology, 88*. https://doi.org/10.1016/j.ntt.2021.107032

Velez, M. L., Jordan, C. J., & Jansson, L. M. (2021b). Reconceptualizing nonpharmacologic approaches to neonatal abstinence syndrome (NAS) and neonatal opioid withdrawal syndrome (NOWS): A theoretical and evidence-based approach. *Neurotoxicology and Teratology, 88*. https://doi.org/10.1016/j.ntt.2021.107020

Velez, M. L., McConnell, K., Spencer, N., Montoya, L., Tuten, M., & Jansson, L. M. (2018). Prenatal buprenorphine exposure and neonatal neurobehavioral functioning. *Early Human Development, 117*, 7–14. https://doi.org/10.1016/j.earlhumdev.2017.11.009

Vignochi, C. M., Teixeira, P. P., & Nader, S. S. (2010). Effect of aquatic physical therapy on pain and state of sleep and wakefulness among stable preterm newborns in neonatal intensive care units. *Revista Brasileira de Fisioterapia, 14*(3), 214–220.

Weller, A. E., Crist, R. C., Reiner, B. C., Doyle, G. A., & Berrettini, W. H. (2021). Neonatal opioid withdrawal syndrome (NOWS): A transgenerational echo of the opioid crisis. *Cold Spring Harbor Perspectives in Medicine, 11*(3). https://doi.org/10.1101/cshperspect.a039669

White-Traut, R. C., Nelson, M. N., Silvestri, J. M., Vasan, U., Littau, S., Meleedy-Rey, P., Gu, G., & Patel, M. (2002). Effect of auditory, tactile, visual, and vestibular intervention on length of stay, alertness, and feeding progression in preterm infants. *Developmental Medicine and Child Neurology, 44*(2), 91–97. https://doi.org/10.1017/s0012162201001736

Yeoh, S. L., Eastwood, J., Wright, I. M., Morton, R., Melhuish, E., Ward, M., & Oei, J. L. (2019). Cognitive and motor outcomes of children with prenatal opioid exposure: A systematic review and meta-analysis. *JAMA Network Open, 2*(7). https://doi.org/10.1001/jamanetworkopen.2019.7025

10 Long-Term Outcomes of Children After Prenatal Opioid Exposure

Ju Lee Oei

10.1 Introduction

For centuries, the long-term outcomes of infants of opioid-using mothers were difficult to appreciate because many babies died soon after birth. Chronic exposure to opioids and other drugs of addiction during pregnancy leads to fetal tolerance. At birth, with cessation of maternal drug supply, many opioid-exposed infants undergo acute withdrawal and need prompt treatment to prevent serious complications. During the 19th and early 20th centuries, neonatal opioid withdrawal syndrome (NOWS) was known as "Congenital Morphinism" because morphine was the most common opioid used by pregnant women. Congenital Morphinism was first described in Western literature in 1875 (Perlstein, 1947) as a condition associated with dire outcomes. In one report, 15 of 16 infants from an opioid-using mother died soon after birth. The sole survivor was given a few drops of morphine which led to rapid resolution of symptoms and saved the infant's life. Without treatment, irritability, poor feeding, diarrhea, failure to thrive, and other complications such as seizures may result in the death of many infants, usually within a few days to weeks of birth (Petty, 1912).

As recently as the 1950s, NOWS continued to have a high mortality rate (Cobrinik et al., 1959). In the 1970s, the term "neonatal abstinence syndrome" (NAS) was proposed to describe the withdrawal syndrome experienced by babies of narcotic-using mothers. Using observations from full-term, bottle-fed, narcotic-exposed infants, Loretta Finnegan and her colleagues developed a detailed 21-point assessment tool, the Finnegan Neonatal Abstinence Severity Scale (FNAS), to standardize diagnosis, assessment, and treatment of infant withdrawal from narcotic drugs. The purpose of the FNAS was to allow withdrawing infants to be differentiated from those experiencing normal newborn behaviors or problems secondary to other pathologies such as infections. The use of this standardized assessment tool increased awareness and refined the prompt

DOI: 10.4324/9781003397267-10

treatment of infants at risk of withdrawal. This led to decreased risk of death from undiagnosed and untreated NAS. Today, NAS and, more specifically, NOWS have become uncommon direct causes of infant death and most babies with one or the other will survive to leave their hospital of birth (Abdel-Latif et al., 2007; Uebel et al., 2015).

The long-term consequences of prenatal opioid exposure are therefore a relatively new concern, made all the more critical to address because of the massive increase in opioid use around the world (McCarthy, 2016). There is increasing evidence that withdrawal is not the only problem faced by children after prenatal opioid exposure, and many children are impacted by adverse circumstances associated with parental drug use disorders, including poor parenting knowledge, parental psychiatric co-morbidities, intergenerational vulnerabilities, and socioeconomic adversities that include poverty, trauma, stress, poor nutrition, and poor education (Casado-Flores, 1990). In the end, all these, including the potential biological impact of opioids on the developing fetus, work to prevent the child from reaching his/her full potential as an adult (Lifschitz et al., 1985).

Elucidating the long-term impact of opioids on a child is made more difficult by the fact that few drugs of addiction, except for alcohol, are structural teratogens. Many children exposed to prenatal opioids are difficult to identify after resolution of withdrawal. The problems affecting children with a history of prenatal opioid exposure may also take several years to emerge (see Figure 10.1). Many of these, such as mental health issues, poor cognitive development, and other physical health problems, are insidious and go unrecognized until a critical event, e.g., when the child enters school. In addition, the eventual presentation may also be considerably altered by other factors such as the child's access to supportive care, and his or her own resilience (Brancato & Cannizzaro, 2018). Nevertheless, in recent years, knowledge about the link between prenatal opioid exposure and risk of neurodevelopmental, mental health, and physical consequences have strengthened and driven many funding and policy directives to investigate and protect the children (United Nations Office of Drug Control, 2022; U.S. Government Accountability Office, 2017).

This is a new paradigm of care which strives to address and understand the "sleeper effects" of prenatal opioid exposure. This is an urgent task because the sheer numbers of infants exposed to opioids are rapidly rising. Each year, 0.5 million deaths are attributed to drug use and 70% of these deaths are related to opioids (World Health Organization, 2021). In the United States alone, 90 infants per day (or one every 15 minutes) are born to an opioid-dependent mother (U.S. Department of Health and Human Services, 2023). Vast resources are spent on optimum NOWS treatment because of the devastating consequences of untreated or unidentified newborn withdrawal. A similar push to understand that intervening

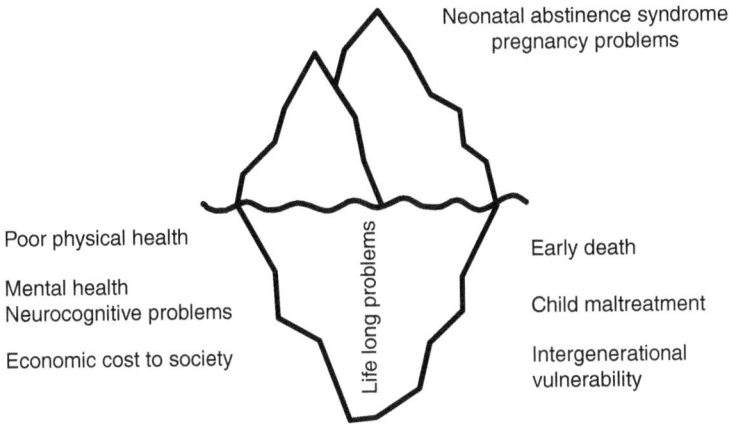

Figure 10.1 Hidden problems associated with opioid exposure that may not emerge for years after birth

in the future problems faced by children who have survived NOWS is now needed.

This chapter will discuss the current understanding of the problems faced by children with a history of prenatal opioid exposure and suggest a pathway of care to address these needs.

10.2 Current Knowledge About the Outcomes of Children After Neonatal Abstinence Syndrome (NAS)

10.2.1 Physical Health

Comprehensive information about the relationship between prenatal opioid exposure and future physical health problems is limited to cohort and population linkage studies. In 1959, Cobrinik et al. (1959) reported on the outcomes of 192 opioid-exposed children born between 1892 and 1956; 25 died (most within the first 2–3 days of life) and three, all of whom were treated with withdrawal medications, became "addicts" at 10, 12, and 58 years of age. Three survivors became "sickly" (n = 1), blind (n = 1), and deaf (n = 1) (Cobrinik et al., 1959).

The fate of people who were at risk of or who underwent withdrawal from maternal drugs in the newborn period remained uncertain for many years, as this was often a marginalized group of people who were otherwise physically healthy. In recent years, the advent of novel population research techniques, such as data linkage, has allowed large-scale tracking of populations that are traditionally elusive or difficult to follow using traditional means. Linking administrative databases with patient identifiers such as names, addresses, dates of birth, and hospital record numbers allows development of people profiles that can be used for research, audit, and administrative purposes.

In 2015, Uebel et al. (2015) used population data linkage techniques to investigate the outcomes of 3,842 children diagnosed with neonatal abstinence syndrome (NAS) or newborn withdrawal. This cohort was born between 2001 to 2011 in the state of New South Wales, Australia. Using birth, death, hospitalization, and education records, Uebel et al. (2015) found that children with a history of NAS were significantly more likely to be re-hospitalized for conditions such as assaults (odds ratio, 95% confidence intervals 15.2, 11.3–20.6), maltreatment (210, 14.3–30.9), mental and behavioral issues (2.6, 2.1–3.2), and infections (Uebel et al., 2015). These findings have since been replicated in other countries, most notably in the United States, emphasizing high use of medical services, most of which are preventable, in children with a history of NAS, even after hospital discharge at birth (Arter et al., 2021; Ko et al., 2021; Milliren et al., 2021; Percy et al., 2020; Shrestha et al., 2021).

The exact causes of these readmissions are multifactorial. Many re-hospitalizations were due to external and preventable causes such as trauma, accidents, and maltreatment and underscore the importance of ensuring that children with a history of prenatal opioid exposure, as well as their parents, are supported adequately, especially during the first difficult few years of life. Uebel et al. (2015) also found that risk of death was as high as eight-fold for children with a history of NAS between 1 month and 1 year of age, compared to other children in the state, mostly from preventable causes such as Sudden Infant Death Syndrome (SIDS), trauma, assault, neglect, and injury (Uebel et al., 2020). In a systematic review and meta-analysis of 16 studies, including 21,726 infants with prenatal opioid exposure, Makarious et al. (2022) found a significantly increased risk of SIDS (RR 11.12, 95% CI 5.97, 20.72) compared to 3,306,180 unexposed infants (Makarious et al., 2022). The cause for this, in the context of decreasing rates of SIDS in the population due to safe sleeping practices, is concerning (Shapiro-Mendoza et al., 2023). Prenatal opioid exposure has been shown to alter infant arousal response to hypercarbia (Olsen & Lees, 1980) and sleep patterns (Rana et al., 2020) which may increase risk of sudden death, especially in the care of parents or guardians with poorer parenting capacity and again, support for the parents and carers of infants with a history of prenatal opioid exposure, especially at peak risk ages of SIDS, is warranted.

Prenatal drug exposure is also one of the strongest predictors of child harm (Taplin & Mattick, 2013). Ensuring that biological parents and other carers are supported enough to provide adequate and safe parenting will be one of the most important societal measures to break stubborn intergenerational cycles of harm and vulnerability (Callaghan et al., 2010). Poor oversight of the physical and emotional needs of the child increases their risk of poorer physical health. For example, as many as 25% of opioid-exposed children do not receive appropriate healthcare within the first crucial 2 years of life (Callaghan et al., 2010), which, not unexpectedly, compounds the risk of many preventable problems including infections, child maltreatment (Raitasalo et al., 2014) and other disorders that have significant impact on long-term health. For example, prenatal drug exposure (not only to opioids) significantly increases risk of visual dysfunction, including reduced acuity, nystagmus, delayed visual maturation, strabismus, refractive errors, and abnormal visual electrophysiology (Gill et al., 2003; Hamilton et al., 2010; McGlone et al., 2008; McGlone et al., 2014; Melinder et al., 2013). If these disorders are unaddressed, the child will have difficulties seeing and progressing through either school or normal daily life. In children, not correcting visual acuity significantly reduces literacy scores from as early as age 4–5 by 1.7 points (95% CI −2.2 to −1.1) for every 1 line reduction in vision (Bruce et al., 2016). Children with uncorrected visual problems have significant psychological and mental health risks (DeCarlo et al., 2012) with major impact on quality of life even until adulthood (Chadha & Subramanian, 2011).

How opioids impact on the child's biological development and function must also be considered. Prenatal opioid exposure is associated with a significant risk of prematurity and low birthweight (Brogly et al., 2021; Sujan et al., 2019), the most important global causes of death in children under 5 years of age (World Health Organization, 2023). In a pooled analysis of 80 studies, Graeve et al. (2022) found that opioid-exposed neonates had lower birthweight (standardized mean difference, SMD −0.77, 95% CI −0.90), head circumferences (SMD −0.67, 95% CI −0.86), shorter birth lengths (SMD −0.97, 95% CI −1.24), and higher risk of neonatal death (risk ratio (RR) 4.05, 95% CI 2.12, 7.72) and preterm birth (RR 1.92, 95% CI 1.57, 2.35) (Graeve et al., 2022). As per the Developmental Origins of Health and Disease (DOHAD) principle (Wadhwa et al., 2009), where future health, including cardiovascular and renal function, is strongly governed by intra-uterine events, further evaluation of the impact of poor intra-uterine growth and gestation on the long-term outcomes of children with a history of prenatal opioid exposure needs to be urgently evaluated (D'Agostin et al., 2023).

The cause for poor fetal growth, increased risk of preterm births, and poorer childhood health in those exposed to prenatal opioids is uncertain but may be due to inflammatory dysregulation. Opioids are potent pro-inflammatory mediators that are underlying biological drivers for poor pregnancy outcomes in a complex of conditions caused by maternal immune activation. For example, opioids modulate T cell function, including inhibition of NF Kappa B, a protein complex that controls DNA transcription, cytokine production, and cell survival (Börner & Kraus, 2013). Children with NOWS have a transient decrease in the number of T cells (Adatia et al., 2021) which may increase risk of the infant to childhood infections such as paronychia (Flanagan et al., 2021), but whether prenatal opioid exposure increases childhood risk to serious infections and increased use of antibiotics remains unclear (Mahic et al., 2020).

10.2.2 Mental Health Disorders (MHD)

MHDs are intertwined with drug abuse. People with MHDs are more likely to use drugs, and vice versa. In a longitudinal examination of 2,000,118 patient records from the Taiwan National health Insurance Research Database between 2000 and 2009, 124,423 people with selected mental health disorders, including affective psychoses, neurotic disorders, schizophrenia, personality disorders, and adjustment reactions, were up to 5 times (Hazard Ratio (HR) 5.09, 95% CI 4.74–5.48) more likely to develop substance use disorders. The risk increased to 14.55 times if patients were aged between 10 and 19 years (Chiu et al., 2018).

Parental drug use is associated with an increased risk of MHD, including anxiety and affective disorders in children (Dean et al., 2010) and in young adulthood (Clark et al., 2004). Eventual outcomes are modified considerably by genetic and environmental influences. Offspring of drug users, for example, are at increased risk of attention-deficit/hyperactivity disorder (ADHD), but this risk is mitigated by adoption into stable home environments from an early age (Kendler et al., 2016). A study of 94 opioid-exposed children found an increased risk of ADHD with maternal but not paternal opioid use even though all parents had a higher genetic risk for ADHD (Ornoy et al., 2016).

Using claims information from the Truven Health Analytics Multi-State Medicaid Database from 2008 to 2010, half of 1,046 children with NAS in the USA were diagnosed with a mental health disorder compared to 30% of other children (Sherman et al., 2019). In a linked study of 65,117 children born in Finland in 1991, Jääskeläinen et al. (2016) noted a 5.5-fold increased risk of MHD if a child had multiple parental risk factors including maternal substance use, mental disorders, non-intact family, and social welfare need. Girls were at higher risk than boys and risk was only ameliorated slightly by improved maternal education (Jääskeläinen et al., 2016). Linked data analysis by Uebel et al. (2015) of an Australian cohort demonstrated more specifically that children with a history of NAS were significantly more likely to be hospitalized for "mental and behavioral disorders," including mental retardation (OR 2.8), psychological disorders (OR 2.9), including speech and language disorders (OR 3.6), autism (OR 3.6), and behavioral and emotional disorders (OR 4.1) (Uebel et al., 2015).

The etiology of MHD and cognitive problems in the context of prenatal opioid exposure is most likely multifactorial. Infants of opioid-using mothers are exposed to opioids during critical periods of very rapid brain growth across fetal life and in early infancy. Associated lifestyle problems causing stress also compound disruption to developing cortical structures, particularly in areas of the brain governing social behavior and anxiety, such as the parahippocampal gyri and middle temporal gyrus (Walhovd et al., 2012).

However, what is also increasingly appreciated now are the indirect effects of opioids on other biological functions, including inflammation that may significantly impair brain development and function (Jantzie et al., 2020). Opioids are potent inflammatory dysregulators. They bind to the MD2 molecule of Toll Like Receptors (TLR) 4, one of 13 TLR that are upstream gatekeepers of the innate defense system. This activates TLR4 and an inflammatory response (Jantzie et al., 2020). In pregnant rat models, inflammation from opioid exposure lasts for weeks, with increased levels of interleukin (IL)-1β (1954%), tumor necrosis factor (TNF)-α (36%), and IL-6 (225%). In the brain, opioids increase TLR4 expression by 42%, MyD88 MRNA by 87%, and microglia, the immune cells of the brain, are activated, leading to loss of axonal integrity, myelin expression, and adult functional deficits including learning and executive dysfunction (Cunha-Oliveira et al., 2010).

In addition to inflammation, opioids also directly impact on CNS function and structure through neurotransmitter dysregulation, oxidative stress, and injury (Fatima et al., 2019; Récamier-Carballo et al., 2017). Indirect stressors, including psychosocial and environmental disorders, modulate hypothalamic axis (HPA) function (Récamier-Carballo et al., 2017), neurogenic regulators, e.g., brain derived neurotrophic factors (BDNF), and epigenetic expression, even in the placenta (Borrelli et al., 2022), which ultimately influences resilience and vulnerability. In adults with opioid use disorders (OUD), cortisol and other anti-inflammatory agents such as N-acetyl aspartate decrease craving and withdrawal symptoms (Walter et al., 2015). In children exposed specifically to maternal opioids, MRI scans show reduced brain volume sizes, especially of the basal ganglia, cerebellum, and whole brain (Yuan et al., 2014) and altered maturation of connective tracts, which may be associated with cognitive, learning, and behavioral difficulties (Koga et al., 2014).

10.2.3 Neurocognitive Function and School Performance

Opioid exposure is associated with poor neurodevelopment. The exact impact of opioids on neurogenesis and function is unclear but opioids induce apoptosis of human brain cell cultures in vitro (Hu et al., 2002), impair synaptosomal uptake of neurotransmitters like dopamine and norepinephrine (Pattison et al., 2014), and impair cognitive function, even after a few days of exposure (Seip-Cammack & Shapiro, 2014). Children exposed to prenatal opioids have smaller volume brains (Sirnes et al., 2017; Yuan et al., 2014) and head circumferences (Sirnes et al., 2017) that persist until adolescence and may even be permanent (Chin et al., 2023), but there is still no firm relationship between neuroanatomical changes and cognitive testing after opioid exposure.

In a meta-analysis of 26 studies comprising 1,455 children exposed to prenatal opioids and 2,982 controls, Yeoh et al. (2019) found that prenatal opioid exposure was significantly associated with poorer mental and physical development from as early as 6 months. Cognitive differences persisted until adolescence with standardized mean differences (95% Confidence Intervals) in test scores varying between 0.52 (0.31–0.74) at ages 0–2 years, 0.38 (0.07–0.69) at ages 2–6 years, and 0.44 (–0.28–1.16) at ages 6–18 years (not significant at this age). These differences were equivalent to a difference in IQ of 7.8 points at population level and a three-fold risk of intellectual disability (Tiffin & Asher, 1948; Yeoh et al., 2019).

Children with a history of NAS, indicating prenatal drug exposure, not only to opioids, have worse school outcomes. Oei et al. (2017) used linked analysis to determine performance in Australian curriculum-based tests until the first year of high school (ages 12–13) for 2,234 children with a previous diagnosis of NAS. Compared to socioeconomically matched controls (n=4,330) and to other children (n = 598,265), children with NAS scored significantly lower in standardized testing than other children from as early as grade 3 (ages 8–9 years). By grade 7, their scores were lower than other children in grade 5 (average 2 years younger). The risk of not meeting minimum standards was independently associated with NAS (adjusted odds ratio, 95% confidence interval, 2.5, 2.2–2.7), indigenous status (2.2, 2.2–2.3), male gender (1.3, 1.3–1.4), and low parental education (1.5, 1.1–1.6). See Figure 10.2 (Oei et al., 2017).

The association between school failure and poor adult outcomes is clear. Children who fail at school or who do not read at grade level, even from as early as ages 8–9 (grade 3) are more likely to use drugs, engage in criminal activity, be incarcerated, be unemployed, and earn less (Van Whitlock & Lubin, 1998). These results suggest that children with a known history of NAS, especially if they have other risk factors such as having younger

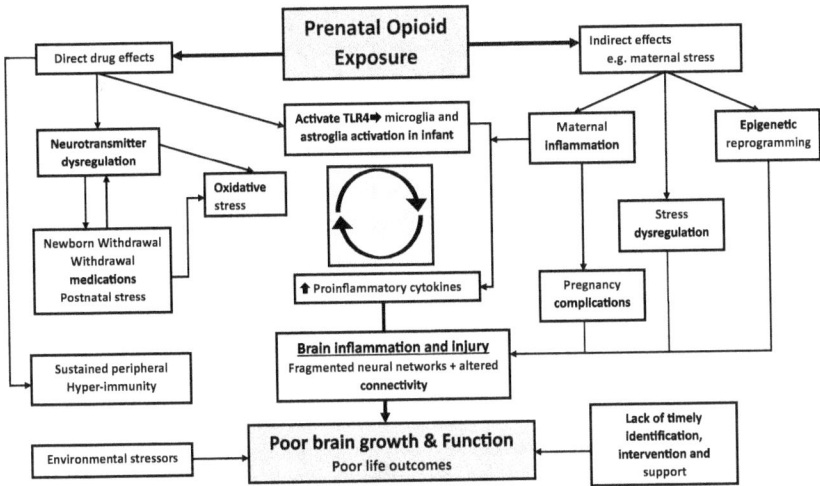

Figure 10.2 The associations between drug, life, and other factors leading to poor life outcomes for children with a history of prenatal opioid exposure

Indigenous mothers, male gender, or being a rural resident, should be targeted for specific neurodevelopmental intervention in a similar manner to children with other risk factors, e.g., prematurity. Such intervention has been shown to be cost-effective and have effects that transcend generations, even in the highest risk communities. Intervention, however, must include the family. The ABCDERIAN project randomized 111 high-risk (98% African-American) infants to an intervention problem of early childhood education. At age 30, 101 of the original subjects demonstrated significant benefits, including higher years of education (Campbell et al., 2012). In addition, the cost-effectiveness of these programs cannot be denied. A review of programs focusing on 3–4-year-old high-risk children found a return for up to US $10 for every dollar spent on the programs, with benefits lasting up to the third decade of life (Reynolds et al., 2011).

10.2.4 *The Risk of Future Addiction and Other Adverse Social Outcomes*

Addiction is a form of MHD and prenatal substance exposure predicts future drug use by up to 50% (O'Brien & Hill, 2014). This is not new information. Of the 192 opioid-exposed infants reviewed by Cobrinik et al. (1959), three patients who had been treated for withdrawal as newborn infants became "addicts" at age 10, 12, and 58 years (Cobrinik et al., 1959). The neuropathology associated with an increased risk of drug-seeking behaviors is unclear, but lower basal ganglia volumes (Yuan et al., 2014) are also noted in patients with poor impulse control and addictive behaviors (O'Brien & Hill, 2014), possibly due to lower levels of dopamine and other neurotransmitters (O'Brien & Hill, 2017).

These inter-connecting traits are common to families affected by drug use: parenting behavior, environmental deprivation, and peer influence (Bushman et al., 2017). Almost half (45%) of child laborers aged 5–15 years in Surat City, India used drugs including tobacco, snuff, alcohol, cannabis, and opium, but this was done mainly to negate the negative aspects of daily life (Bansal & Banerjee, 1993). Drug-using parents are less adaptive and responsive towards the needs of their children and generally have harsher parenting behaviors (Dawe et al., 2003) which, along with environmental deprivation and stress, could lead to early-life physical and mental health issues including social disorientation and adverse behavior such as drug use.

Deviant behavior may start young but is often not noticed until later life. In an interview of 285 predominantly African-American children of addicted mothers aged 12–17 years, 64% had committed a deviant act (e.g., fighting, disobeying parents and police officers, shoplifting, trespassing, damaging property, stealing, carrying a deadly weapon, dealing in stolen goods) by 11 years of age (mean 8.3 (2.2) years), 21% had used illicit drugs (mostly marijuana) (mean 13.1 (1.5) years), and 37% had used alcohol (mean 12.3 (2.6) years), with 16% reporting drinking to intoxicated states. Negative behaviors were compounded by a lack of family structure and positive home atmosphere. Only 39% had an intact family (continuous presence of both birth parents) and only 18% reported a positive and encouraging home environment (Parolin et al., 2016).

Psychological issues, including hostility, depression, and impulsivity, are recognized in adults with a history of intra-uterine drug exposure (Herranz, 2014) and consistently predict early drug use. This suggests that multi-focused programs with a trauma-focused approach are needed to best address the continuum of emotional needs of children of drug users. Certainly, any intervention needs to take in the whole family and not the child because parental modelling is crucial in the lead-up to future addiction and other divisive behaviors.

10.2.5 Adulthood

Currently, there is limited information about the relationship between prenatal opioid exposure and adult outcomes. Herranz (2014) conducted a series of interviews with 30 heroin-exposed adults (mean age 22.3 years) with a postnatal diagnosis of NAS from Spain. Adverse problems in this cohort were evident from early childhood. Of the original cohort of 151 children, 5 had died (4 from AIDS, 1 of unknown reasons), and 94 were not contactable. Up to 40% of their mothers and 30% of fathers had died, 23% were adopted/fostered before childhood, and emotional and physical abuse were reported by 25%. One in 5 were diagnosed with ADHD, 87% had used cannabis, and 47% had used cocaine. Half were educated beyond school but 37% were unemployed, and 57% had received psychiatric treatment during childhood (Herranz, 2014).

10.3 Summary

10.3.1 Unifying the Problem

Complex relationships exist between prenatal substance exposure and the eventual outcomes of the children. Although it is difficult to disentangle the multiple adverse associations with prenatal opioid use and long-term complications, it is imperative that a coordinated and visionary approach be made. Extraordinary resources are spent on ensuring prompt, timely, and safe treatment of infants with prenatal opioid exposure and a risk of NAS, but little effort is made to understand, prevent, and mitigate any problems that they may have later in life. The scant data we have show that a combination of adverse factors, including direct drug effects, genetic influences, and environmental issues, have the potential to lead to extremely poor outcomes for most opioid-exposed children, including future drug use.

Unlike many childhood problems that have no identifiable link to an etiology, we are in the enviable position of providing support and intervention to children with known prenatal opioid exposure and to treat this condition with the respect and support that is given to other childhood problems that do not resolve with infancy, such as prematurity. Addressing this issue, including input from end users such as adults with NAS, must be addressed as an urgent global priority to stop the inexorable and intergenerational disadvantage for millions of children around the world.

10.3.2 Suggested Pathways of Care

Just like any other infant and family impacted by prenatal problems, an infant affected by prenatal opioid exposure should be offered long-term support, ideally until school age. Whilst prompt identification and treatment of NOWS is life-saving, the consequences of prenatal opioid exposure as well as treatment with the same types of drugs that caused the child's withdrawal must be addressed. After resolution of withdrawal treatment, longer-term follow-up, with support for parenting and care of the infant, is vital. The following provides a suggested pathway until the child reaches school age:

1. Ensure adequate growth and nutrition with regular weighs until at least 6 months of age. Many children with NOWS are hyperphagic, but this settles with adequate treatment of withdrawal (Martinez et al., 1999). Restricting feeds may make the infant irritable, which may be met by increased treatment with withdrawal medications, while overfeeding may increase risk of reflux, and future obesity.

2. Develop a well-defined follow-up pathway for high-risk health complications, including surveillance of blood-borne viruses (e.g. Hepatitis C), eye checks, and developmental assessments.

3. Provide support for parents and foster families, especially during the first year of life, when the infant may need more than the usual care due to difficulties caused by withdrawal, feeding behavior, and the other stressors associated with new parenthood.

4. Provide information for parents and foster families, educators, and other services involved in the care of the child about the impact of prenatal opioid exposure on child development, including risk of mental health and behavioral issues.

5. Recognize that support and intervention services may change as the child ages. Young adults may benefit from employment support, addressing social issues such as housing and opportunities for further education if formal schooling is disrupted due to unpreventable circumstances.

References

Abdel-Latif, M. E., Bajuk, B., Lui, K., & Oei, J. (2007). Short-term outcomes of infants of substance-using mothers admitted to neonatal intensive care units in New South Wales and the Australian Capital Territory. *Journal of Paediatrics and Child Health, 43*(3), 127–133. https://doi.org/10.1111/j.1440-1754.2007.01031.x

Adatia, A., Ling, L., Chakraborty, P., Brick, L., & Brager, R. (2021). Neonatal abstinence syndrome is a potential cause of low TREC copy number. *Allergy, Asthma & Clinical Immunology, 17*(1), 115. https://doi.org/10.1186/s13223-021-00617-3

Arter, S., Lambert, J., Brokman, A., & Fall, N. (2021). Diagnoses during the first three years of life for children with prenatal opioid exposure and neonatal abstinence syndrome using a large maternal infant data hub. *Journal of Pediatric Nursing, 61,* 34–39. https://doi.org/10.1016/j.pedn.2021.03.011

Bansal, R., & Banerjee, S. (1993). Substance use by child labourers. *Indian Journal of Psychiatry, 35*(3), 159–161.

Börner, C., & Kraus, J. (2013). Inhibition of NF-KB by opioids in T cells. *The Journal of Immunology, 191*(9), 4640–4647. https://doi.org/10.4049/jimmunol.1300320

Borrelli, K. N., Wachman, E. M., Beierle, J. A., Taglauer, E. S., Jain, M., Bryant, C. D., & Zhang, H. (2022). Effect of prenatal opioid exposure on the human placental methylome. *Biomedicines*, *10*(5), 1150. https://doi.org/10.3390/biome dicines10051150

Brancato, A., & Cannizzaro, C. (2018). Mothering under the influence: How perinatal drugs of abuse alter the mother-infant interaction. *Reviews in the Neurosciences*, *29*(3), 283–294. https://doi.org/10.1515/revneuro-2017-0052

Brogly, S. B., Velez, M. P., Werler, M. M., Li, W., Camden, A., & Guttmann, A. (2021). Prenatal opioid analgesics and the risk of adverse birth outcomes. *Epidemiology*, *32*(3), 448–456. https://doi.org/10.1097/ede.000000000 0001328

Bruce, A., Fairley, L., Chambers, B., Wright, J., & Sheldon, T. A. (2016). Impact of visual acuity on developing literacy at age 4–5 years: A cohort-nested cross-sectional study. *BMJ Open*, *6*(2). https://doi.org/10.1136/bmjopen-2015-010434

Bushman, G., Victor, B. G., Ryan, J. P., & Perron, B. E. (2017). In utero exposure to opioids: An observational study of mothers involved in the child welfare system. *Substance Use & Misuse*, *53*(5), 844–851. https://doi.org/10.1080/10826084.2017.1388406

Callaghan, T., Crimmins, J., & Schweitzer, R. D. (2010). Children of substance-using mothers: Child health engagement and child protection outcomes. *Journal of Paediatrics and Child Health*, *47*(4), 223–227. https://doi.org/10.1111/j.1440-1754.2010.01930.x

Campbell, F. A., Pungello, E. P., Burchinal, M., Kainz, K., Pan, Y., Wasik, B. H., Barbarin, O. A., Sparling, J. J., & Ramey, C. T. (2012). Adult outcomes as a function of an early childhood educational program: An abecedarian project follow-up. *Developmental Psychology*, *48*(4), 1033–1043. https://doi.org/10.1037/a0026644

Casado-Flores, J. (1990). Social and medical problems in children of heroin-addicted parents. *American Journal of Diseases of Children*, *144*(9), 977. https://doi.org/10.1001/archpedi.1990.02150330037017

Chadha, R. K., & Subramanian, A. (2011). The effect of visual impairment on quality of life of children aged 3–16 years. *British Journal of Ophthalmology*, *95*(5), 642–645. https://doi.org/10.1136/bjo.2010.182386

Chin, E. M., Kitase, Y., Madurai, N. K., Robinson, S., & Jantzie, L. L. (2023). In utero methadone exposure permanently alters anatomical and functional connectivity: A preclinical evaluation. *Frontiers in Pediatrics*, *11*. https://doi.org/10.3389/fped.2023.1139378

Chiu, M.-L., Cheng, C.-F., Liang, W.-M., Lin, P.-T., Wu, T.-N., & Chen, C.-Y. (2018). The temporal relationship between selected mental disorders and substance-related disorders: A nationwide population-based cohort study. *Psychiatry Journal*, *2018*, 1–12. https://doi.org/10.1155/2018/5697103

Clark, D. B., Cornelius, J., Wood, D. S., & Vanyukov, M. (2004). Psychopathology risk transmission in children of parents with substance use disorders. *American Journal of Psychiatry*, *161*(4), 685–691. https://doi.org/10.1176/appi.ajp.161.4.685

Cobrinik, R. W., Hood, R. T., & Chusid, E. (1959). The effect of maternal narcotic addiction on the newborn infant. *Pediatrics*, 24(2), 288–304. https://doi.org/10.1542/peds.24.2.288

Cunha-Oliveira, T., Rego, A. C., Garrido, J., Borges, F., Macedo, T., & Oliveira, C. R. (2010). Neurotoxicity of heroin–cocaine combinations in rat cortical neurons. *Toxicology*, 276(1), 11–17. https://doi.org/10.1016/j.tox.2010.06.009

D'Agostin, M., Di Sipio Morgia, C., Vento, G., & Nobile, S. (2023). Long-term implications of fetal growth restriction. *World Journal of Clinical Cases*, 11(13), 2855–2863. https://doi.org/10.12998/wjcc.v11.i13.2855

Dawe, S., Harnett, P. H., Rendalls, V., & Staiger, P. (2003). Improving family functioning and child outcome in methadone maintained families: The Parents Under Pressure Programme. *Drug and Alcohol Review*, 22(3), 299–307. https://doi.org/10.1080/0959523031000154445

Dean, K., Stevens, H., Mortensen, P. B., Murray, R. M., Walsh, E., & Pedersen, C. B. (2010). Full spectrum of psychiatric outcomes among offspring with parental history of mental disorder. *Archives of General Psychiatry*, 67(8), 822–829. https://doi.org/10.1001/archgenpsychiatry.2010.86

DeCarlo, D. K., McGwin, G., Bixler, M. L., Wallander, J., & Owsley, C. (2012). Impact of pediatric vision impairment on daily life. *Optometry and Vision Science*, 89(9), 1409–1416. https://doi.org/10.1097/opx.0b013e318264f1dc

Fatima, M., Srivastav, S., Ahmad, M. H., & Mondal, A. C. (2019). Effects of chronic unpredictable mild stress induced prenatal stress on neurodevelopment of neonates: Role of gsk-3β. *Scientific Reports*, 9(1). https://doi.org/10.1038/s41598-018-38085-2

Flanagan, K. E., Lal, K., Blankenship, K., Gorji, N., Rork, J., & Wiss, K. (2021). Nail disease in neonatal abstinence syndrome. *Pediatric Dermatology*, 38(4), 787–793. https://doi.org/10.1111/pde.14632

Gill, A., Oei, J., Lewis, N., Younan, N., Kennedy, I., & Lui, K. (2003). Strabismus in infants of opiate-dependent mothers. *Acta Paediatrica*, 92(3), 379–385. https://doi.org/10.1111/j.1651-2227.2003.tb00561.x

Graeve, R., Balalian, A. A., Richter, M., Kielstein, H., Fink, A., Martins, S. S., Philbin, M. M., & Factor-Litvak, P. (2022). Infants' prenatal exposure to opioids and the association with birth outcomes: A systematic review and meta-analysis. *Paediatric and Perinatal Epidemiology*, 36(1), 125–143. https://doi.org/10.1111/ppe.12805

Hamilton, R., McGlone, L., MacKinnon, J. R., Russell, H. C., Bradnam, M. S., & Mactier, H. (2010). Ophthalmic, clinical and visual electrophysiological findings in children born to mothers prescribed substitute methadone in pregnancy. *British Journal of Ophthalmology*, 94(6), 696–700. https://doi.org/10.1136/bjo.2009.169284

Herranz, G. S. (2014). Children born to heroin-addicted mothers: What's the outcome 25 years later? *Journal of Addiction Research & Therapy*, 5(2). https://doi.org/10.4172/2155-6105.1000180

Hu, S., Sheng, W. S., Lokensgard, J. R., & Peterson, P. K. (2002). Morphine induces apoptosis of human microglia and neurons. *Neuropharmacology*, 42(6), 829–836. https://doi.org/10.1016/s0028-3908(02)00030-8

Jääskeläinen, M., Holmila, M., Notkola, I.-L., & Raitasalo, K. (2016). Mental disorders and harmful substance use in children of substance abusing parents: A Longitudinal Register-based study on a complete birth cohort born in 1991. *Drug and Alcohol Review*, *35*(6), 728–740. https://doi.org/10.1111/dar.12417

Jantzie, L. L., Maxwell, J. R., Newville, J. C., Yellowhair, T. R., Kitase, Y., Madurai, N., Ramachandra, S., Bakhireva, L. N., Northington, F. J., Gerner, G., Tekes, A., Milio, L. A., Brigman, J. L., Robinson, S., & Allan, A. (2020). Prenatal opioid exposure: The next neonatal neuroinflammatory disease.*Brain, Behavior, and Immunity*, *84*, 45–58. https://doi.org/10.1016/j.bbi.2019.11.007

Kendler, K. S., Ohlsson, H., Sundquist, K., & Sundquist, J. (2016). Cross-generational transmission from drug abuse in parents to attention-deficit/hyper-activity disorder in children. *Psychological Medicine*, *46*(6), 1301–1309. https://doi.org/10.1017/s0033291715002846

Ko, J. Y., Yoon, J., Tong, V. T., Haight, S. C., Patel, R., Rockhill, K. M., Luck, J., & Shapiro-Mendoza, C. (2021). Maternal opioid exposure, neonatal abstinence syndrome, and infant healthcare utilization: A retrospective cohort analysis. *Drug and Alcohol Dependence*, *223*. https://doi.org/10.1016/j.drugalcdep.2021.108704

Koga, K., Izumi, G., Mor, G., Fujii, T., & Osuga, Y. (2014). Toll-like receptors at the maternal-fetal interface in normal pregnancy and pregnancy complications. *American Journal of Reproductive Immunology*, *72*(2), 192–205. https://doi.org/10.1111/aji.12258

Lifschitz, M. H., Wilson, G. S., Smith, E. O., & Desmond, M. M. (1985). Factors affecting head growth and intellectual function in children of drug addicts. *Pediatrics*, *75*(2), 269–274. https://doi.org/10.1542/peds.75.2.269

Mahic, M., Hernandez-Diaz, S., Wood, M., Kieler, H., Odsbu, I., Nørgaard, M., Öztürk, B., Bateman, B. T., Hjellvik, V., Skurtveit, S., & Handal, M. (2020). In utero opioid exposure and risk of infections in childhood: A multinational Nordic Cohort Study. *Pharmacoepidemiology and Drug Safety*, *29*(12), 1596–1604. https://doi.org/10.1002/pds.5088

Makarious, L., Teng, A., & Oei, J. L. (2022). SIDS is associated with prenatal drug use: A meta-analysis and systematic review of 4 238 685 infants. *Archives of Disease in Childhood – Fetal and Neonatal Edition*, *107*(6), 617–623. https://doi.org/10.1136/archdischild-2021-323260

Martinez, A., Kastner, B., & Taeusch, H. W. (1999). Hyperphagia in neonates withdrawing from methadone. *Archives of Disease in Childhood – Fetal and Neonatal Edition*, *80*(3), 178–182. https://doi.org/10.1136/fn.80.3.f178

McCarthy, M. (2016). Incidence of neonatal abstinence syndrome triples in US. *BMJ*, *354*. https://doi.org/10.1136/bmj.i4476

McGlone, L., Hamilton, R., McCulloch, D. L., MacKinnon, J. R., Bradnam, M., & Mactier, H. (2014). Visual outcome in infants born to drug-misusing mothers prescribed methadone in pregnancy. *British Journal of Ophthalmology*, *98*(2), 238–245. https://doi.org/10.1136/bjophthalmol-2013-303967

McGlone, L., Mactier, H., Hamilton, R., Bradnam, M. S., Boulton, R., Borland, W., Hepburn, M., & McCulloch, D. L. (2008). Visual evoked potentials in infants exposed to methadone in utero. *Archives of Disease in Childhood, 93*(9), 784–786. https://doi.org/10.1136/adc.2007.132985

Melinder, A., Konijnenberg, C., & Sarfi, M. (2013). Deviant smooth pursuit in preschool children exposed prenatally to methadone or buprenorphine and tobacco affects integrative visuomotor capabilities. *Addiction, 108*(12), 2175–2182. https://doi.org/10.1111/add.12267

Milliren, C. E., Melvin, P., & Ozonoff, A. (2021). Pediatric hospital readmissions for infants with neonatal opioid withdrawal syndrome, 2016–2019. *Hospital Pediatrics, 11*(9), 979–988. https://doi.org/10.1542/hpeds.2021-005904

National Institutes of Health. (2023, August 22). Novel technologies for infants with neonatal opioid withdrawal syndrome. https://heal.nih.gov/news/stor ies/technologies-neonatal-opioid-withdrawal#:~:text=In%20other%20wo rds%2C%20about%2090,wean%20them%20from%20the%20drugs

O'Brien, J. W., & Hill, S. Y. (2014). Effects of prenatal alcohol and cigarette exposure on offspring substance use in multiplex, alcohol-dependent families. *Alcoholism: Clinical and Experimental Research, 38*(12), 2952–2961. https://doi.org/10.1111/acer.12569

O'Brien, J. W., & Hill, S. Y. (2017). Neural predictors of substance use disorders in young adulthood. *Psychiatry Research: Neuroimaging, 268*, 22–26. https://doi.org/10.1016/j.pscychresns.2017.08.006

Oei, J. L., Melhuish, E., Uebel, H., Azzam, N., Breen, C., Burns, L., Hilder, L., Bajuk, B., Abdel-Latif, M. E., Ward, M., Feller, J. M., Falconer, J., Clews, S., Eastwood, J., Li, A., & Wright, I. M. (2017). Neonatal abstinence syndrome and high school performance. *Pediatrics, 139*(2). https://doi.org/10.1542/peds.2016-2651

Olsen, G. D., & Lees, M. H. (1980). Ventilatory response to carbon dioxide of infants following chronic prenatal methadone exposure. *The Journal of Pediatrics, 96*(6), 983–989. https://doi.org/10.1016/s0022-3476(80)80622-6

Ornoy, A., Finkel-Pekarsky, V., Peles, E., Adelson, M., Schreiber, S., & Ebstein, P. R. (2016). ADHD risk alleles associated with opiate addiction: Study of addicted parents and their children. *Pediatric Research, 80*(2), 228–236. https://doi.org/10.1038/pr.2016.78

Parolin, M., Simonelli, A., Mapelli, D., Sacco, M., & Cristofalo, P. (2016). Parental substance abuse as an early traumatic event. preliminary findings on neuropsychological and personality functioning in young drug addicts exposed to drugs early. *Frontiers in Psychology, 7*. https://doi.org/10.3389/fpsyg.2016.00887

Pattison, L. P., Mcintosh, S., Sexton, T., Childers, S. R., & Hemby, S. E. (2014). Changes in dopamine transporter binding in nucleus accumbens following chronic self-administration cocaine: Heroin combinations. *Synapse, 68*(10), 437–444. https://doi.org/10.1002/syn.21755

Percy, Z., Brokamp, C., McAllister, J. M., Ryan, P., Wexelblatt, S. L., & Hall, E. S. (2020). Subclinical and overt newborn opioid exposure: Prevalence and first-year healthcare utilization. *The Journal of Pediatrics, 222*, 52–58. https://doi.org/10.1016/j.jpeds.2020.03.052

Perlstein, M. A. (1947). Congenital morphinism: A rare cause of convulsions in the newborn. *Journal of the American Medical Association, 135*(10), 633. https://doi.org/10.1001/jama.1947.62890100006006c

Petty, G. (1912). Congenital morphinism, with report of cases. *Texas Medical Journal, 27*(9), 337–343.

Raitasalo, K., Holmila, M., Autti-Rämö, I., Notkola, I.-L., & Tapanainen, H. (2014). Hospitalisations and out-of-home placements of children of substance-abusing mothers: A register-based Cohort Study. *Drug and Alcohol Review, 34*(1), 38–45. https://doi.org/10.1111/dar.12121

Rana, D., Pollard, L., Rowland, J., Dhanireddy, R., & Pourcyrous, M. (2020). Amplitude-integrated EEG in infants with neonatal abstinence syndrome. *Journal of Neonatal-Perinatal Medicine, 12*(4), 391–397. https://doi.org/10.3233/npm-1834

Récamier-Carballo, S., Estrada-Camarena, E., & López-Rubalcava, C. (2017). Maternal separation induces long-term effects on monoamines and brain-derived neurotrophic factor levels on the frontal cortex, amygdala, and hippocampus: Differential effects after a stress challenge. *Behavioural Pharmacology, 28*(7), 545–557. https://doi.org/10.1097/fbp.0000000000000324

Reynolds, A. J., Temple, J. A., White, B. A., Ou, S., & Robertson, D. L. (2011). Age 26 cost–benefit analysis of the child–parent center early education program. *Child Development, 82*(1), 379–404. https://doi.org/10.1111/j.1467-8624.2010.01563.x

Seip-Cammack, K. M., & Shapiro, M. L. (2014). Behavioral flexibility and response selection are impaired after limited exposure to oxycodone. *Learning & Memory, 21*(12), 686–690. https://doi.org/10.1101/lm.036251.114

Shapiro-Mendoza, C. K., Woodworth, K. R., Cottengim, C. R., Erck Lambert, A. B., Harvey, E. M., Monsour, M., Parks, S. E., & Barfield, W. D. (2023). Sudden unexpected infant deaths: 2015–2020. *Pediatrics, 151*(4). https://doi.org/10.1542/peds.2022-058820

Sherman, L. J., Ali, M. M., Mutter, R., & Larson, J. (2019). Mental disorders among children born with neonatal abstinence syndrome. *Psychiatric Services, 70*(2), 151. https://doi.org/10.1176/appi.ps.201800341

Shrestha, S., Roberts, M. H., Maxwell, J. R., Leeman, L. M., & Bakhireva, L. N. (2021). Post-discharge healthcare utilization in infants with neonatal opioid withdrawal syndrome. *Neurotoxicology and Teratology, 86*. https://doi.org/10.1016/j.ntt.2021.106975

Sirnes, E., Oltedal, L., Bartsch, H., Eide, G. E., Elgen, I. B., & Aukland, S. M. (2017). Brain morphology in school-aged children with prenatal opioid exposure: A structural MRI study. *Early Human Development, 106–107*, 33–39. https://doi.org/10.1016/j.earlhumdev.2017.01.009

Sujan, A. C., Quinn, P. D., Rickert, M. E., Wiggs, K. K., Lichtenstein, P., Larsson, H., Almqvist, C., Öberg, A. S., & D'Onofrio, B. M. (2019). Maternal prescribed opioid analgesic use during pregnancy and associations with adverse birth outcomes: A population-based study. *PLoS Medicine, 16*(12). https://doi.org/10.1371/journal.pmed.1002980

Taplin, S., & Mattick, R. P. (2013). Mothers in methadone treatment and their involvement with the child protection system: A replication and extension study. *Child Abuse & Neglect, 37*(8), 500–510. https://doi.org/10.1016/j.chiabu.2013.01.003

Tiffin, J., & Asher, E. J. (1948). The Purdue Pegboard: Norms and studies of reliability and validity. *Journal of Applied Psychology, 32*(3), 234–247. https://doi.org/10.1037/h0061266

Uebel, H., Wright, I. M., Burns, L., Hilder, L., Bajuk, B., Breen, C., Abdel-Latif, M. E., Falconer, J., Clews, S., Ward, M., Eastwood, J., & Oei, J. L. (2020). Characteristics and causes of death in children with neonatal abstinence syndrome. *Journal of Paediatrics and Child Health, 56*(12), 1933–1940. https://doi.org/10.1111/jpc.15091

Uebel, H., Wright, I. M., Burns, L., Hilder, L., Bajuk, B., Breen, C., Abdel-Latif, M. E., Feller, J. M., Falconer, J., Clews, S., Eastwood, J., & Oei, J. L. (2015). Reasons for rehospitalization in children who had neonatal abstinence syndrome. *Pediatrics, 136*(4), 811–820. https://doi.org/10.1542/peds.2014-2767

United Nations Office on Drug and Crime. (2022, May 27). *Neonatal abstinence syndrome: UNODC and experts discuss support for mothers and infants exposed prenatally to synthetic drugs.* https://www.unodc.org/unodc/frontpage/2022/May/neonatal-abstinence-syndrome_-unodc-and-experts-discuss-support-for-mothers-and-infants-exposed-prenatally-to-synthetic-drugs.html

U.S. Department of Health and Human Services. (2023, August 22). *Novel technologies for infants with neonatal opioid withdrawal syndrome.* National Institutes of Health. https://www.heal.nih.gov/news/stories/technologies-neonatal-opioid-withdrawal

U.S. Government Accountability Office. (2017, October 4). Newborn health: Federal action needed to address neonatal abstinence syndrome. https://www.gao.gov/products/gao-18-32

Van Whitlock, R., & Lubin, B. (1998). Psychometric properties of the grade 4 reading level multiple affect adjective check list-revised with offenders. *Perceptual and Motor Skills, 86*(2), 551–560. https://doi.org/10.2466/pms.1998.86.2.551

Wadhwa, P., Buss, C., Entringer, S., & Swanson, J. (2009). Developmental origins of health and disease: Brief history of the approach and current focus on epigenetic mechanisms. *Seminars in Reproductive Medicine, 27*(5), 358–368. https://doi.org/10.1055/s-0029-1237424

Walhovd, K. B., Watts, R., Amlien, I., & Woodward, L. J. (2012). Neural tract development of infants born to methadone-maintained mothers. *Pediatric Neurology, 47*(1), 1–6. https://doi.org/10.1016/j.pediatrneurol.2012.04.008

Walter, M., Bentz, D., Schicktanz, N., Milnik, A., Aerni, A., Gerhards, C., Schwegler, K., Vogel, M., Blum, J., Schmid, O., Roozendaal, B., Lang, U. E., Borgwardt, S., & de Quervain, D. (2015). Effects of cortisol administration on craving in heroin addicts. *Translational Psychiatry, 5*(7), 610. https://doi.org/10.1038/tp.2015.101

World Health Organization. (2021, August 4). *Opioid overdose.* https://www.who.int/news-room/fact-sheets/detail/opioid-overdose

World Health Organization. (2023, May 11) *Preterm birth.* https://www.who.int/news-room/fact-sheets/detail/preterm-birth#:~:text=Globally%2C%20prematurity%20is%20the%20leading,around%20the%20world%20are%20stark

Yeoh, S. L., Eastwood, J., Wright, I. M., Morton, R., Melhuish, E., Ward, M., & Oei, J. L. (2019). Cognitive and motor outcomes of children with prenatal opioid exposure. *JAMA Netw Open, 2*(7). https://doi.org/10.1001/jamanetw orkopen.2019.7025

Yuan, Q., Rubic, M., Seah, J., Rae, C., Wright, I. M., Kaltenbach, K., Feller, J. M., Abdel-Latif, M. E., Chu, C., Oei, J. L., Pham, M., Lees, S., Nanan, R., Fonseca, B., Lovett, A., Abdel-Latif, M., Sinn, J., Maher, C., Stack, J., ... Lee Oei, J. (2014). Do maternal opioids reduce neonatal regional brain volumes? A pilot study. *Journal of Perinatology, 34*(12), 909–913. https://doi.org/10.1038/jp.2014.111

11 Support for Mothers and Children Impacted by Substance Use: Being Effective and Addressing Challenges

Lynn Kemp and Stacy Blythe

11.1 Introduction

There is substantial evidence that children of mothers who use harmful and addictive substances have significant negative long-term challenges. Recent literature reveals that these children have the potential to experience adverse developmental outcomes, including cognitive, executive functioning, and language delay (Hatzis et al., 2017; Joseph et al., 2020; Neger & Prinz, 2015; Niccols et al., 2012; Peacock-Chambers et al., 2022; Renk et al., 2016); impaired physical growth (Cataldo et al., 2019; Joseph et al., 2020; Niccols et al., 2012); poor health and congenital abnormalities that vary by the type and timing of fetal substance exposure (Cataldo et al., 2019; Joseph et al., 2020; Niccols et al., 2012); mental health problems (McGovern et al., 2022; Neger & Prinz, 2015); injuries (McGovern et al., 2022); poor school performance and achievement (Joseph et al., 2020; Niccols et al., 2012; Peacock-Chambers et al., 2022); emotional and behavioral and maladjustment issues, including inattention, hyperactivity, and internalizing and externalizing disorders (Hatzis et al., 2017; McGovern et al., 2023; McGovern et al., 2022; Neger & Prinz, 2015; Niccols et al., 2012; Parolin & Simonelli, 2016; Peacock-Chambers et al., 2022; Renk et al., 2016), with substance-using fathers also significantly impacting on child internalizing and externalizing problems (McGovern et al., 2023); and impairments in social behavior and poor social outcomes (Joseph et al., 2020; McGovern et al., 2022; Neger & Prinz, 2015; Renk et al., 2016).

When seeking to understand the "causes" of these child outcomes, it can be difficult to separate the physiological impacts of fetal exposure and its teratogenic and epigenetic impacts, from the impacts of toxic stress. Toxic stress is chronically elevated cortisol levels experienced by substance-using mothers during pregnancy due to concurrent issues such as mental illness, intimate partner and family violence, homelessness, and isolation,

DOI: 10.4324/9781003397267-11

and the quality of parenting particularly in the early years of the child's life (Hatzis et al., 2017; Joseph et al., 2020; Renk et al., 2016). There is increasing evidence that the neural circuitry affected by substances, particularly the dopaminergic and oxytonic systems, reduces maternal ability to experience feelings of reward from interaction with their baby and read and interpret their baby's cues (Cataldo et al., 2019; Parolin & Simonelli, 2016; Renk et al., 2016). These impacts, however, are also associated with stress and elevated cortisol levels (Flykt et al., 2021).

Regardless of the mechanisms of action which may be biological, behavioral, or stress-related, these children are more likely to experience demanding or coercive parenting, rigidity, and authoritarianism (Milligan et al., 2020); less parental supervision (Neger & Prinz, 2015; Parolin & Simonelli, 2016; Renk et al., 2016); punitive discipline and parental anger (Neger & Prinz, 2015; Parolin & Simonelli, 2016); parental intrusiveness and over-involvement (Parolin & Simonelli, 2016); accelerated autonomy and reversal of parent/child roles (Parolin & Simonelli, 2016); and insecure or disordered attachment (Hatzis et al., 2017). It is also clear that they are more likely to live in circumstances with severe economic problems/poverty (Moreland & McRae-Clark, 2018; Neger & Prinz, 2015; Niccols et al., 2012); poor housing or homelessness (Moreland & McRae-Clark, 2018; Neger & Prinz, 2015; Niccols et al., 2012); parental mental illness (Niccols et al., 2012); intimate partner and family violence; all potentially at a level that would be deemed abuse with subsequent engagement with the child protection system (Moreland & McRae-Clark, 2018; Niccols et al., 2012). Furthermore, as these children become adolescents, they are likely to go on to engage in risky behavior and substance use themselves (Neger & Prinz, 2015; Renk et al., 2016), with substance use by fathers as well as mothers significantly impacting their children's subsequent drug or alcohol use.

This chapter is focused on how the biological, ecological, and behavioral pathways from maternal substance use to poor child outcomes can be disrupted through effective support. Neger and Prinz (2015) summarized the evidence by conceptualizing five interacting and overlapping pathways of influence, namely deficits in parental emotional regulation; psychosocial factors; deficits in knowledge of parenting and child development; preoccupation with drug-seeking; and decreased pleasure in parenting. In light of these multiple "causal pathways" to child outcomes, we will identify the elements of effective support and challenges to provision of this support for substance impacted children and their mothers, partners, and families during pregnancy and after the baby comes home, with an emphasis on children's early years when they are most vulnerable (Renk et al., 2016). Pregnancy and early childhood can provide a unique "window of opportunity" to engage parents in interventions to improve outcomes for children impacted by substance use (Milligan et al., 2020).

We consider children "impacted by substance use" to not just be those with neonatal opioid withdrawal syndrome (NOWS), or other teratogenic effects from maternal fetal substance use, but rather all children who are at risk from exposure to patterns of parenting and social circumstances within their early life environment that results from their interactions with parents and/or significant others who are misusing substances. A focus solely on the mother can result in underestimating the impacts for children. For example, in a study of the risks impacting children enrolled in a sustained nurse home visiting program commencing in pregnancy and completing at child age 2 years, 10.6% of mothers disclosed they were using addictive substances, and 18.7% of the mothers disclosed that significant others in their lives (e.g., partner and/or other family) were using addictive substances (Kemp et al., 2022). All these people impact on the health and wellbeing of children.

11.2 Comprehensive Parenting Support

There have been many programs developed and much debate about the most effective way to improve outcomes for children impacted by substance use, including those with NOWS. Interventions vary from those aiming to reduce parental substance use and treating and managing associated risks such as mental illness or violence, to those targeting parenting behaviors and skills, to population and service system approaches, some supportive and some punitive (Barrett et al., 2023). Management or treatment of parental substance use can include psychosocial and/or pharmacological interventions. However, there is evidence that psychosocial interventions are not effective in reducing frequency of substance use in mothers, although psychoeducational interventions for fathers who use alcohol have been shown to have modest effects in reducing the level of drinking and substance use (Barrett et al., 2023).

Recently there has been increasing consensus about what is most likely to work to improve both parental and child outcomes, built around a strong body of evidence of what makes interventions effective for high-risk families more broadly, with consideration of the particular complexity experienced by parents of children impacted by substance use (Neger & Prinz, 2015; Parolin & Simonelli, 2016; West et al., 2020). This evidence shows that a bi-generational response is needed that integrates management or treatment of the parental substance use, harnesses the role of the infant/child in facilitating parents' motivation to change, and is combined with parenting support and provision of services to address the families' contexts, such as housing or financial support, mental health, or intimate partner violence. Such comprehensive approaches necessitate interprofessional collaboration.

Findings about the effectiveness of integrated parenting and substance use treatment programs are as mixed as the different program foci and content. Most show that parents who participate in comprehensive, integrated interventions that address parental substance use and provide parenting education and support generally have better parenting and child outcomes, as well as reductions in substance use, than programs that focus on either parenting or substance use alone (Herron & Isgro, 2014; McGovern et al., 2022; Moreland & McRae-Clark, 2018; Neo et al., 2021; Niccols et al., 2012). The variation in reported impacts related to the complexity of the families and whether the intervention and measures focused on parenting, substance use, child, or other outcomes such as parental mental health (Barrett et al., 2023; Moreland & McRae-Clark, 2018; Ward et al., 2022). For example, for parents impacted by substance use, intimate partner violence, and child maltreatment, integrated programs grounded in interdisciplinary collaboration and teamwork are essential as standard individual treatments often have approaches that are incompatible, such as child welfare interventions that are compliance-based, violence interventions that are based on empowerment, and parenting programs based on relational approaches. Bosk et al. (2022) suggest that when a mother is exposed to these competing approaches, each individual approach is likely to be ineffective, when compared to an integrated, comprehensive program with a clear singular approach. This clarity is also needed in understanding who the client is, as well as understanding the family as a unit, the mother, the father, and the children (Peacock-Chambers et al., 2022).

The general consensus is that comprehensive, integrated programs are likely to be more effective in both improving child and parenting outcomes and reducing substance use. As noted by Neger and Prinz (2015),

> Treating SA [substance abuse] without addressing parenting leaves parents with insufficient skills for handling child behaviour issues and makes them more vulnerable to drug relapse as a coping mechanism. Additionally, addressing parenting without addressing SA is likely futile as effective parenting requires a significant amount of emotional-regulation and intrinsic motivation, both of which are incompatible with drug and withdrawal state.
>
> (p. 74)

Despite the variations between integrated programs, there are common elements of comprehensive integrated programs that are more likely to be successful for both parents and children. These have been identified as programs that:

- start prenatally;
- focus on parenting skills, emotional regulation, and reflective functioning;
- are attachment-based and trauma-informed; and
- are salutogenic and strengths-based, focusing on the building blocks of positive childhood experiences.

Box 11.1 details the reflections of a clinician providing, and a mother engaging with, an integrated, comprehensive, and sustained intervention. The Maternal Early Childhood Sustained Home-visiting (MECSH) program (Kemp et al., 2017) was followed for this case. MECSH commences nurse home visiting prenatally, integrates parent skills education with psychological support for emotional regulation, and is aspirational and strengths-based (Goldfeld et al., 2018; Goldfeld et al., 2019; Kemp et al., 2011). In addition, to be maximally effective interventions should attend to the complex issues faced by families impacted by substance use and address the needs of fathers and other family members as well as mothers.

Box 11.1 Comprehensive integrated program element impacts (MECSH)

Clinician Reflection

Maddie* was initially assessed and recruited onto the MECSH programme during antenatal contact. After discussion about the level of commitment required from both the client and practitioner, Maddie decided that MECSH may be the right programme for her.

Maddie is an only child born and raised overseas until age 19 years, who explained her life experience as good until she made "bad choices" to include serious drug use and addiction to heroin. Maddie admitted to using drugs for more than 10 years but based on a desire to change her lifestyle and marrying her husband, enrolled onto the methadone programme when she found out she was pregnant.

At each contact, Maddie remains excited and committed to having in depth support in helping her to become a proactive, responsive and loving parent despite her past behaviours. To date, Maddie continues to engage well with her nurse home visitor and drug support adviser. She independently reduced her medication and has discussed with medical professionals her aspiration to be completely off methadone by the end of this year.

Maddie continues to keep her daughter at the heart of her daily activities and continues to engage in activities focusing on child communication and development and is growing in confidence daily, with regards to her parenting skills and potential.

Maddie's Reflection

So far, I have thoroughly enjoyed the MECSH programme and I believe it has been very beneficial to both my baby and I. Having the possibility to see my nurse home visitor regularly has helped me become a more confident parent to [my daughter], especially since my mum and the rest of my family live abroad. Her psychological support and practical advice have been outstanding.

Moreover, the handbook I was given as part of the programme has proven to be a very interesting read, providing a very useful insight on how to communicate with my daughter and what to expect from her in terms of physical and psychological development. During visits, I also get to focus on and discuss what my priorities and aspirations are both as a person and as a parent.

* pseudonym

11.2.1 Start Prenatally

The "window of opportunity" for intervention or support commences in pregnancy. Pregnancy is recognized as a critical period as expectant parents reassess their priorities and are commonly motivated to minimize harmful effects of drug use on and create the optimal environment for their child (Parolin & Simonelli, 2016; Peacock-Chambers et al., 2022). Attachment is now understood to begin in pregnancy, with women becoming increasingly focused on the baby as pregnancy progresses. However, for women who are using substances, pregnancy can be exceptionally stressful, including fear and guilt about the impact of the substance on the child, heightened socioeconomic stressors, social isolation, and risk for intimate partner violence (Flykt et al., 2021; Hyysalo et al., 2022). Further, the neurophysiological impacts of substance use can prove a challenge as the usual reward patterns experienced by pregnant women as they increasingly attach to and experience the excitement of pregnancy may be either not experienced, or neurologically affected (Cataldo et al.,

2019; Hyysalo et al., 2022). Pregnancy can also be a time when parents' own adverse childhood experiences (ACE) can be remembered and trigger trauma-related emotions and dysregulation (Flykt et al., 2021).

Intervention and support in pregnancy can provide an opportunity to maximize the motivation to cease or reduce substance use and support women to develop and access new reward systems and mechanisms for emotional regulation. Integrated prenatal services have been shown to improve fetal growth, reduce prematurity and birth complications, as well as improve care attendance (Flykt et al., 2021; Milligan et al., 2020). For Maddie, pregnancy motivated her to change her drug use behavior; however, the provision of MECSH (Kemp et al., 2017) was essential for supporting her ongoing engagement with parenting and drug treatment services. It is essential to also recognize that the stresses of pregnancy, such as the family isolation that Maddie was experiencing, can trigger craving and relapses (Rutherford et al., 2015), in the absence of support at this time. This should include actions to address issues causing stress such as poverty and associated risks such as homelessness. Often families with young children living in poverty in high-income countries are unaware of their financial entitlements and services that can assist with housing and debt management. Partnerships between health services accessed by nearly all pregnant women and income maximization services can improve access to financial resources and reduce stress (Burley et al., 2022).

11.2.2 Build Parenting Skills

Parents who have problematic substance use may have a number of difficulties in parenting due commonly (although not for Maddie) to exposure to adverse experiences in their own childhood and/or current adverse social environments and social networks (Milligan et al., 2020). These difficulties include limited understanding and expectations of their child's development; less sensitive, more passive, and disengaged interactions with infants; and an inability to identify what their children are/are not able to do. This lack of understanding regarding their children's development and capacities may cause parents to expect too much or misattribute their children's behavioral intentions and thus engage in inappropriate discipline (Milligan et al., 2020; Neger & Prinz, 2015; West et al., 2020).

Structured programs that build parenting skills, particularly focusing on reading children's cues and "serve and return" interactions (Komanchuk et al., 2023), where the parent is supported to build their knowledge of children's development and interpret and respond to their child's cues and behaviors in developmentally appropriate ways, are useful for parents impacted by substance use and associated complexities such as mental illness, intimate partner violence, and involvement with the child protection system. For example, structured sustained nurse home visiting programs that commence prenatally and focus on parent–infant/child interaction, supported by tools such as video feedback, are reported by parents to support positive child development outcomes (Kemp, Elcombe, et al., 2022). Such serve and return–based programs move beyond a cognitive or educational approach focused on "correction of maladaptive attitudes and the learning of behavioural parenting skills" (Parolin & Simonelli, 2016, p. 5) to address the key emotional elements of parent–child interactions (Renk et al., 2016), as the MECSH program (Kemp et al., 2017) is clearly doing for Maddie. This is particularly important for parents with substance use whose altered neural states and reward systems may negatively affect their ability to read and respond to their infant/child's emotional cues (Lowell et al., 2021).

11.2.3 Support Emotional Regulation, Reflective Functioning, and Parent–Child Attachment

The ability to respond to infants' and children's emotional cues requires parents to regulate their own emotions and reflect on their responses. Emotional regulation and difficulties in the interactions between substance-using mothers and their infants and children have been posited as two of the primary mechanisms by which substance use impacts parenting (Hyysalo et al., 2022; Milligan et al., 2020). The altered neural states of parents who use substances can limit emotional reflection on the parent's own internal states, and negatively impact their ability to attune to their infant/child's emotions or understand them appropriately, interpreting them as intrusive or even hostile, particularly in the context of infant crying and distress (Cataldo et al., 2019; Flykt et al., 2021; Parolin & Simonelli, 2016). These states and responses can subsequently result in insecure attachment in children, as the mothers experience less reward and increased stress in interactions with their infants and provide unpredictable, rejecting, or unresponsive care (Hyysalo et al., 2022; Parolin & Simonelli, 2016; Peacock-Chambers et al., 2022), which can be exacerbated by the high irritability in substance-exposed infants (depending on the substance and the age of fetal exposure) (Heimdahl & Karlsson, 2016).

Emotional regulation is particularly important for parents to manage the psychosocial and infant/child behavior stressors that may trigger maladaptive responses including drug use (Neger & Prinz, 2015). This may be particularly challenging as parents who use substances have often experienced trauma and poor attachment in their own childhood and may have other mental health problems (Hatzis et al., 2017; Hyysalo et al., 2022; Parolin & Simonelli, 2016). Building emotional regulation in parents impacted by substance use is best achieved by reflective interventions based in the concept of mentalization, that is, the ability to make sense of and organize their own and others' feelings and corresponding behaviors (Lowell et al., 2021; Renk et al., 2016). Comprehensive programs that first address parents' emotional regulation through learning emotional coping strategies prior to addressing parenting skills have beneficial outcomes for parents such as Maddie who valued the combination of "psychological support and practical advice" and "insight on how to communicate with [her] daughter" through understanding her child's emotional cues or signals and responding to their needs, building the emotional bond between parents and their children, and fostering positive attachment.

11.2.4 Trauma-Informed, Salutogenic, and Strengths-Based

As mentioned above, mothers with substance use disorders often have high rates of adverse experiences and trauma in their own childhood, and co-occurring mental health disorders that impact their emotional regulation and caregiving for their own children (Flykt et al., 2021; Hyysalo et al., 2022; West et al., 2020). When clinicians working with parents with a history of substance use provide trauma-informed care that recognizes the impact of unresolved childhood trauma, then care is less judgmental of parents as unmotivated or deficient, thus improving service engagement and parent self-efficacy, and reducing trauma symptoms (Bosk et al., 2022; Flykt et al., 2021).

A key strategy to use in trauma-informed care is engagement with parents with substance use issues using strategies that identify and build on their strengths. Such engagement should focus on salutogenic factors, that is, those that build health and wellbeing, rather than pathogenic factors, that is, those that cause deficits and problems (Antonovsky, 1987). Neurologically, chronic substance use can dampen the activity of the brain's reward centers and impact parents' capacity to derive pleasure from their parenting (Milligan et al., 2020; Neger & Prinz, 2015). Strength and health focusing can help parents to identify sources of pleasure in their life and parenting and be future-oriented and aspirational for themselves and their children. As expressed by Maddie, through the use of this salutogenic approach in the MECSH program (Kemp et al., 2017), she was able to "focus on and discuss what my priorities and aspirations are both as a person and as a parent." In this way, Maddie could both minimize any exposure of her child to adverse childhood experiences and provide the positive experiences essential for healthy child outcomes. Healthy outcomes from positive experiences (HOPE) in nurturing, supportive relationships, safe, protective, and equitable environments, social engagement and connectedness, and opportunities for social and emotional growth, can both prevent and mitigate the effects of adverse childhood experiences and environments (Sege & Harper Browne, 2017). There is clear and growing evidence that comprehensive and positively focused supports that start prenatally (ideally) to build parenting skills and support parent–child relationship development can be effective in reducing maternal substance use and improving mother and child outcomes. However, these families are also impacted by other adversities that need addressing.

11.3 Addressing the Contextual Ecology

The previous section outlined the components of effective substance use and parenting interventions that are essential for improving outcomes for parents and children. However, there is evidence that, for many parents impacted by substance use, this may still be insufficient to address the complex needs of this population (Hatzis et al., 2017; West et al., 2020). The following section discusses the importance of addressing parents' co-occurring needs and engaging with partners, family, and friends.

11.3.1 Addressing Co-Occurring Needs

It is not uncommon for parents impacted by substance use to have multiple issues and psychosocial stressors, often deriving from a history of trauma, that will impact their ability to engage with substance use and parenting interventions and achieve positive health outcomes for themselves and their children, including mental health issues, intimate partner violence (IPV), poverty, homelessness, and engagement with the child welfare system (Barrett et al., 2023; Cataldo et al., 2019; Heimdahl & Karlsson, 2016; Hyysalo et al., 2022; Milligan et al., 2020; Neger & Prinz, 2015; Peacock-Chambers et al., 2022). "Research suggests that when co-occurring needs remain either unacknowledged or unmet, clients are less likely to remain in treatment, follow treatment recommendations, and develop strong relationships with treatment providers" (Bosk et al., 2022, p. 3). Thus, substance use and parenting interventions should occur within a context of a comprehensive, interdisciplinary service response that addresses the broader life factors impacting these families, particularly financial hardship (Barrett et al., 2023; Burley et al., 2022; Heimdahl & Karlsson, 2016).

For women like Maddie, this means that whilst the MECSH nurse home visiting intervention focuses on supporting her to "parent effectively despite" the adversities in her life, an interdisciplinary response is required to concurrently address "the despites" (Kemp et al., 2016, p. 43). To be effective, responses must be complex, engaging diverse professionals and organizations, community supports, child welfare services, and others to meet the complex needs of children and families (Colvin et al., 2020).

Where interventions address multiple needs, connect families to community supports, and build parent capacity and skills, child and parent outcomes are improved (Barrett et al., 2023). This should include the engagement of the family and social systems that can be potentially helpful if engaged, or harmful if ignored (Salonen et al., 2023).

11.3.2 Engaging Partners, Family, and Friends

Most interventions for substance-using parents have focused on mothers and the mother–child dyad, ignoring the role of the partner, family, friends, and social networks (Barrett et al., 2023; Flykt et al., 2021; Salonen et al., 2023). Positive relationships and social and civic engagement are two of the key domains of positive experiences that can mitigate the impact of adversity (Sege & Harper Browne, 2017), and "Socially rewarding experiences and relationships are protective factors against drug-seeking behaviours" (Cataldo et al., 2019, p. 5), yet currently there is little evidence that interventions include these components. There is also evidence that in the context of mothers experiencing adversity, substance use by partners and other family members may be more prevalent than that of mothers in the perinatal period (Kemp, Bruce, et al., 2022), and the substance use of both parents and significant others in the family's life impacts on child outcomes (Salonen et al., 2023). Fathers, however, have been largely absent from the focus of interventions for parents (Heimdahl & Karlsson, 2016), or actively excluded as negative influences on their children (Bell et al., 2020), despite evidence that fathers would be open to interventions that would support their parenting role (Stover et al., 2018).

It has been suggested that interventions that include family members and significant others might be more successful, particularly in supporting parents to continue with positive parenting and reduced substance use following the completion of intervention programs (Neger & Prinz, 2015). Somewhat paradoxically, to date interventions that focus on the substance use of fathers have been more intensive than those provided to mothers, and shown positive impacts on reduction of alcohol and drug use in fathers but not mothers. This confirms the evidence that, for mothers, comprehensive integrated substance use and intensive parenting programs, such as sustained nurse home visiting commencing prenatally as described above, are required, combined with alcohol and drug use–targeted programs specifically tailored for fathers who are often excluded from settings designed for women and children (Cioffi & DeGarmo, 2021; McGovern et al., 2022; Salonen et al., 2023). Others are suggesting, however, that fatherhood can motivate a reduction of substance use in the same way as motherhood (as demonstrated by Maddie), and that men feel positively about comprehensive interventions and they, their partner, and children could benefit from comprehensive interventions that address substance use whilst also building parenting skills and improved family relationships (Bell et al., 2020; Cioffi & DeGarmo, 2021; Flykt et al., 2021). Comprehensive supports that address the context of the lives of mothers and children impacted by substance use, their partners, families, and friends are critical for effective outcomes.

11.4 Challenges

There is increasing evidence, presented above, on what works well to improve outcomes for parents and children impacted by substance use. However, significant challenges remain to be addressed in providing effective interventions, particularly around the identification and engagement of families in programs, and the capacity of the service system to respond to these families' complex needs. How to identify and respond to mothers and infants impacted by substance use and issues related to accessing services are discussed below.

11.4.1 Identifying and Responding to Impacted Mothers and Children

It has been estimated that about one in ten children worldwide live in households impacted by alcohol or other substance use and dependence (Penny & Pratt, 2011), and identification as early as possible to provide effective support is critical to achieving the best outcomes for the child. For infants experiencing neonatal opioid withdrawal syndrome (NOWS) that is clinically discernible, early identification is clear. However, many infants impacted by substance use in pregnancy (or afterwards) do not present with NOWS. The mother may have used substances early in pregnancy but have ceased in sufficient time prior to birth for the baby to not experience active withdrawal, or the child may be impacted by a substance (e.g., methamphetamine) that does not present with perinatal withdrawal.

For these infants and children, identification requires disclosure of substance use by the mother. Parents with substance use histories are reluctant to disclose their substance use for fear of losing their child to child welfare, criminal prosecution, and stigmatization (Flykt et al., 2021; Neger & Prinz, 2015). Disclosure requires three conditions:

- confidentiality: belief that the person to whom the disclosure is made will keep the information private;
- trust: a trusting relationship between the parent and person to whom they are disclosing; and
- action: the belief that the person to whom the disclosure is made has the willingness and capacity to enact change/improve the situation.

It is rare for women in the perinatal period to feel that professional services provide these three conditions (Parolin & Simonelli, 2016; Rollans et al., 2013). In a study of risk disclosure by women with psychosocial adversity (poverty, unemployment, poor educational level, isolation) who were enrolled in a sustained nurse home visiting program (Kemp, Bruce, et al., 2022), only one in five women who reported substance use disclosed this at commencement of the program (in the first or second visit), with most requiring on average 11 visits by the same nurse over a period of four to six months to feel safe to disclose (see Figure 11.1). In the absence of services such as sustained nurse home visiting that creates the conditions for disclosure, "evidence suggests that most adults who need substance use treatment do not receive it," nor perceive the need for treatment (West et al., 2020, p. 138).

There is also evidence that even when parents disclose substance use, services struggle to respond. Services have been shown to lack capacity, knowledge, and skills in engaging parents with substance use (Peacock-Chambers et al., 2022; Penny & Pratt, 2011). In our research (Kanda et al., 2022) we found nurses delivering a sustained home visiting program were significantly less likely to provide a service response in relation to a disclosure of substance use than, for example, a disclosure of mental health issues. Thus, it is recommended that specific training is needed to build nurses' skills in addressing substance use (Kanda et al., 2022).

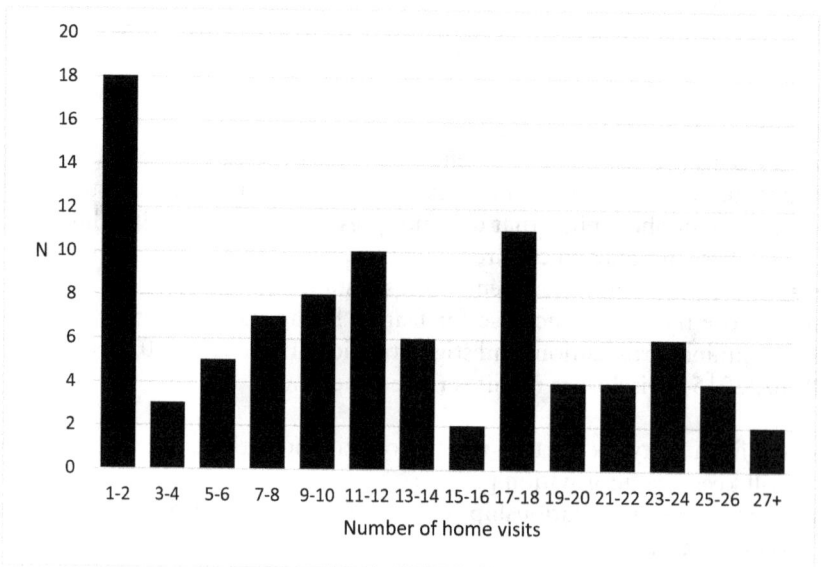

Figure 11.1 Number of home visits conducted at time of disclosure

11.4.2 Access and Engagement Issues

Once identified, parents face considerable issues in accessing and engaging with effective services and support, experiencing program, psychological, and practical barriers. Program barriers include the requirement for parents to attend multiple, uncoordinated appointments (Flykt et al., 2021; Milligan et al., 2020) in multiple locations (Milligan et al., 2020; Niccols et al., 2012). Parents have, often from experience, poor expectations of treatment efficacy (Parolin & Simonelli, 2016), particularly related to programs that are unresponsive to clients' needs (Peacock-Chambers et al., 2022) and have content that is seen by parents as lacking relevance (Moreland & McRae-Clark, 2018).

Psychologically, parents who have substance use issues are often prevented from seeking services and support due to feelings of stigma, guilt, and shame (Herron & Isgro, 2014; Lowell et al., 2021; Milligan et al., 2020; Neger & Prinz, 2015; Niccols et al., 2012; Ward et al., 2022). These feelings can be exacerbated by services that are perceived as judgmental, uncaring, and punitive (Flykt et al., 2021; Lowell et al., 2021; Neger & Prinz, 2015; Niccols et al., 2012). Fear of child welfare involvement and being separated from or losing custody of their children is also a major barrier (Herron & Isgro, 2014; Milligan et al., 2020; Niccols et al., 2012; Parolin & Simonelli, 2016; Ward et al., 2022).

Even when families are motivated to engage with services and supports, they can be prevented from engaging due to lack of transport (Herron & Isgro, 2014; Milligan et al., 2020; Neger & Prinz, 2015), lack of child care/child supervision (Bosk et al., 2022; Herron & Isgro, 2014; Milligan et al., 2020; Neger & Prinz, 2015), and poverty and/or unemployment preventing their ability to meet service costs (Herron & Isgro, 2014). These practical challenges, together with the issues in identifying mothers and children and responding appropriately to their needs, can negatively impact engagement and require addressing to support positive outcomes.

11.5 Addressing Challenges

Three key principles of service practice can support addressing the challenges of providing effective comprehensive programs for parents impacted by substance use. According to Bosk et al. (2022), these are engaging families where they are at, psychologically, contextually, and physically; working with parents in partnership, in relationship-based practice that builds trust through consistency and continuity of engagement; and providing adaptable, flexible, and relevant content.

There is mixed evidence about the relative effectiveness of inpatient and outpatient programs, and both can be used to deliver comprehensive substance use and parenting interventions. No matter the setting, the key to engagement is that the children remain with their parent/s and parenting support, practical support, parent–child attachment, and therapeutic care are included in the program (Flykt et al., 2021; Neger & Prinz, 2015; Parolin & Simonelli, 2016). Home-based programs, such as the home visiting program that Maddie received, have the added benefit of engaging families within the real-world context of their lives, providing opportunity to observe and address the other challenges and co-occurring needs in their lives, and positively engage partners, family, and friends for support.

To address challenges of parent concerns and experiences of stigma, judgmental and punitive responses, and their potential histories of trauma and adverse childhood experiences, services need to use relationship-based practices and consistent engagement that build trusting and secure relationships. This needs to commence with a warm, welcoming, and accepting environment that empowers parents and fosters regulation and reflective functioning (Bosk et al., 2022; Flykt et al., 2021; Health Resources and Services Administration, 2018; Parolin & Simonelli, 2016). The relationship built with one consistent service provider can facilitate retention with treatment and support, and warm handoffs, that is provider-facilitated connections to other needed services (Moreland & McRae-Clark, 2018).

Finally, programs that are adaptable, flexible, and tailored to address the broad range of families' needs are more likely to have good engagement and retention and achieve the desired outcomes (West et al., 2020). Clear clinical pathways aid in keeping families engaged with services (Penny & Pratt, 2011). Efforts to ensure that services are designed as described here would increase the likelihood that mothers and children impacted by substance use can access, engage with, and gain benefit from the support provided.

11.6 Discussion

Evidence about the effectiveness of support for mothers and children impacted by substance use has grown significantly in the past decade, with emerging clarity about the pathways to poorer outcomes and the elements of programs that can disrupt those pathways. What is now needed are clearer statements of and greater coherence in the theories of change of programs that identify the negative pathways that are being disrupted by the intervention for parents with children of what age impacted by which substance (Neger & Prinz, 2015). Neger and Prinz (2015) helpfully presented their model of pathways to poorer outcomes. Based on the evidence reviewed in this chapter, and the effective components identified, Figure 11.2 re-presents their model with the components of effective

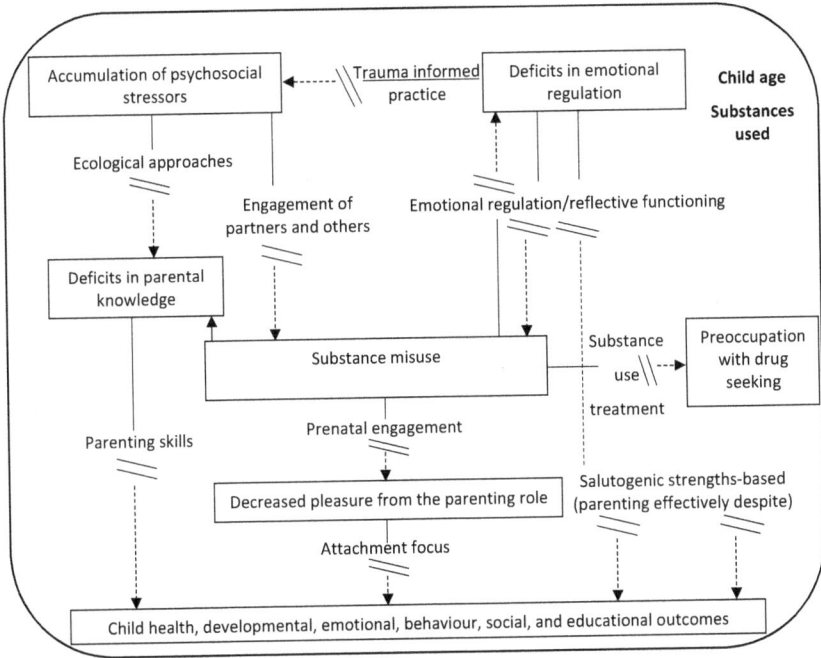

Figure 11.2 Effective interventions and supports to disrupt the pathways between parental substance use, parenting difficulties, and child outcomes, modelled on Neger and Prinz (2015)

interventions mapped onto the pathways they disrupt, within the broader contexts of the children's ages and the substances used.

The model in Figure 11.2 provides a mandate for comprehensive, inter-disciplinary, integrated programs of interventions that address multiple pathways, clearly indicating that interventions addressing single pathways are unlikely to be successful for mothers, parents, and families with children who are impacted by substance use. Parental skill building and substance use treatment provide a core of intervention activity to alter the two pathways of parent knowledge deficit and preoccupation with drug seeking. Support for emotional regulation and reflective functioning are key to mitigating the negative feedback loop between substance use and deficits in emotional regulation, whilst trauma-informed practice can help services to support families experiencing an accumulation of psycho-social stressors. Addressing these stressors requires program and system approaches that meet the broad ecology of needs of these families and engage fathers and significant others. Prenatal engagement can support parents to find their role pleasurable and rewarding; further enhanced by attachment-focused support both pre- and postnatally. Finally, salutogenic strengths-based approaches that support families to "parent effectively despite" provide immediate remedy where there is emotional dysregulation and ongoing drug seeking.

Addressing the challenges in current programs and service systems suggests this is best achieved by providing comprehensive parenting interventions such as sustained nurse home visiting (such as the MECSH (Kemp et al., 2017) program that Maddie received) that are relationship- and trust-based, with continuity of provider and strengths-based approaches, which are integrated within an interdisciplinary service system that connects families with the support needed for their broad range of needs, including substance use treatment, financial support, housing and child care, mitigating the "accumulation of psychosocial stressors" experienced by parents.

11.7 Summary

What has become clear in the evidence developed over the past decade is that comprehensive programs for parents that integrate substance use treatment with building parenting skills, emotional regulation, and reflective functioning, and are attachment- and trauma-informed and use salutogenic and strengths-based approaches, are most successful. Successful programs also need to address co-occurring needs and engage partners, family, and friends. Systems are required that have the capacity to identify impacted mothers, infants, and children; the ability to facilitate parents' access to and engagement with non-stigmatizing, non-judgmental support services; and a focus on achieving healthy outcomes from positive experiences (HOPE) for mothers and children impacted by substance use, including NOWS.

References

Antonovsky, A. (1987). *Unraveling The Mystery of Health – How People Manage Stress and Stay Well*. Jossey-Bass Publishers.

Barrett, S., Muir, C., Burns, S., Adjei, N., Forman, J., Hackett, S., Hirve, R., Kaner, E., Lynch, R., Taylor-Robinson, D., Wolfe, I., & McGovern, R. (2023). Interventions to reduce parental substance use, domestic violence and mental health problems, and their impacts upon children's well-being: A systematic review of reviews and evidence mapping. *Trauma, Violence, and Abuse*. https://doi.org/10.1177/15248380231153867

Bell, L., Herring, R., & Annand, F. (2020). Fathers and substance misuse: A literature review. *Drugs and Alcohol Today*, 20(4), 353–369. https://doi.org/10.1108/DAT-06-2020-0037

Bosk, E. A., Van Scoyoc, A., Mihalec-Adkins, B., Conrad, A., Hanson, K., & Chaiyachati, B. H. (2022). Integrating responses to caregiver substance misuse, intimate partner violence and child maltreatment: Initiatives and policies that support families at risk for entering the child welfare system. *Aggression and Violent Behavior, 65*, https://doi.org/10.1016/j.avb.2021.101637

Burley, J., Samir, N., Price, A., Parker, A., Zhu, A., Eapen, V., Contreras-Suarez, D., Schreurs, N., Lawson, K., Lingam, R., Grace, R., Raman, S., Kemp, L., Bishop, R., Goldfeld, S., & Woolfenden, S. (2022). Connecting healthcare with income maximisation services: A systematic review on the health, wellbeing and financial impacts for families with young children. *International Journal of Environmental Research and Public Health, 19*(11), https://doi.org/10.3390/ije rph19116425

Cataldo, I., Azhari, A., Coppola, A., Bornstein, M. H., & Esposito, G. (2019). The influences of drug abuse on mother-infant interaction through the lens of the biopsychosocial model of health and illness: A review. *Frontiers in Public Health, 7*(45). https://doi.org/10.3389/fpubh.2019.00045

Cioffi, C. C., & DeGarmo, D. S. (2021). Improving parenting practices among fathers who misuse opioids: Fathering through change intervention. *Frontiers in Psychology, 12*, https://doi.org/10.3389/fpsyg.2021.683008

Colvin, M. L., Thompson, H. M., & Cooley, M. E. (2020). The "cost" of collaborating and other challenges in inter-organizational child welfare practice: A community-wide perspective. *Journal of Public Child Welfare, 15*(5), 617–651. https://doi.org/10.1080/15548732.2020.1778597

Flykt, M. S., Salo, S., & Pajulo, M. (2021). "A window of opportunity": Parenting and addiction in the context of pregnancy. *Current Addiction Reports, 8*(4), 578–594. https://doi.org/10.1007/s40429-021-00394-4

Goldfeld, S., Price, A., & Kemp, L. (2018). Designing, testing, and implementing a sustainable nurse home visiting program: Right@home. *Annals of the New York Academy of Sciences, 1419*(1), 141–159. https://doi.org/10.1111/nyas.13688

Goldfeld, S., Price, A., Smith, C., Bruce, T., Bryson, H., Mensah, F., Orsini, F., Gold, L., Hiscock, H., Bishop, L., Smith, A., Perlen, S., & Kemp, L. (2019). Nurse home visiting for families experiencing adversity: A randomized trial. *Pediatrics, 143*(1). https://doi.org/10.1542/peds.2018-1206

Hatzis, D., Dawe, S., Harnett, P., & Barlow, J. (2017). Quality of caregiving in mothers with illicit substance use: A systematic review and meta-analysis. *Substance Abuse: Research and Treatment, 11*. https://doi.org/10.1177/11782 21817694038

Health Resources and Services Administration. (2018). *HRSA's home visiting program: Supporting families impacted by opioid use and neonatal abstinence syndrome.* U.S. Department of Health and Human Services. https://mchb.hrsa. gov/sites/default/files/mchb/programs-impact/miechv-opioid-nas-resource.pdf

Heimdahl, K., & Karlsson, P. (2016). Psychosocial interventions for substance-abusing parents and their young children: A scoping review. *Addiction Research and Theory, 24*(3), 236–247. https://doi.org/10.3109/16066359.2015.1118064

Herron, A. J., & Isgro, M. (2014). Substance use disorders and motherhood. In N. Benders-Hadi & M. E. Barber (Eds.), *Motherhood, mental illness and recovery* (pp. 73–87). Springer International Publishing. https://doi.org/10.1007/ 978-3-319-01318-3_6

Hyysalo, N., Gastelle, M., & Flykt, M. (2022). Maternal pre- and postnatal substance use and attachment in young children: A systematic review and meta-analysis. *Development and Psychopathology*, *34*(4), 1231–1248. https://doi. org/10.1017/S0954579421000134

Joseph, R., Brady, E., Hudson, M. E., & Moran, M. M. (2020). Perinatal substance exposure and long-term outcomes in children: A literature review. *Pediatric Nursing*, *46*(4), 163–173. https://www.scopus.com/inward/record. uri?eid=2-s2.0-85098597415&partnerID=40&md5=f9554e076649df4c1118c 6284acbb541

Kanda, K., Blythe, S., Grace, R., Elcombe, E., & Kemp, L. (2022). Variations in sustained home visiting care for mothers and children experiencing adversity. *Public Health Nursing*, *39*(1), 71–81. https://doi.org/10.1111/phn.13014

Kemp, L., Bruce, T., & Byrne, F. (2016). Parenting effectively despite: The Maternal Early Childhood Sustained Home-visiting program. *Australian Nursing & Midwifery Journal*, *24*(2), 43. https://www.scopus.com/inward/record.uri?eid= 2-s2.0-85040644152&partnerID=40&md5=f40c3d61097eca25ef29b60c9 368f8de

Kemp, L., Bruce, T., Elcombe, E. L., Byrne, F., Scharkie, S. A., Perlen, S. M., & Goldfeld, S. R. (2022). Identification of families in need of support: Correlates of adverse childhood experiences in the right@home sustained nurse home visiting program. *PLoS ONE*, *17*(10). https://doi.org/10.1371/journal.pone.0275423

Kemp, L., Cowley, S., & Byrne, F. (2017). Maternal Early Childhood Sustained Home-visiting (MECSH): A UK update. *Journal of Health Visiting*, *5*(8), 392–397. https://doi.org/10.12968/johv.2017.5.8.392

Kemp, L., Elcombe, E., Sumpton, W., Hook, B., Cowley, S., & Byrne, F. (2022). Evaluation of the impact of the MECSH programme in England: A mixed methods study. *Journal of Health Visiting*, *10*(5), 200–215. https://doi.org/ 10.12968/johv.2022.10.5.200

Kemp, L., Harris, E., McMahon, C., Matthey, S., Impani, G. V., Anderson, T., Schmied, V., Aslam, H., & Zapart, S. (2011). Child and family outcomes of a long-term nurse home visitation programme: A randomised controlled trial. *Archives of Disease in Childhood*, *96*(6), 533–540. https://doi.org/10.1136/ adc.2010.196279

Komanchuk, J., Letourneau, N., Duffett-Leger, L., & Cameron, J. L. (2023). History of "Serve and Return" and a synthesis of the literature on its impacts on children's health and development. *Issues in Mental Health Nursing*, *44*(5), 406–417. https://doi.org/10.1080/01612840.2023.2192794

Lowell, A. F., Peacock-Chambers, E., Zayde, A., DeCoste, C. L., McMahon, T. J., & Suchman, N. E. (2021). Mothering from the inside out: Addressing the intersection of addiction, adversity, and attachment with evidence-based parenting intervention. *Current Addiction Reports*, *8*(4), 605–615. https://doi. org/10.1007/s40429-021-00389-1

McGovern, R., Bogowicz, P., Meader, N., Kaner, E., Alderson, H., Craig, D., Geijer-Simpson, E., Jackson, K., Muir, C., Salonen, D., Smart, D., & Newham,

J. J. (2023). The association between maternal and paternal substance use and child substance use, internalizing and externalizing problems: A systematic review and meta-analysis. *Addiction, 118*(5), 804–818. https://doi.org/10.1111/add.16127

McGovern, R., Newham, J., Addison, M., Hickman, M., & Kaner, E. (2022). The effectiveness of psychosocial interventions at reducing the frequency of alcohol and drug use in parents: Findings of a Cochrane Review and meta-analyses. *Addiction, 117*(10), 2571–2582. https://doi.org/10.1111/add.15846

Milligan, K., Meixner, T., Tremblay, M., Tarasoff, L. A., Usher, A., Smith, A., Niccols, A., & Urbanoski, K. A. (2020). Parenting interventions for mothers with problematic substance use: A systematic review of research and community practice. *Child Maltreatment, 25*(3), 247–262. https://doi.org/10.1177/1077559519873047

Moreland, A. D., & McRae-Clark, A. (2018). Parenting outcomes of parenting interventions in integrated substance-use treatment programs: A systematic review. *Journal of Substance Abuse Treatment, 89*, 52–59. https://doi.org/10.1016/j.jsat.2018.03.005

Neger, E. N., & Prinz, R. J. (2015). Interventions to address parenting and parental substance abuse: Conceptual and methodological considerations. *Clinical Psychology Review, 39*, 71–82. https://doi.org/10.1016/j.cpr.2015.04.004

Neo, S. H. F., Norton, S., Kavallari, D., & Canfield, M. (2021). Integrated treatment programmes for mothers with substance use problems: A systematic review and meta-analysis of interventions to prevent out-of-home child placements. *Journal of Child and Family Studies, 30*(11), 2877–2889. https://doi.org/10.1007/s10826-021-02099-8

Niccols, A., Milligan, K., Sword, W., Thabane, L., Henderson, J., & Smith, A. (2012). Integrated programs for mothers with substance abuse issues: A systematic review of studies reporting on parenting outcomes. *Harm Reduction Journal, 9*(14). https://doi.org/10.1186/1477-7517-9-14

Parolin, M., & Simonelli, A. (2016). Attachment theory and maternal drug addiction: The contribution to parenting interventions. *Frontiers in Psychiatry, 7*(152). https://doi.org/10.3389/fpsyt.2016.00152

Peacock-Chambers, E., Buckley, D., Lowell, A., Clark, M. C., Friedmann, P. D., Byatt, N., & Feinberg, E. (2022). Relationship-based home visiting services for families affected by substance use disorders: A qualitative study. *Journal of Child and Family Studies, 31*(8), 2121–2133. https://doi.org/10.1007/s10826-022-02313-1

Penny, R., & Pratt, J. (2011). The trial and evaluation of a clinical pathway for parents with substance use issues. *Neonatal, Paediatric and Child Health Nursing, 14*(3), 14–20. http://www.scopus.com/inward/record.url?eid=2-s2.0-84870866879&partnerID=40&md5=a57f9092be69ce26062b525d0392f5c2

Renk, K., Boris, N. W., Kolomeyer, E., Lowell, A., Puff, J., Cunningham, A., Khan, M., & McSwiggan, M. (2016). The state of evidence-based parenting interventions for parents who are substance-involved. *Pediatric Research, 79*(1–2), 177–183. https://doi.org/10.1038/pr.2015.201

Rollans, M., Schmied, V., Kemp, L., & Meade, T. (2013). Digging over that old ground: An Australian perspective of women's experience of psychosocial assessment and depression screening in pregnancy and following birth. *BMC Women's Health*, *13*(1). https://doi.org/10.1186/1472-6874-13-18

Rutherford, H. J. V., Gerig, G., Gouttard, S., Potenza, M. N., & Mayes, L. C. (2015). Investigating maternal brain structure and its relationship to substance use and motivational systems. *Yale Journal of Biology and Medicine*, *88*(3), 211–217. https://www.scopus.com/inward/record.uri?eid=2-s2.0-84940764 619&partnerID=40&md5=853c196eca5aaa214743737ecef4c91c

Salonen, D., McGovern, R., Sobo-Allen, L., Adams, E., Muir, C., Bourne, J., Herlihy, J., Tasker, F., Hunter, D., & Kaner, E. (2023). Being and becoming a father in the context of heavy drinking and other substance use – a qualitative evidence synthesis. *Drugs: Education, Prevention and Policy*. https://doi.org/10.1080/09687637.2023.2167650

Sege, R. D., & Harper Browne, C. (2017). Responding to ACEs with HOPE: Health Outcomes from Positive Experiences. *Academic Pediatrics*, *17*(7), 79–85. https://doi.org/10.1016/j.acap.2017.03.007

Stover, C. S., Carlson, M., Patel, S., & Manalich, R. (2018). Where's dad? The importance of integrating fatherhood and parenting programming into substance use treatment for men. *Child Abuse Review*, *27*(4), 280–300. https://doi.org/10.1002/car.2528

Ward, B., Moller, C., Maybery, D., Weimand, B., Krause, M., Dietze, P., Harvey, P., Kippen, R., McCormick, F., Lloyd-Jones, M., & Reupert, A. (2022). Interventions to support parents who use methamphetamine: A narrative systematic review. *Children and Youth Services Review*, *139*. https://doi.org/10.1016/j.childyouth.2022.106525

West, A. L., Dauber, S., Gagliardi, L., Correll, L., Lilli, A. C., & Daniels, J. (2020). Systematic review of community- and home-based interventions to support parenting and reduce risk of child maltreatment among families with substance-exposed newborns. *Child Maltreatment*, *25*(2), 137–151. https://doi.org/10.1177/1077559519866272

12 Support Foster/Kinship and Adoptive Parents of Children With a History of Prenatal Substance Exposure

Stacy Blythe and Lynn Kemp

12.1 Introduction

Neonatal opioid withdrawal syndrome (NOWS), sometimes also referred to as neonatal abstinence syndrome (NAS), is but one outcome associated with maternal drug use during pregnancy. Parental substance use is a common factor in child welfare cases as it increases children's risk for neglect and maltreatment (Kepple, 2018; Turney & Goodsell, 2018). Recent data from the United States indicates that child maltreatment cases associated with parental substance abuse are increasing (Boyd, 2019). In this context, when intervention and support are ineffective, or untenable (or unavailable), children may be placed into out-of-home care (OOHC). Unfortunately, child removal from parental care due to parental substance use is on the rise (Meinhofer & Angleró-Díaz, 2019), and it has been suggested that parental substance use is a contributing factor for as many as 80% of the children living in out-of-home care (McGlade et al., 2009). In some jurisdictions, maternal substance use during pregnancy can even result in unborn child reports (Wise & Corrales, 2023), and in some cases may result in maternal criminal charges (Faherty et al., 2019). Unsurprisingly, maternal substance use during pregnancy is one of the most common reasons for infant removal (Boyd, 2019; Sieger & Becker, 2020). Consequently, infants, children, and young people with a history of prenatal substance exposure (PSE) are over-represented in OOHC (Marcellus & Badry, 2023; Sieger & Becker, 2020). The purpose of this chapter is to provide health care professionals with some understanding of the OOHC context and how to best support the individuals caring for infants with NOWS and children with a history of PSE.

OOHC provides an alternate living arrangement to children who are unable to live safely with their parents. Most children in OOHC reside in home-based care with a foster or kinship carer (Luke & Sebba, 2013).

DOI: 10.4324/9781003397267-12

These carers undergo a training, assessment, and screening process prior to being authorized to provide care. Typically, kinship carers have a pre-existing relationship with the children (e.g., relative or close family friend), whereas foster carers are strangers to the children prior to their placement into care. These carers assume the day-to-day responsibility of providing a safe, stable, family-like environment within their own home, on a short- or long-term basis, but are not considered the legal guardians of the children placed into their care (Blythe et al., 2014). Although there is variability between countries and jurisdictions, generally, the legal parental responsibility for children in OOHC remains with the relevant judicial and government authorities, or their delegates (e.g., foster care agencies) (Gribble et al., 2022).

With increasing numbers of children requiring care on a long-term basis, more and more children are being adopted from OOHC. This is particularly true in the United States where federal incentives have long been in place to encourage adoption and ease the financial burden on the OOHC system (Hansen, 2007; Zill, 2011). Increasingly, adoption is being viewed as the preferred avenue to securing permanency for children requiring long-term care (Gribble et al., 2022; Skivenes & Benbenishty, 2023). Parallel to this, more and more pregnant women are using harmful and addictive substances, resulting in increasing numbers of infants being placed with adoption agents. There is emergent evidence that children removed from home due to parental substance use are more likely to achieve permanency through adoption rather than reunification with their families (Akin et al., 2015). This particularly applies to infants and young children (<3 years) (Boyd, 2019; Lloyd et al., 2017).

Box 12.1 presents a case study of the typical trajectory of prenatal and hospital experience of children with PSE whose pathway is into OOHC. Given the increasing numbers of children with a history of PSE being adopted and/or requiring foster or kinship care there is a need to understand how best to engage with these parents and carers to achieve optimal outcomes for the children in their care.

Box 12.1 Case study Emily, part one

Emily's mother (21 years) struggled with addiction throughout her teenage years. At 16 years she moved in with her boyfriend when her parents asked her to leave the family home. At 17 years she became pregnant but miscarried. At 19, she gave birth to a little girl who was removed from her care at six weeks of age due to her substance use issues, which were reported to child welfare services by health care professionals during the prenatal period. As a result, when she became pregnant with Emily, she did not seek prenatal care.

Emily was born prematurely (34 weeks) at a public hospital. Health professionals immediately informed child welfare services as her mother was deemed to be "under the influence" when she presented to the hospital. Upon investigation, child welfare determined it was unsafe for Emily to remain in her mother's care. Subsequently, Emily's mother was restricted to three, one-hour, supervised visits a week with Emily. Hospital security was called when she attempted the first visit, as her behavior was deemed "aggressive" towards staff. After that, she did not attempt another visit. Emily's father was unknown and did not visit her in the hospital.

Emily remained in the hospital for three weeks receiving treatment for withdrawal. When discharged, a caseworker collected her from the hospital and delivered her to the home of Imran (56 years), a full-time motor mechanic, and his wife Jodie (53 years), a part-time teaching assistant. Imran and Jodie were "empty nesters" now that both their adult sons (26 and 29) had moved out of their home. Having recently completed their foster care training, Emily was the first child placed into their care.

Emily arrived with only the clothes on her back, one blanket and a can of formula. Imran and Jodie were told she had experienced withdrawal, but that had resolved, and she was now healthy.

12.2   Special Considerations for Children in Out-of-Home Care

Infants, children, and young people with a history of PSE have increased caregiving needs. However, these needs are compounded for those who are adopted or reside in out-of-home care. Many infants experience withdrawal that requires specialist medical and pharmacological treatment for symptom management necessitating an extended hospital stay. As a result, these infants are predisposed to poor attachment and significant developmental delays. Consequently, these infants, children, and young people have increased caregiving needs that required targeted interventions. Moreover, many parents and carers report being unaware of children's PSE and its potential impact on the child. As a result, many parents and carers are unprepared for the multiple, sometimes persistent, challenges children experience due to their PSE. A select number of these challenges are discussed below.

12.2.1 Withdrawal

While not all infants with PSE experience withdrawal, those exposed to opioids are more likely to withdraw (Liu et al., 2010; Ruwanpathirana et al., 2015) and experience NOWS. Many of these infants require specialized medical care and management during withdrawal (Whalen et al., 2019). This often necessitates additional time in the hospital's Neonatal Intensive or Special Care Units for pharmacological treatment and monitoring. In this context, nurses assess infants' withdrawal symptoms and titrate their pharmacological treatment according to a pre-set protocol under the supervision of a neonatologist. As infants' symptoms ease, their medication is reduced. The period of time infants remain in the hospital is influenced by a number of factors, including the severity of withdrawal symptoms, the type and amount of substance exposure, and the medical management provided. The discharge destination, whether into parental or foster care, may also influence the length of hospital stay. A recent cross-sectional study of 1,377 infants diagnosed with NOWS at 30 hospitals found infants' length of stay varied from 2–49 days, with approximately a quarter of the infants being discharged into foster or kinship care (Young et al., 2021). Furthermore, a study by Johnson (2014) found substance-exposed infants discharged into OOHC spent, on average, nearly eight days longer in the hospital compared to substance-exposed infants discharged into parental care (17.5 vs. 9.6 days). This resonates with the work of Blythe et al. (2022) who report that some infants remain in the hospital while child welfare services identify appropriate carers to receive the infant at discharge. Emily's story is typical of the extended length of hospitalization and subsequent placement directly into OOHC once "healthy" and a suitable placement has been found. Her story is also characteristic of the limited amount of information and level of preparation commonly provided for carers with whom these children are placed. For example, in a recent study of 232 foster and kinship carers, 52 indicated the infant in their care had been prenatally exposed to substances. However, only 14 of these carers reported receiving information about the care of an infant who had experienced prenatal substance exposure (Blythe et al., 2022).

More recently, home-based pharmacotherapy has been implemented to decrease an infant's length of hospital stay and associated costs (Whalen et al., 2019). This requires parents and carers to be trained to assess, score, and manage infant withdrawal symptoms and administer medication (Johnson, 2014). Home-based pharmacotherapy is proving effective in shortening the length of infant hospital stays; however, research indicates these infants require significantly longer periods of treatment compared to those pharmacologically managed in the hospital (Murphy-Oikonen &

McQueen, 2019). This may, however, be particularly difficult to manage for infants in OOHC who have frequent visits with their parents. The time away from the carer, which could also include significant travel time (Humphreys & Kiraly, 2011), confounds carers' ability to appropriately assess and manage infants' withdrawal symptoms. This could result in the infant receiving an inaccurate dose of medication, thereby causing the infant undue distress (too little) or extending the period of pharmacological management (too much). The implications of home-based pharmacotherapy over this extended period are not yet known.

Nonpharmacological treatment of withdrawal symptoms for infants with NOWS is common practice (Patrick et al., 2020; Whalen et al., 2019). In a recent review of the literature, Ryan et al. (2017) found commonly implemented nonpharmacological interventions to encompass five categories. These include environmental control, feeding methods, social integration, soothing techniques, and therapeutic modalities. However, there is a lack of rigorous research supporting the effectiveness of many of these interventions (Pahl et al., 2020; Ryan et al., 2017). For example, the reduction of noxious stimuli is thought to reduce infant arousal, but there are no studies which have demonstrated this to be the case. Swaddling has been found to decrease arousal and prolong sleep in infants (van Sleuwen et al., 2007). While this practice is widely used, there is no research demonstrating its effectiveness for infants with NOWS. Similarly, the use of pacifiers, infant positioning, and music therapy lack a robust evidence base (Ryan et al., 2017), but are commonly used for infants with NOWS.

There is consistent evidence that rooming-in (MacMillan et al., 2018), skin-to-skin contact (Grossman et al., 2017), and breastfeeding (Wu & Carre, 2018) reduce infants' need for pharmacologic treatment and their length of hospital stay. A retrospective study by Howard et al. (2017) found parental presence at the infant's bedside was also associated with less medication and a shorter hospital stay. Unfortunately, infants who have been removed from maternal care to be placed into OOHC do not generally have access to these effective, nonpharmacological interventions as they often have no primary caregiver during their hospitalization (Shannon et al., 2021; Whalen et al., 2019). This increases their likelihood of requiring pharmacological treatment, longer lengths of hospitalization, and poor attachment.

12.2.2 Attachment

Attachment in early infancy is crucial for healthy child development and lays the foundation for emotional, social, and cognitive wellbeing throughout life (Zeanah, Berlin, et al., 2011). Healthy attachment is a strong bond between the infant and their primary caregiver (most often their mother) that provides the infant with a sense of security, comfort, and trust that the caregiver is available, capable, and responsive to their needs. Healthy attachment positively impacts brain development. Infancy and early childhood are critical periods when the brain is rapidly developing. Responsive caregiving and nurturing interactions during this time support the development of neural pathways involved in emotional regulation, stress response, and social skills. Poor attachment in infancy negatively impacts the infant's mental health and neurologic development (Zeanah, Berlin, et al., 2011).

Infant mental health refers to the developing capacity of an infant to experience, express, and regulate emotions; form close and secure relationships; explore their environment; and learn (Osofsky & Thomas, 2012). Infants residing in OOHC are predisposed to poor mental health due to their initial placement into care and subsequent frequent disruptions to care to facilitate visits with their birth families (Zeanah, Berlin, et al., 2011; Zeanah, Schauffer, et al., 2011). Generally, infants in OOHC have frequent visits with their parents (Zeanah, Schauffer, et al., 2011) as it is often considered, somewhat controversially, an important factor for successful family reunification (Humphreys & Kiraly, 2011; Sen & Broadhurst, 2011). This practice may result in inconsistent caregiving as the infant is retrieved from the carer by a transport worker who delivers the infant to the care of the parents who are supervised by a professional for a specified period of time. The infant is then retrieved by a transport worker (not necessarily the same one) and subsequently returned to the carer. While these visits are often viewed as essential to family reunification, they also disrupt the infant's ability to form healthy attachments with their primary caregivers. Poorly attached infants experience difficulties in regulating their emotions. They may have heightened levels of distress, display excessive crying or fussiness, and struggle to self-soothe. They may also experience cognitive and developmental delays and are at an increased risk of developing behavioral problems, poor executive function, and mental health issues such as anxiety and depression (Cassidy & Shaver, 2002). These difficulties and delays require increased caregiving.

Infant hospitalization in the first few days of life is also known to disrupt attachment between the infant and primary caregiver (Fegran et al., 2008). As such, infants who have experienced PSE have an increased risk of developing poor attachment due to hospitalization for treatment of withdrawal symptoms. This is especially relevant for infants discharged to OOHC, given their length of hospital stay is often longer (Johnson, 2014). Moreover, as portrayed in Emily's case study (see Box 12.1), research has shown that when an infant who experienced PSE is removed from parental care after birth, there is often no alternate primary caregiver provided for the infant until they are discharged from the hospital (Blythe et al.,

2022; Shannon et al., 2021). Consequently, the absence of a primary caregiver during this period of hospitalization in early infancy significantly compromises the infant's ability to form healthy attachments.

There is much evidence that disruptions to attachment in infants, as well as the teratogenic and epigenetic impacts of PSE, can have long-term negative impacts on children's physical, cognitive, emotional, and behavioral development (Joseph et al., 2020). Box 12.2 follows Emily's story to five years of age, demonstrating an all-too-common pattern of delay, disadvantage, and lack of early intervention for children in OOHC.

Box 12.2 Case study Emily, part two

Following a lengthy series of legal proceedings, it was determined that Emily (now 2 ½ years old) would not be returned to the care of her mother. Imran and Jodie agreed to care for Emily on a long-term basis, as they had become quite fond of her, and were also considering adoption.

Around the time Emily turned 3, she began to exhibit aggressive and troubling behaviors both at home and at preschool. She had severe temper tantrums and seemed inconsolable when she didn't get her way. Not having experienced this with their sons, Imran and Jodie felt quite embarrassed and overwhelmed by Emily's behavior, particularly in public. This caused Imran and Jodie to spend more time at home, and less time pursuing hobbies or socializing with family and friends.

During this time, it became apparent that Emily's speech was not developing in a typical fashion, and she was experiencing visual difficulties (nystagmus). Specialist services were sought, but reliance on the public health system meant there were lengthy waiting periods.

When she was five, Emily's kindergarten teacher contacted Imran and Jodie to voice concerns regarding Emily's short attention span and inability to follow simple instructions. The teacher also noted that Emily was easily upset and difficult to console. She suggested Emily may need further specialist intervention if she was to remain in the classroom.

Imran and Jodie did not understand why Emily was having so many issues. Emily's case worker did not seem to have any insights either. Now in their late 50s and early 60s, Imran and Jodie felt exhausted by the multiple medical appointments and weary from Emily's poor emotion regulation and aggressive behavior. Due to her increased caregiving needs, they began to question whether they were the right carers for Emily.

12.2.3 Developmental Delays

Research suggests many children with a history of PSE are at an increased risk for developmental and cognitive delays (Fucile et al., 2021; Maguire et al., 2016). Often these difficulties are compounded for children residing in OOHC, as they are undetected and/or remain untreated (Jee et al., 2010). This may be due to several factors, including focus on child safety, placement, and prioritization of legal proceedings. Heavy caseloads and high case-worker turnover may also result in poor monitoring of children's health and developmental status. Long waiting lists for services and/or multiple foster/kinship placements in different geographical locations may lead to missed medical appointments. Moreover, Blythe et al. (2022) report that children's history of PSE is often minimized or not communicated to carers, particularly if the children are older at the time of placement into OOHC. This may be due to children not being formally diagnosed with NAS (or NOWS) after birth or because there is no enduring diagnosis once withdrawal has resolved (Oei et al., 2023). Irrespective of the reason, omitting this information disadvantages the child and may even put the placement at risk as the carers are unprepared for children's increased caregiving needs, as can be seen in Emily's case study (see Box 12.2).

It has long been acknowledged that early intervention is the most effective way to support healthy child and family development (Guralnick, 2011). During hospitalization, infants often receive or are referred for a range of early intervention services, provided by occupational and physical therapists, speech-language pathologists, pediatric nurses, and social workers, among others. However, research suggests that infants with NAS who are placed into foster care are less likely to be referred or enrolled into early intervention services after discharged from the hospital (Peacock-Chambers et al., 2019). The reason for this is unclear, but potentially it may be due to poor communication between the hospital, child welfare services, and the foster carer. Children in care may also move multiple times to different locations and carers, further complicating the referral process or access to services. However, without early intervention and ongoing support, children are less likely to achieve optimal outcomes.

Nurse home-visiting programs, a key publicly funded child and family health, development, and wellbeing strategy, which is focused on prevention, early intervention, and connection to indirect support and the broader resource system (e.g., playgroups, parent groups, etc.), are an example of early intervention and have the potential to improve child outcomes, but are not consistently available to foster carers (Blythe et al., 2022). These nurses work with infants and young children (<5 years) and their parents to promote and monitor children's healthy development and wellbeing while providing parental support and referral where necessary

(Rossiter et al., 2017; Schmied et al., 2014). This includes activities that facilitate attachment as well as increase parental sensitivity and responsiveness, creating a home environment conducive to healthy development. To date, however, this core model of support for families has been predominantly limited to birthing mothers with access ceasing when children are moved into alternative care arrangements. Such support was not available to Imran and Jodie. Consequently, infants and young children like Emily in OOHC and adoptive families often miss out on the essential support for improved child and family outcomes that can be provided by home-visiting nurses (Blythe et al., 2021; Blythe et al., 2022; Schmied et al., 2018).

12.3 Foster/Kinship and Adoptive Parents' Needs

Foster/kinship and adoptive parents are a marginalized group, representative of deviant parenting discourses (Goodwin & Huppatz, 2010). Despite increasing acceptance of, and advocacy for, diverse family constructs (e.g., single-parent families, same-sex parents, etc.), foster/kinship and adoptive families continue to challenge societal stereotypes and expectations. Inaccurate and sensationalized media portrayals (Lonne & Parton, 2014) perpetuate misconceptions regarding the motivation of these parents and carers and the legitimacy of the families they form. As a result, many experience stigma and marginalization and have poor access to education and practical support.

12.3.1 Reducing Stigma and Marginalization

There is an increasing body of evidence that suggests foster and kinship carers are poorly supported in their caregiving role (Blythe et al., 2014; Harding et al., 2020), feel misunderstood (Blythe, Halcomb, et al., 2012), and experience stigma (Blythe, Jackson, et al., 2012). For Imran and Jodie, their concerns and embarrassment over Emily's behavior marginalized and isolated them. It is therefore not surprising that recruitment and retention of carers is a persistent issue (Gouveia et al., 2021). This is most concerning as research has demonstrated foster and kinship carers to be a key determinant in children's long-term outcomes (Li et al., 2019).

As the day-to-day care providers, foster carers have a key role in facilitating health care for the children in their care. However, research consistently demonstrates that stigmatized populations are less likely to access health care services (Amon et al., 2022). One important issue with stigmatization is that the individuals being stigmatized are often looked at as though they have brought it on themselves (Halter, 2008). This may be one factor contributing to carers' difficulty accessing health care services for the children in their care (McLean et al., 2020; York & Jones,

2017). Becoming a foster or kinship carer is a conscious choice, most often based on altruistic motivations (Sebba, 2012) like in Imran and Jodie's case, with an expectation of support from the child welfare system (Randle et al., 2017).

There are several supports available to parents with substance use disorders; however, these same supports are not generally available to carers and adoptive parents. Unfortunately, there is consistent evidence that carers are poorly supported (Blythe et al., 2014, Gouveia et al., 2021). Carers report receiving minimal or inaccurate information regarding the children placed into their care. This impacts their ability to confidently engage with health care professionals (Blythe et al., 2013; Blythe, Halcomb, et al., 2012). Moreover, carers also report receiving minimal or irrelevant training as it relates to the care of infants and children with increased caregiving needs (Miller et al., 2019), including those with a history of PSE (Blythe et al., 2022). This lack of support leads to poor outcomes for children, resulting in multiple foster care placements (Lockwood et al., 2015), and adoption breakdown (Palacios et al., 2019). Furthermore, feeling marginalized and unsupported in their caregiving role is a common factor leading to foster carer attrition (Randle et al., 2017), which results in multiple placements for children in care (Konijn et al., 2019) – a potential scenario for Emily. This instability and lack of a consistent, stable, nurturing home are known to result in poor overall outcomes for children (Lewis et al., 2007).

Health care professionals should engage in reflective practice to identify any personal bias toward carers and/or adoptive parents. When health care professionals have biased feelings towards a patient, it can result in devaluation of the patient as an individual and inequitable treatment or suboptimal care. Although carers and adoptive parents may have minimal knowledge of children's health history, they can provide valuable current information as it relates to children's health and development. Moreover, as the day-to-day care providers, carers and adoptive parents are most likely to engage children in therapeutic activities within the home. As such, clinicians should endeavor to work in partnership with carers and adoptive parents. This will help alleviate their fear of being stigmatized and ultimately result in a therapeutic relationship that benefits the children in care.

12.3.2 *Education and Practical Support*

Research related to best practice for children with PSE largely focuses on infant and early childhood and generally caters to birthing families. This lack of evidence, and inconsistency and inequity in practice offerings to birthing parents and other carers, negatively impacts children, carers, and adoptive parents. There is a clear need to provide similar services to foster, kinship, and adoptive families caring for children with PSE. Such services, however, will also need to address the specific needs of carer and adoptive parents like Imran and Jodie who are caring for children like Emily who are impacted by PSE and the associated health and developmental issues and disrupted early attachment.

Carers and adoptive parents need education and training specific to the care of infants, children, and young people with PSE. Although some jurisdictions provide training, like the Safe Babies Program in Canada (Marcellus, 2000), others do not (Blythe et al., 2022). Training is deemed most valuable when it provides an understanding of the impact of PSE on children, practical caregiving strategies from birth through to adulthood, and insights into the concepts of trauma-informed care (Marcellus & Badry, 2023).

There is also a need for practical supports for carers and adoptive parents of infants with NOWS and children who have experienced PSE. This includes specific supports for carers and adoptive parents which reduce their isolation and concerns (Mukherjee et al., 2013), including support for carers and adoptive parents to manage their own psychosocial stressors. Where tenable, carers and adoptive parents should be present during an infant's hospitalization. This will enable them to engage directly with health care professionals, thereby developing a better understanding of PSE and how it impacts the infant, as well as learn and practice the strategies which are most effective for symptom management during withdrawal. This knowledge and skill development will likely increase carers and adoptive parents' confidence to care for the infant. Further, the presence of a consistent primary caregiver during infant hospitalization will help to facilitate infant attachment, resulting in better infant mental health. For those carers and adoptive parents who receive infants post hospital or later in the child's life, special attention to developing skills and strategies to manage disordered attachment and build positive relationships is needed.

12.4 Summary

Increasing numbers of infants with NOWS and children who have experienced prenatal substance exposure to harmful and addictive substances are being adopted or requiring foster/kinship care. These infants and children have increased caregiving needs. Their experiences of withdrawal and hospitalization predispose them to poor attachment and subsequent negative mental health outcomes, as well as other health and developmental issues. Their carers and adoptive parents do not routinely receive training or supports related to the care of infants with NOWS or children with a history of PSE, and, indeed, may not even know that the child they care for had PSE. Moreover, the stigma and marginalization experienced by carers and adoptive parents can preclude children's access to health care services. Health services, such as nurse home visiting, that are available to birthing parents are usually not available to carers and adopting parents, and, if available, require further development to meet the attachment and relationship needs of children in OOHC and their carers or adopting parents. Reflective practice and working in partnership with carers and adoptive parents, and providing training and practical supports are ways to best support children with PSE in care and adoptive families.

References

Akin, B. A., Brook, J., & Lloyd, M. H. (2015). Examining the role of methamphetamine in permanency: A competing risks analysis of reunification, guardianship, and adoption. *American Journal of Orthopsychiatry*, *85*(2), 119. https://doi.org/10.1037/ort0000052

Amon, J. J., Sun, N., Iovita, A., Jurgens, R., & Csete, J. (2022). Addressing stigma is not enough. *Health and Human Rights*, *24*(2), 111.

Blythe, S., Elcombe, E., Carter, R., & Stacpoole, M. (2022). Caring for infants in out-of-home care in New South Wales: Carers' perspectives. Western Sydney University. https://doi.org/10.26183/9SQ0-FA56

Blythe, S., Elcombe, E., Peters, K., Burns, E., & Gribble, K. (2021). Australian foster carers' views of supporting maternal breastfeeding and attachment in out-of-home care. *Child Abuse & Neglect*. https://doi.org/10.1016/j.chiabu.2021.105360

Blythe, S. L., Halcomb, E. J., Wilkes, L., & Jackson, D. (2012). Perceptions of long-term female foster-carers: I'm not a carer, I'm a mother. *British Journal of Social Work*, *43*(6). https://doi.org/10.1093/bjsw/bcs047

Blythe, S., Halcomb, E., Wilkes, L., & Jackson, D. (2013). Caring for vulnerable children: Challenges of mothering in the Australian foster care system. *Contemporary Nurse*, *44*(1), 87–98. https://doi.org/10.5172/conu.2013.44.1.87

Blythe, S. L., Jackson, D., Halcomb, E. J., & Wilkes, L. (2012). The stigma of being a long-term foster carer. *Journal of Family Nursing*, *18*(2), 234–260. https://doi.org/10.1177/107484071142391

Blythe, S. L., Wilkes, L., & Halcomb, E. J. (2014). The foster carer's experience: An integrative review. *Collegian*, *21*(1), 21–32. https://doi.org/10.1016/j.colegn.2012.12.001

Boyd, R. (2019). Foster care outcomes and experiences of infants removed due to substance abuse. *Journal of Public Child Welfare*, *13*(5), 529–555. https://doi.org/10.1080/15548732.2018.1536627

Cassidy, J., & Shaver, P. R. (2002). *Handbook of attachment: Theory, research, and clinical applications*. Rough Guides.

Faherty, L. J., Kranz, A. M., Russell-Fritch, J., Patrick, S. W., Cantor, J., & Stein, B. D. (2019). Association of punitive and reporting state policies related to substance use in pregnancy with rates of neonatal abstinence syndrome. *JAMA Network Open*, *2*(11). https://doi.org/10.1001/jamanetworkopen.2019.14078

Fegran, L., Helseth, S., & Fagermoen, M. S. (2008). A comparison of mothers' and fathers' experiences of the attachment process in a neonatal intensive care unit. *Journal of Clinical Nursing, 17*(6), 810–816. https://doi.org/10.1111/j.1365-2702.2007.02125.x

Fucile, S., Gallant, H., & Patel, A. (2021). Developmental outcomes of children born with neonatal abstinence syndrome (NAS): A scoping review. *Physical & Occupational Therapy in Pediatrics, 41*(1), 85–98. https://doi.org/10.1080/01942638.2020.1766637

Goodwin, S., & Huppatz, K. (2010). *The good mother: Contemporary motherhoods in Australia.* University Of Sydney, N.S.W. Sydney University Press.

Gouveia, L., Magalhães, E., & Pinto, V. S. (2021). Foster families: A systematic review of intention and retention factors. *Journal of Child and Family Studies, 30*(11), 2766–2781. https://doi.org/10.1007/s10826-021-02051-w

Gribble, K., Villarosa, A., Ghimire, P., & Blythe, S. (2022). Enduring familial relationships and identity preservation make simple adoption the preferred permanency option for children in out-of-home care. *Australian Social Work*, 1–15. https://doi.org/10.1080/0312407X.2022.2105163

Grossman, M. R., Berkwitt, A. K., Osborn, R. R., Xu, Y., Esserman, D. A., Shapiro, E. D., & Bizzarro, M. J. (2017). An initiative to improve the quality of care of infants with neonatal abstinence syndrome. *Pediatrics, 139*(6). https://doi.org/10.1542/peds.2016-3360

Guralnick, M. J. (2011). Why early intervention works: A systems perspective. *Infants and Young Children, 24*(1), 6. https://doi.org/10.1097/IYC.0b013e3182002cfe

Halter, M. J. (2008). Perceived characteristics of psychiatric nurses: Stigma by association. *Archives of Psychiatric Nursing, 22*(1), 20–26. https://doi.org/10.1016/j.apnu.2007.03.003

Hansen, M. E. (2007). Using subsidies to promote the adoption of children from foster care. *Journal of Family and Economic Issues, 28*, 377–393. https://doi.org/10.1007/s10834-007-9067-6

Harding, L., Murray, K., Shakespeare-Finch, J., & Frey, R. (2020). The wellbeing of foster and kin carers: A comparative study. *Children and Youth Services Review, 108.* https://doi.org/10.1016/j.childyouth.2019.104566

Howard, M. B., Schiff, D. M., Penwill, N., Si, W., Rai, A., Wolfgang, T., Moses, J. M., & Wachman, E. M. (2017). Impact of parental presence at infants' bedside on neonatal abstinence syndrome. *Hospital Pediatrics, 7*(2), 63–69. https://doi.org/10.1542/hpeds.2016-0147

Humphreys, C., & Kiraly, M. (2011). High-frequency family contact: A road to nowhere for infants. *Child & Family Social Work, 16*(1), 1–11. https://doi.org/https://doi.org/10.1111/j.1365-2206.2010.00699.x

Jee, S. H., Szilagyi, M., Ovenshire, C., Norton, A., Conn, A.-M., Blumkin, A., & Szilagyi, P. G. (2010). Improved detection of developmental delays among young children in foster care. *Pediatrics, 125*(2), 282–289. https://doi.org/10.1542/peds.2009-0229

Johnson, K. (2014). A foster carers' training package for home treatment of neonatal abstinence syndrome: Facilitating early discharge. *Infant, 10*(6), 191–193.

Joseph, R., Brady, E., Hudson, M. E., & Moran, M. M. (2020). Perinatal substance exposure and long-term outcomes in children: A literature review [Review]. *Pediatric Nursing*, 46(4), 163–173. https://www.scopus.com/inward/record.uri?eid=2-s2.0-85098597415&partnerID=40&md5=f9554e076649df4c1118c6284acbb541

Kepple, N. J. (2018). Does parental substance use always engender risk for children? Comparing incidence rate ratios of abusive and neglectful behaviors across substance use behavior patterns. *Child Abuse & Neglect*, 76, 44–55. https://doi.org/10.1016/j.chiabu.2017.09.015

Konijn, C., Admiraal, S., Baart, J., van Rooij, F., Stams, G.-J., Colonnesi, C., Lindauer, R., & Assink, M. (2019). Foster care placement instability: A meta-analytic review. *Children and Youth Services Review*, 96, 483–499. https://doi.org/10.1016/j.childyouth.2018.12.002

Lewis, E. E., Dozier, M., Ackerman, J., & Sepulveda-Kozakowski, S. (2007). The effect of placement instability on adopted children's inhibitory control abilities and oppositional behavior. *Developmental Psychology*, 43(6), 1415–1427. https://doi.org/10.1037/0012-1649.43.6.1415

Li, D., Chng, G. S., & Chu, C. M. (2019). Comparing long-term placement outcomes of residential and family foster care: A meta-analysis. *Trauma, Violence, & Abuse*, 20(5), 653–664. https://doi.org/10.1177/1524838017726427

Liu, A. J., Jones, M. P., Murray, H., Cook, C. M., & Nanan, R. (2010). Perinatal risk factors for the neonatal abstinence syndrome in infants born to women on methadone maintenance therapy. *Australian and New Zealand Journal of Obstetrics and Gynaecology*, 50(3), 253–258. https://doi.org/10.1111/j.1479-828X.2010.01168.x

Lloyd, M. H., Akin, B. A., & Brook, J. (2017). Parental drug use and permanency for young children in foster care: A competing risks analysis of reunification, guardianship, and adoption. *Children and Youth Services Review*, 77, 177–187. https://doi.org/10.1016/j.childyouth.2017.04.016

Lockwood, K. K., Friedman, S., & Christian, C. W. (2015). Permanency and the foster care system. *Current Problems in Pediatric and Adolescent Health Care*, 45(10), 306–315. https://doi.org/10.1016/j.cppeds.2015.08.005

Lonne, B., & Parton, N. (2014). Portrayals of child abuse scandals in the media in Australia and England: Impacts on practice, policy, and systems. *Child Abuse & Neglect*, 38(5), 822–836.

Luke, N., & Sebba, J. (2013). *How are foster carers selected. An international literature review of instruments used within foster carer selection.* University of Oxford: Rees Centre. https://www.researchgate.net/publication/260798445_How_are_foster_carers_selected_An_international_literature_review_of_instruments_used_within_foster_carer_selection#fullTextFileContent

MacMillan, K. D. L., Rendon, C. P., Verma, K., Riblet, N., Washer, D. B., & Volpe Holmes, A. (2018). Association of rooming-in with outcomes for neonatal abstinence syndrome: A systematic review and meta-analysis. *JAMA Pediatrics*, 172(4), 345–351. https://doi.org/10.1001/jamapediatrics.2017.5195

Maguire, D. J., Taylor, S., Armstrong, K., Shaffer-Hudkins, E., Germain, A. M., Brooks, S. S., Cline, G. J., & Clark, L. (2016). Long-term outcomes of infants with neonatal abstinence syndrome. *Neonatal Network, 35*(5), 277–286. https://doi.org/10.1891/0730-0832.35.5.277

Marcellus, L. (2000). Safe babies: One community's response. *The Canadian Nurse, 96*(10), 22.

Marcellus, L., & Badry, D. (2023). Infants, children, and youth in foster care with prenatal substance exposure: A synthesis of two scoping reviews. *International Journal of Developmental Disabilities, 69*(2), 265–290. https://doi.org/10.1080/20473869.2021.1945890

McGlade, A., Ware, R., & Crawford, M. (2009). Child protection outcomes for infants of substance-using mothers: A matched-cohort study. *Pediatrics, 124*(1), 285–293. https://doi.org/10.1542/peds.2008-0576

McLean, K., Clarke, J., Scott, D., Hiscock, H., & Goldfeld, S. (2020). Foster and kinship carer experiences of accessing healthcare: A qualitative study of barriers, enablers and potential solutions. *Children and Youth Services Review, 113.* https://doi.org/10.1016/j.childyouth.2020.104976

Meinhofer, A., & Angleró-Díaz, Y. (2019). Trends in foster care entry among children removed from their homes because of parental drug use, 2000 to 2017. *JAMA Pediatrics, 173*(9), 881–883. https://doi.org/10.1016/j.childyouth.2020.104976

Miller, L., Randle, M., & Dolnicar, S. (2019). Carer factors associated with foster-placement success and breakdown. *The British Journal of Social Work, 49*(2), 503–522. https://doi.org/10.1093/bjsw/bcy059

Mukherjee, R., Wray, E., Commers, M., Hollins, S., & Curfs, L. (2013). The impact of raising a child with FASD upon carers: Findings from a mixed methodology study in the UK. *Adoption & Fostering, 37*(1), 43–56. https://doi.org/10.1177/0308575913477331

Murphy-Oikonen, J., & McQueen, K. (2019). Outpatient pharmacologic weaning for neonatal abstinence syndrome: A systematic review. *Primary Health Care Research & Development, 20*, 76. https://doi.org/10.1017/S1463423618000270

Oei, J. L., Blythe, S. L., Dicair, L., Didden, D., Preisz, A., & Lantos, J. (2023). What's in a name?: The ethical implications and opportunities in diagnosing an infant with neonatal abstinence syndrome (NAS). *Addiction*, 4–6. https://doi.org/10.1111/add.16022

Osofsky, J. D., & Thomas, K. (2012). What is infant mental health? *Zero to Three Journal, 33*(2), 9.

Pahl, A., Young, L., Buus-Frank, M. E., Marcellus, L., & Soll, R. (2020). Non-pharmacological care for opioid withdrawal in newborns. *Cochrane Database of Systematic Reviews*, (12). https://doi.org/10.1002/14651858.CD013217.pub2

Palacios, J., Rolock, N., Selwyn, J., & Barbosa-Ducharne, M. (2019). Adoption breakdown: Concept, research, and implications. *Research on Social Work Practice, 29*(2), 130–142. https://doi.org/10.1177/1049731518783852

Patrick, S. W., Barfield, W. D., Poindexter, B. B., Committee on Fetus and Newborn, Committee on Substance Use and Prevention, Cummings, J., Hand, I., Adams-Chapman, I., Aucott, S. W., Puopolo, K. M., Goldsmith, J. P., Kaufman, D., Martin, C., Mowitz, M., Gonzalez, L., Camenga, D. R., Quigley, J., Ryan, S. A., & Walker-Harding, L. (2020). Neonatal opioid withdrawal syndrome. *Pediatrics, 146*(5). https://doi.org/10.1542/peds.2020-029074

Peacock-Chambers, E., Leyenaar, J. K., Foss, S., Feinberg, E., Wilson, D., Friedmann, P. D., Visintainer, P., & Singh, R. (2019). Early intervention referral and enrollment among infants with neonatal abstinence syndrome. *Journal of Developmental & Behavioral Pediatrics, 40*(6), 441–450. https://doi.org/ 10.1097/DBP.0000000000000679

Randle, M., Ernst, D., Leisch, F., & Dolnicar, S. (2017). What makes foster carers think about quitting? Recommendations for improved retention of foster carers. *Child & family social work, 22*(3), 1175–1186. https://doi.org/10.1111/ cfs.12334

Rossiter, C., Schmied, V., Kemp, L., Fowler, C., Kruske, S., & Homer, C. S. (2017). Responding to families with complex needs: A national survey of child and family health nurses. *Journal of Advanced Nursing, 73*(2), 386–398. https://doi. org/10.1111/jan.13146

Ruwanpathirana, R., Abdel-Latif, M. E., Burns, L., Chen, J., Craig, F., Lui, K., & Oei, J. L. (2015). Prematurity reduces the severity and need for treatment of neonatal abstinence syndrome. *Acta Paediatrica, 104*(5), 188–194. https://doi. org/10.1111/apa.12910

Ryan, G., Dooley, J., Gerber Finn, L., & Kelly, L. (2019). Nonpharmacological management of neonatal abstinence syndrome: A review of the literature. *The Journal of Maternal-fetal & Neonatal Medicine, 32*(10), 1735–1740. https:// doi.org/10.1080/14767058.2017.1414180

Schmied, V., Fowler, C., Rossiter, C., Homer, C., & Kruske, S. (2014). Nature and frequency of services provided by child and family health nurses in Australia: Results of a national survey. *Australian Health Review, 38*(2), 177– 185. https://doi.org/10.1071/AH13195

Schmied, V., Kearney, E., Dahlen, H. G., Hay, P., Kemp, L. A., Liamputtong, P., Meade, T., Smith, C., Possamai-Inesedy, A., & Sheehan, A. (2018). Tackling maternal anxiety in the perinatal period: Reconceptualising mothering narratives. https://doi.org/10.26183/5e69a1713ac58

Sebba, J. (2012). *Why do people become foster carers? An international literature review on the motivation to foster.* University of Oxford. Rees Centre. https:// www.researchgate.net/publication/260798440_Why_Do_People_Become_ Foster_Carers_An_International_Literature_Review_on_the_Motivation_to_ Foster#fullTextFileContent

Sen, R., & Broadhurst, K. (2011). Contact between children in out-of-home placements and their family and friends networks: A research review. *Child & Family Social Work, 16*(3), 298–309. https://doi.org/10.1111/ j.1365-2206.2010.00741.x

Shannon, J., Peters, K., & Blythe, S. (2021). The challenges to promoting attachment for hospitalised infants with NAS. *Children, 8*(2), 167. https://doi. org/10.3390/children8020167

Sieger, M. H. L., & Becker, J. (2020). Neonatal abstinence syndrome and trends in infant foster care admissions. *Child Welfare, 98*(3), 121–144.

Skivenes, M., & Benbenishty, R. (2023). Securing permanence for children in care: A cross-country analysis of citizen's view on adoption versus foster care. *Child & Family Social Work, 28*(2), 432–442. https://doi.org/10.1111/cfs.12974

Turney, K., & Goodsell, R. (2018). Parental incarceration and children's wellbeing. *The Future of Children*, 28(1), 147–164. https://www.jstor.org/stable/26641551

van Sleuwen, B. E., Engelberts, A. C., Boere-Boonekamp, M. M., Kuis, W., Schulpen, T. W., & L'Hoir, M. P. (2007). Swaddling: A systematic review. *Pediatrics*, 120(4), 1097–1106. https://doi.org/10.1542/peds.2006-2083

Whalen, B. L., Holmes, A. V., & Blythe, S. (2019). Models of care for neonatal abstinence syndrome: What works? *Seminars in Fetal and Neonatal Medicine*, 24(2), 121–132. https://doi.org/10.1016/j.siny.2019.01.004

Wise, S., & Corrales, T. (2023). Discussion of the knowns and unknowns of child protection during pregnancy in Australia. *Australian Social Work*, 76(2), 173–185. https://doi.org/10.1080/0312407X.2021.2001835

Wu, D., & Carre, C. (2018). The impact of breastfeeding on health outcomes for infants diagnosed with neonatal abstinence syndrome: A review. *Cureus*, 10(7). https://doi.10.7759/cureus.3061

York, W., & Jones, J. (2017). Addressing the mental health needs of looked after children in foster care: The experiences of foster carers. *Journal of Psychiatric and Mental Health Nursing*, 24(2–3), 143–153. https://doi.org/10.1111/jpm.12362

Young, L. W., Hu, Z., Annett, R. D., Das, A., Fuller, J. F., Higgins, R. D., Lester, B. M., Merhar, S. L., Simon, A. E., & Ounpraseuth, S. (2021). Site-level variation in the characteristics and care of infants with neonatal opioid withdrawal. *Pediatrics*, 147(1). https://doi.org/10.1542/peds.2020-008839

Zeanah, C. H., Berlin, L. J., & Boris, N. W. (2011). Practitioner review: Clinical applications of attachment theory and research for infants and young children. *Journal of Child Psychology and Psychiatry*, 52(8), 819–833. https://doi.org/10.1111/j.1469-7610.2011.02399.x

Zeanah, C. H., Shauffer, C., & Dozier, M. (2011). Foster care for young children: Why it must be developmentally informed. *Journal of the American Academy of Child and Adolescent Psychiatry*, 50(12), 1199–1201. https://doi.org/10.1016/j.jaac.2011.08.001

Zill, N. (2011). *Adoption from foster care: Aiding children while saving public money*. Washington, DC: Brookings Institution, Center on Children and Families. https://www.brookings.edu/articles/adoption-from-foster-care-aiding-children-while-saving-public-money/

Index

Note: Page numbers in *italics* indicate figures and page numbers in **bold** indicate tables in the text.

For Product Safety Concerns and Information please contact our EU
representative GPSR@taylorandfrancis.com
Taylor & Francis Verlag GmbH, Kaufingerstraße 24, 80331 München, Germany

* 9 7 8 1 0 3 2 5 0 1 8 9 5 *